Studying a Study and Testing a Test
How to Read the Medical Evidence

Fourth Edition

Studying a Study and Testing a Test
How to Read the Medical Evidence

Fourth Edition

Richard K. Riegelman, M.D., M.P.H., PH.D.
Dean, The George Washington University
School of Public Health and Health Services
Professor of Epidemiology-Biostatistics, Medicine,
and Health Services Management and Policy
Washington, D.C.

LIPPINCOTT WILLIAMS & WILKINS
A **Wolters Kluwer** Company
Philadelphia · Baltimore · New York · London
Buenos Aires · Hong Kong · Sydney · Tokyo

Acquisitions Editor: Richard Winters
Developmental Editors: Brian Brown and Sonya Seigafuse
Manufacturing Manager: Kevin Watt
Production Editor: Brandy Mui
Cover Designer: David Levy
Compositor: Circle Graphics
Printer: Maple-Vail

© 2000 by Joseph G. Rubenson and Kenneth A. Wasch, Trustees of the Riegelman Children's Trust
Published by Lippincott Williams & Wilkins
530 Walnut Street
Philadelphia, PA 19106-3780 USA
LWW.com

Printed in the USA

Library of Congress Cataloging-in-Publication Data

Riegelman, Richard K.
    Studying a study and testing a test : how to read the medical evidence / Richard K.
    Riegelman—4th ed.
        p.   cm.
    Includes bibliographical references and index.
    ISBN 0-7817-1860-0
    1. Medical literature—Evaluation.   2. Medicine—Research—Evaluation.   I. Title.
R118.6.R537 1999
610′.7′2—dc21   99-056118

ISBN: 0-7817-1860-0

10 9 8 7 6 5 4

Contents

IV. Considering Costs and Evaluating Effectiveness

V. Selecting a Statistic

Preface

Faced with the onslaught of health research articles, what is the busy student or practitioner to do? This question takes on increasing importance every day as the communications revolution brings us a deluge of data. We are truly faced with information overload. How can we identify the valid and the valuable in that mountain of material?

That is the goal of the fourth edition of *Studying a Study and Testing a Test: How to Read the Medical Evidence*. The aim is to teach a practical, enjoyable, step-by-step approach to thoughtful, critical, and ultimately more efficient reading of the health research literature.

The fourth edition builds on the approaches successfully used in the first three editions: the step-by-step approach of the Uniform Framework, scenarios to demonstrate what can go wrong, checklists of questions to ask, and new flaw-catching exercises providing practice using what you have learned. A new section entitled "Considering Costs and Evaluating Effectiveness" uses the step-by-step process incorporated in the Uniform Framework to walk you through decision analysis and cost-effectiveness analysis.

The fourth edition includes, for the first time, a CD-ROM with interactive questions and answers that parallel each of the first four sections of the text: Studying a Study, Testing a Test, Rating a Rate, and Considering Costs. *These questions and answers can be used for self-study or Continuing Education credit.*

Statistical concepts are presented without reliance on mathematics. The emphasis is on understanding what questions statistics ask and what the answers imply. To make this easier, a flowchart of statistics summarizes the selection and helps with the interpretation of statistical methods. Extensive footnotes are intended for the statistically oriented reader or for formal classroom use. The basic book, however, remains oriented to practitioners who wish to read the literature on their own or as part of a journal club.

Practicing clinicians including physicians, physician assistants, and nurses, as well as residents and students, should see this edition as a practical guide. In addition, the population perspective built into the approach should appeal to public health students and practitioners. The emphasis on cost-effectiveness analysis and the institutional perspective should also make *Studying a Study and Testing a Test* useful to health care managers.

The uniform frameworks, hypothetical illustrations of what can go wrong, and flaw-catching exercises are designed to provide hands-on experience using the "Studying a Study" approach. By the time you are done, you should be able to efficiently review journal articles and feel comfortable finding flaws in the articles you read. It is important to remember, however, that the goal is not just finding flaws but finding truth. Thus, it is important to recognize that not every flaw is fatal or every error avoidable. The goal is to recognize problems and take them into account as you put research into practice.

Health care today constantly puts us out on a limb. We should not be afraid to venture forth. However, we need to be on the lookout for data that challenge our basic assumptions. We live in an era when miracles are ever more miraculous and hazards ever more horrendous. Practitioners who can critically read the health literature are better able to bring the benefits and head off the harms. Gaining confidence in your ability to read the health research literature should make you less afraid to crawl out on that limb. Beware, however, that reading the health literature can be habit-forming. You might even find it enjoyable.

After completing *Studying a Study and Testing a Test*, you may want practice applying your skills to real journal articles. For practice and academic distance education programs using the *Studying a Study and Testing a Test* approach to reading the health research literature, take a look at the George Washington University School of Public Health and Health Services website at http://www.gwumc.edu/spphs/

Acknowledgments

The fourth edition of *Studying a Study and Testing a Test* is built upon my experience teaching and learning from students in-person in the classroom and on the computer via distant education. I am especially grateful to the public health students, medical students, and residents at The George Washington University School of Public Health and Health Services and School of Medicine and Health Sciences, who have shared their ideas, their critiques, and their encouragement.

Faculty, students, and residents throughout the world have provided invaluable input and stimulated the new "Considering Cost" section and the CD-ROM. They have also encouraged me to aim the fourth edition at clinicians, administrators, and public health professions, incorporating the individual perspective of the clinician, the institutional perspective of the manager, and the population perspective of public health.

The translation of the previous edition into Spanish and Japanese has enlarged the audience and given me an international perspective. Learning how to cross cultures is a challenge for all who read the health research literature. I hope that the fourth edition helps address these issues.

I am most grateful to Richard Winters and his colleagues at Lippincott Williams & Wilkins for their commitment to *Studying a Study and Testing a Test*. Their encouragement to pursue the CD-ROM and the new "Considering Cost" section have made the effort most worthwhile.

Let me give special thanks to Karyn Pomerantz and Ann Goldman, who have helped me think through changes in the fourth edition based on their growing experience teaching these approaches to a world-wide audience.

Studying a Study and Testing a Test continues to be a labor of love. I can only hope that this edition continues to reach an ever expanding audience who find reading the health research literature relevant and rewarding.

Studying a Study

1 Introduction and Sample Test

The traditional course in reading the health literature consists of "Here's the *New England Journal of Medicine.* Read it!" This approach is analogous to learning to swim by the total immersion method. Some persons can learn to swim this way, of course, but a few drown, and many learn to fear the water.

In contrast to the method of total immersion, a step-by-step, active-participation approach to reviewing the health research literature is presented here. With these analytic techniques, you should be able to read a journal article critically and efficiently. Considerable emphasis will be placed on the errors that can occur in the various kinds of studies, but try to remember that not every flaw is fatal. The goal of literature reading is to recognize the limitations of a study and then to put them into perspective. This is essential before putting the results into practice.

Before developing and illustrating the elements of critical analysis, however, let us begin with a flaw-catching exercise, using a simulated journal article, and see how well you can do. Read the following study and then try to answer the accompanying questions.

Cries Syndrome: Caused by Television or Just Bad Taste?

A medical condition known as Cries syndrome has been described as occurring among children ages 7 to 9 years old. The condition is characterized by episodes of uninterrupted crying lasting at least an hour per day for 3 consecutive days. The diagnosis also includes symptoms of sore throat, runny nose, and fever which precedes the onset of the crying and are severe enough to keep the child out of school.

Investigators studying this condition identified 100 children with Cries syndrome. For each of these children, a control child was identified from among classmates of the same gender who remained in school. The study was conducted over a month period after the onset of symptoms. The investigators examined 20 variables, which included all the characteristics they could think of as being potentially associated with Cries syndrome. They collected data on all medication use, number of spankings, hours of television viewing, number of hours at home, as well as 16 other variables.

Using pictures, they asked the children to identify the medications they had taken while they had Cries syndrome. Their classmates without Cries syndrome were also asked to identify medications taken during the same time period using the same pictures. The investigators then asked each child to classify each medication taken as good-tasting or bad-tasting medications. The data on spankings were obtained from the primary caregiver. The investigators found the following data:

Percentage of children who reported taking bad-tasting medication
Cries syndrome: 90%
Controls: 10%

3

Average number of spankings per day
Cries syndrome: 1
Controls: 2
Average number of television viewing hours per day
Cries syndrome: 8 (range 5 to 12)
Controls: 2 (range 0 to 4)

Among the 20 variables, analyzed one at a time, these were the only ones, which were statistically significant using the usual statistical methods. The P values were 0.05 except for the hours of television, which had a P value of 0.001. The investigators drew the following conclusions. Bad-tasting medication is a contributory cause of Cries syndrome since it was strongly associated with Cries syndrome. Spanking protects children from Cries syndrome since the controls had an increased frequency of being spanked. Television viewing at least 4 hours per day is a necessary cause of Cries syndrome since all children with Cries syndrome and none of the controls watched television more than 4 hours per day during the period under investigation.

Since Cries syndrome patients have a relative risk of 9 of taking bad-tasting medication, the investigators concluded that removing bad-tasting medication from the market would eliminate almost 90% of Cries syndrome cases among children like those in this investigation. In addition, regular spanking of all children 7 to 9 years old should be widely used as a method of preventing Cries syndrome.

Now to get an idea of what you will be learning in the Studying a Study section see if you can answer the following questions:

- What type of investigation is this?
- What is the hypothesis?
- Was the control group correctly assigned?
- Was the pairing of cases and controls performed correctly?
- Are reporting or recall biases likely to be present?
- Does the method of data collection raise issues of precision?
- Was the statistical significance testing or inference testing performed correctly?
- Was the estimate of the strength of the relationship performed correctly?
- Was an adjustment procedure used?
- Was an association established between the use of bad-tasting medicine and Cries syndrome?
- Was it established that the spankings occurred prior to the development of Cries syndrome or that altering spanking will alter the frequency of Cries syndrome?
- Was it established that TV viewing is a necessary cause of Cries syndrome?
- Did the investigators correctly extrapolate regarding medication?
- Did the investigators correctly extrapolate regarding spanking?

For answers to these questions go to The George Washington University School of Public Health and Health Services website at http://www.gwumc.edu/spphs/

2 Uniform Frameworks

Uniform Framework

Three basic types of investigations are found in the health research literature: CASE-CONTROL STUDIES, COHORT STUDIES, and RANDOMIZED CLINICAL TRIALS. Each of these types of investigations attempts to address a defined question or hypothesis by comparing one or more study groups with one or more control groups.[1]

A uniform framework can be used to evaluate each of these three types of studies. The uniform framework is divided into *six* components:

- Study design
- Assignment
- Assessment
- Analysis
- Interpretation
- Extrapolation

Figure 2.1 outlines the application of the uniform framework to a research study. Study design issues are common to all types of health research. They require the investigators to clarify exactly what they are attempting to achieve by defining what they will investigate, who they will investigate, and how many they will investigate. The uniform framework divides each of the six components into three specific issues. For study design, the issues and key questions are as follows:

- **Study hypothesis:** What is the study question?
- **Study population:** What are the inclusion and exclusion criteria for the subjects included in the investigation?
- **Sample's size and statistical power:** How many individuals are included in the study and in the control groups, and how great is the ability to demonstrate statistical significance if the study hypothesis is true?

Before investigators can decide which and how many individuals to include in an investigation, they need to define the study hypothesis or the study question. Then, they can focus on the question of which individuals or population should be included in the investigation. Health research is not generally conducted by including everyone in the population of interest, or TARGET POPULATION. Rather, health

---

[1]The investigations discussed in this "Studying a Study" section are sometimes called ANALYTICAL STUDIES. Analytical studies compare study groups with control groups. Investigations do not always have comparison groups. *Descriptive studies* obtain data on a group of individuals without comparing them to another group. Sometimes, descriptive studies may use data external to the investigation to compare those in the investigation with other groups or to the same group at an earlier period of time. These comparison groups are sometimes called HISTORICAL CONTROLS. These types of investigations will be discussed in the "Rating a Rate" section later in this book. In special situations, descriptive studies may also be called *case-series,* DESCRIPTIVE EPIDEMIOLOGY STUDIES, or NATURAL HISTORY STUDIES.

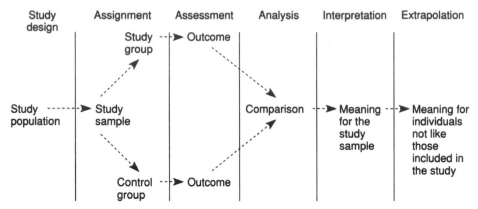

Figure 2.1. Uniform framework for studying a study.

research is generally performed using only a subgroup, or SAMPLE, of all individuals who could in theory be included. For all types of health research, choosing who to include and how many to include in an investigation are basic issues of study design.

Thus, study design, the first component of the uniform framework, defines the study question and sets the rules for selecting or drawing the study and control samples. For now, simply keep these issues regarding study design in mind. After we provide an overview of the other components of the uniform framework, we will examine each component in more detail.

The uniform framework continues with the following additional components:

Assignment: Selection of individuals for study and control groups
Assessment: Determination of the results of the investigation in the study and the control groups
Analysis: Comparison of the results of the study and the control groups
Interpretation: Drawing conclusions about the meaning of any difference found between the study and control groups for those included in the investigation
Extrapolation: Drawing conclusions about the meaning of the study, for individuals not included in the investigation or situations unlike those addressed by the study

To illustrate the application of the uniform framework to case-control, cohort, and randomized clinical trials, let us outline the essential features of each type of study and then see how we could apply each study type to the question of birth-control pill use and potential risk of stroke. The study design components differ according to the type of study, as we will discuss in this chapter.

We discuss each type of investigation, assuming that there is one study and one control group. However, in all types of studies, more than one study and more than one control group can be included.

Case-Control Study

The unique feature of case-control studies of disease is that they begin after individuals already have developed or failed to develop the disease being investigated. They go back in time to determine the characteristics of individuals before the onset of disease. In case-control studies, "cases" are the individuals who have developed the disease already, and the controls are the individuals who have not developed the disease. To use a case-control study to examine the relationship between birth-control pill use and stroke, an investigator would proceed as follows:

Assignment: Select a study group of women who have had a stroke (cases) and a group of otherwise similar women who have not had a stroke (controls). Because the development of the disease has occurred without the investigator's intervention, this process is called OBSERVED ASSIGNMENT.

Assessment: Determine whether each woman in the study group and in the control group previously took birth control pills.

Analysis: Calculate the odds that the group of women with a stroke had used birth-control pills versus the odds that the group of women without stroke had used birth-control pills.

Interpretation: Draw conclusions about the meaning of birth-control pill use for women included in the study.

Extrapolation: Draw conclusions about the meaning of birth-control pill use for categories of women not like those included in the study, such as women on newer low-dose birth-control pills.

Figure 2.2 illustrates the application of the uniform framework to this study.

Cohort Study

Cohort studies of disease differ from case-control studies in that they begin by identifying individuals for study and control groups before the investigator is aware of whether they have or will develop the disease. A COHORT is a group of individuals who share a common experience. A cohort study begins by identifying a cohort that possesses the characteristics under study as well as a cohort that does not possess those particular characteristics. Then, the frequency of disease in the two cohorts is obtained and compared. To use a cohort study to examine the relationship between birth-control pill use and stroke, an investigator might proceed as follows:

Assignment: Select a study group of women who are using birth-control pills and an otherwise similar control group of women who have never used birth-control

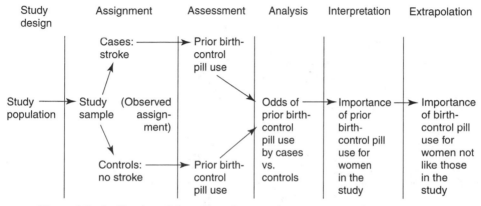

Figure 2.2. Application of the uniform framework to a case-control study.

pills. Because the use of birth-control pills is observed to occur without the investigator's intervention, this process is also called *observed assignment.*

Assessment: Observe the study group and the control group of women to determine who subsequently develops strokes.

Analysis: Calculate the probability of developing a stroke for women using birth-control pills versus women not using birth-control pills.

Interpretation: Draw conclusions about the meaning of birth-control pill use for women included in the study.

Extrapolation: Draw conclusions about the use of birth-control pills for women not included in the study, such as women on newer low-dose birth-control pills.

Figure 2.3. illustrates the application of the uniform framework to a cohort study.

Randomized Clinical Trial (Controlled Clinical Trial)

Randomized clinical trials are also called controlled clinical trials. As in cohort studies, individuals are assigned to study and control groups and are followed forward in time to determine whether they develop the particular disease or condition under investigation. The unique feature of randomized clinical trials, however, is the method for assigning individuals to study and control groups. Ideally, individuals are randomized either to a study group or to a control group.

RANDOMIZATION means that chance is used to assign a person to either the study or control group. This is done so that any one individual has a known, but not necessarily equal, probability of being assigned to the study or the control group. Ideally, the study participants as well as the investigator are not aware of their assigned groups. They are said to be *blinded* or *masked.*

DOUBLE-BLIND ASSIGNMENT, the preferred form of blinding or masking, implies that neither the participants nor the investigators know whether a particular participant has been assigned to a study group or to a control group. To use a randomized clinical trial to examine the relationship between birth-control pills and stroke, an investigator might proceed as follows:

Assignment: Using randomization, women are assigned in a double-blind fashion to a study group that will be prescribed birth-control pills or to a control group that will not be prescribed birth-control pills.

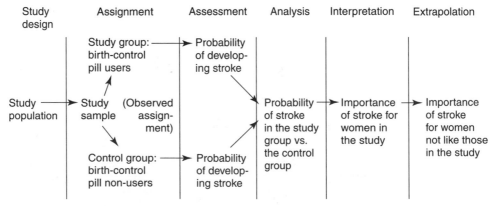

Figure 2.3. Application of the uniform framework to a cohort study.

Assessment: Observe these women to determine who develops stroke.

Analysis: Calculate the probability that women prescribed birth-control pills will develop a stroke versus women not prescribed birth-control pills.

Interpretation: Draw conclusions about the meaning of prescribing birth-control pills for women included in the study.

Extrapolation: Draw conclusions about the meaning of the use of birth-control pills for women not included in the study, such as women on new low-dose birth-control pills.

Figure 2.4 illustrates the application of the uniform framework to a randomized or controlled clinical trial.

This brief presentation of the three basic study types used in health research is intended to show how each type of study can be structured using the uniform framework.

The basic types of comparison studies discussed here are not the only types of studies encountered in the health literature. CROSS-SECTIONAL studies also are frequently performed. In these investigations, the study characteristic and the outcome are measured at the same point in time; in other words, the assignment and assessment are performed at the same point in time. They can be useful when one expects that exposure is not likely to change over time or that the time between exposure and disease is very short. In most respects, the cross-sectional study is a special type of case-control study.

As we have seen, there are three key questions to ask pertaining to study design, the first component of the uniform framework. There are also three key questions to ask regarding each of the other components. These questions are briefly outlined in the following section. We will explain them in more detail in subsequent chapters.

Assignment

The process of assignment asks questions about the characteristics of the study and control groups.

- **Method of Assignment:** What method was used to assign individuals to study and control groups?

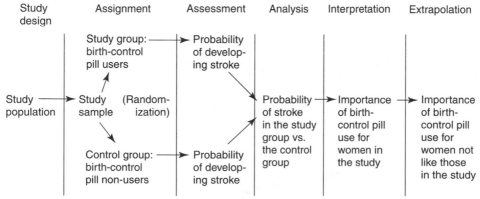

Figure 2.4. Application of the uniform framework to a randomized clinical trial.

- **Confounding Variables:** Are there differences between the study and control groups (other than the characteristic being investigated) that may affect the results of the investigation?
- **Masking (or blinding):** Do the individuals in the investigation and/or the investigators know the results of the assignment?

Assessment

The process of assessment asks questions about the quality of how the investigation's results were measured.

- **Appropriate measurement:** Is the measurement of the results appropriate to address the study question?
- **Precise and accurate measurement:** Is the measurement of the results precise and accurate?
- **Complete and unaffected by observation:** Is the measurement of the results complete and unaffected by the process of conducting the investigation?

Analysis

The process of analysis quantitatively compares the results in the study group with the results in the control group.

- **Estimation:** What methods are used to estimate the magnitude or strength of the associations or relationships observed in the investigation?
- **Inference:** What method is used to perform statistical significance testing to make inferences about populations based on the results of the study's samples?
- **Adjustment:** What methods are used to take into account the differences between the study and control group that may affect the results?

Interpretation

The interpretation portion of health research studies asks us to draw conclusions regarding the subjects in the investigation. Specifically, it asks us to draw conclusions about cause-and-effect relationships, or what we will call CONTRIBUTORY CAUSE, when we are talking about the etiology of a disease or EFFICACY when we are asking whether a treatment or other intervention works to improve outcome. Establishing cause and effect requires that each of the following questions be answered positively. That is, a cause-and-effect relationship requires that we establish all *three* of the following criteria:

1. **Association:** Does the investigation establish a substantial and statistically significant association that provides convincing evidence that the "cause" occurs more frequently together with the "effect" than expected by chance alone?
2. **Prior association:** Does the investigation establish that the "cause" precedes the "effect"?
3. **Altering the "cause" alters the "effect":** Does the investigation establish that altering or modifying the frequency or severity of the "cause" alters the frequency or severity of the disease or other "effect"?

Extrapolation

Extrapolation of health research studies asks how we can go beyond the data and individuals in a particular investigation to draw conclusions about groups and situations that are not specifically included in the investigation. These groups may be your patients, your institution, or your community.

* **Extrapolation to groups similar to the study population:** Has the investigator extrapolated to groups similar to those included in the investigation?
* **Extrapolation beyond the data:** What assumptions were required to extrapolate beyond the data contained in the investigation?
* **Extrapolation to other populations:** What assumptions were required to extrapolate to populations that are not included in the investigation?

Strengths and Weaknesses of the Basic Study Types

The basic components and key questions we've outlined are common to all three basic types of investigations, including the case-control, cohort, and randomized clinical trial. Each type, however, has its own strengths, weaknesses, and role to play in health research.

CASE-CONTROL STUDIES have the distinct advantage of being useful for studying rare conditions or diseases. If a condition is rare, case-control studies can detect differences between groups using far fewer individuals than other study designs require. Much less time is often needed to perform a case control study because the disease has already developed. This method also allows investigators to simultaneously explore multiple characteristics or exposures that are potentially associated with a disease. One could examine, for instance, the many variables that are possibly associated with colon cancer, including prior diet, surgery, ulcerative colitis, polyps, alcohol, cigarettes, family history, and many other variables.

The major objection to case-control studies is that they are prone to various errors and biases that will be explained in the following chapters. Despite these problems, case-control studies are very important for establishing associations. They are often capable of showing that a potential "cause" and a disease or other outcome occur together more often than expected by chance alone.

COHORT STUDIES have the major advantage of demonstrating with greater assurance that a particular characteristic preceded a particular outcome being studied. As we will see, this is a critical distinction when assessing a cause-and-effect relationship. CONCURRENT COHORT STUDIES, which follow patients forward over long periods of time, are expensive and time-consuming. It is possible, however, to perform a cohort study without such a lengthy follow-up period. If reliable data on the presence or absence of the study characteristic are available from an earlier time, these data can be used to perform a NONCONCURRENT COHORT STUDY *or* what is often called a *database study*. In a nonconcurrent cohort study, the assignment of individuals to groups is made on the basis of these past data. However, the groups are identified without the investigator being aware of the results of the outcomes being assessed. After assignment has occurred, the investigator can then look at the data on subsequent disease occurrence.

For instance, if low-density lipoprotein (LDL) readings from a group of adults were available from 15 years before the current study began, those with and those without high LDL could be examined to assess the subsequent development of coronary artery disease, strokes, or other consequences of high LDL cholesterol that might have occurred. The critical element, which characterizes all cohort studies, is the identification of individuals for study and control groups without knowledge of whether the disease or condition under study has developed.

Cohort studies can be used to delineate various consequences that may be produced by a single risk factor. For instance, researchers can simultaneously study the relationship between hypertension and stroke, myocardial infarction, heart failure, or renal disease. Cohort studies can produce more in-depth understanding of the effect of an etiologic factor on multiple outcomes.

Both case-control and cohort studies are OBSERVATIONAL STUDIES; that is, they observe the assignment of individuals rather than impose the characteristics or interventions.

RANDOMIZED CLINICAL TRIALS are distinguished from observational studies by the intervention that occurs when an investigator randomizes individuals to study and control groups. The ability to assign individuals by randomization helps to ensure that the study characteristic, and not some underlying predisposition, produces the study results. When properly performed, randomized clinical trials are able to support all three criteria for contributory cause: association, prior association, and altering the cause alters the effect.

The strengths and weaknesses of controlled clinical trials are explored in-depth in Chapter 9.

3 Study Design

As we have discussed, study design is the process of identifying a study hypothesis as well as study and control samples to investigate a specific question in a defined population. The following are key questions in study design:

- **Study hypothesis:** What is the study question?
- **Study population:** What are the inclusion and exclusion criteria for the subjects included in the investigation?
- **Sample's size and statistical power:** How many individuals are included in the study and in the control groups, and how great is the ability to demonstrate statistical significance if the study hypothesis is true?

Study Hypothesis

The study hypothesis, or study question, provides the starting point from which an investigation is organized. This component is essential for all investigations that compare study and control groups. When reading the health research literature, therefore, the first question to ask is: What is the study question or hypothesis? Investigators usually define a hypothesis. The hypothesis may be an association between a characteristic known as a RISK FACTOR (*e.g.,* birth-control pills) and a DISEASE (*e.g.,* stroke) or between an INTERVENTION (*e.g.,* reduction in blood pressure) and an IMPROVEMENT IN OUTCOME (*e.g.,* reduced frequency of strokes).

It is often important to distinguish between what the investigators would ideally like to study and what they have in fact actually studied. Investigators may want to study the end-organ effects of hypertension, for example, but the inability to perform renal biopsies and cerebral angiograms may force them to carefully study retinal changes. Researchers may wish to investigate the long-term effects of a new drug to prevent osteoporosis, but time, money, and the desire to publish may limit their investigation to its short-term effects on bone metabolism and bone density.

To conduct an investigation, it is important to have a specific study hypothesis rather than a general relationship in mind. Consider the following example:

> An investigator wishes to study the relationship between hypertension and vascular damage. The investigator hypothesizes that the degree of end-organ damage will correlate with the degree of hypertension.

This hypothesis is not specific enough to study. A more specific one might be that an increased degree of narrowing of the retinal arteries, as measured on retinal photographs after 3 years of observation, will be associated with an increased level of diastolic blood pressure taken as the average of three blood pressure measurements at the beginning of the study. This provides a specific study question that can be addressed by an investigation.

Failure to clarify the hypotheses being tested makes it difficult for the researcher to choose and the reader to assess the appropriateness of the study design. For instance, imagine the following situation:

> An investigator wishes to demonstrate that birth-control pills are a contributory cause of strokes. The investigator conducts a case-control study using very careful methods. The results demonstrate a strong relationship between birth-control pills and strokes. The investigator concludes that birth-control pills are a contributory cause of stroke.

This investigator has failed to recognize that the use of a case-control study implies that the investigator is interested in demonstrating that birth-control pills are associated with strokes rather than demonstrating that birth-control pills are a contributory cause of strokes.

Study Population

The population being studied must be defined before beginning an investigation. This includes determining the characteristics of individuals who will be selected as part of the actual study and control samples. In addition, the characteristics of the population being investigated play an important role in helping us to extrapolate the results of the investigation.

To characterize a study population, investigators need to define the INCLUSION CRITERIA and EXCLUSION CRITERIA, which are the explicit requirements for entrance into the investigation. Let us see why inclusion and exclusion criteria are needed by looking at the next example:

> An investigator wanted to study the effect of a new therapy for breast cancer. He selected all available breast cancer patients and found that the treatment, on average, resulted in no improvement in outcome. Later research revealed that the therapy provided a substantial improvement in outcome for women with stage III breast cancer. The therapy, however, was shown to have no benefit if women with breast cancer had undergone previous radiation therapy.

If this investigation had been conducted by requiring stage III breast cancer as inclusion criteria and previous radiation therapy as an exclusion criteria, the results may have been very different. Inclusion criteria serve to identify the types of individuals who should be included in the investigation. Exclusion criteria serve to remove individuals from eligibility because of special circumstances that may complicate their treatment or make interpretation more difficult.

Inclusion and exclusion criteria define the characteristics of those being studied. In addition, they narrow the group to which the results can be immediately applied or extrapolated. For instance, women diagnosed with stage II breast cancer are not included in the study. Thus, it is not clear whether the results of the study apply to them.

Sample Size

Having identified the study hypothesis and population, the reader of the health research literature should focus on the sample size of individuals selected for study and control groups. The question to ask is:

• Is there an adequate number of individuals to allow a reasonable chance of demonstrating a statistically significant difference between the study and control groups if, in fact, a difference actually exists in the larger population from which the study samples were drawn?

The answer to this question is given by the statistical power of an investigation. STATISTICAL POWER is the probability of demonstrating statistical significance if the study hypothesis is true. Research articles often identify the type II error rather than statistical power. TYPE II ERROR is the complement of the statistical power. In other words, type II error is the probability of failing to demonstrate statistical significance if the study hypothesis is true.

Thus, if the type II error is 10%, the statistical power is 90%; if the type II error is 20%, the statistical power is 80%. Well-designed investigations should include enough individuals in the study and the control groups to provide at least an 80% statistical power or 80% probability of demonstrating statistical significance if the study hypothesis is true.

As we will see when we further discuss sample size in Chapter 9, statistical power depends on a series of assumptions. In addition, the number of individuals required to obtain the same statistical power is very different in case-control studies compared to cohort studies or randomized clinical trials. Failure to appreciate this distinction can lead to the follow error:

> Investigators wished to study whether birth-control pills are associated with the rare occurrence of strokes in young women. The researchers monitored 2,000 women on birth-control pills and 2,000 women on other forms of birth control for 10 years. After spending millions of dollars in follow-up, they found two cases of stroke among the pill users and one case among the non-pill users. The differences were not statistically significant.

In case-control studies of birth-control pills and stroke, we are interested in determining whether the use of birth-control pills is greater among those with stroke. Birth-control pill use may be a relatively common characteristic of young women who have experienced a stroke. If so, the sample size required to conduct a case-control study may be quite small, perhaps 100 or less in each group.

On the other hand, when conducting a cohort study or randomized clinical trial, even if there is a strong relationship between birth-control pill use and stroke, it may be necessary to follow a large number of women who have and have not taken birth-control pills to identify the fact that more women on these pills experience strokes. When the occurrence of an outcome such as stroke is rare, say less than 1%, many thousands of women may be required for the study and control groups in cohort and randomized clinical trials to provide an adequate statistical power to demonstrate statistical significance, even if the study hypothesis is true. In Chapter 9, we explore in more depth the implications of sample size.

An evaluation of study design requires that we consider the study hypothesis, the study population being investigated, and the adequacy of the sample size. Equipped with an understanding of these key study design questions, we are ready to turn our attention to the next component of our uniform framework, *i.e.,* assignment.

4 Assignment

Regardless of the type of investigation, there are three basic assignment issues:

- **Method:** What method is being used to assign individuals to study and control groups?
- **Confounding variables:** Are there differences between the study and the control groups, due to either bias or chance, that may affect the results of the investigation?
- **Masking:** Are the results of the assignment known to the study participants or the investigators?

Method

In the next five chapters, we apply our uniform framework to case-control and cohort studies. These two types of studies are known as observational studies. In an observational study, no intervention is attempted, and thus no attempt is made to alter the course of a disease. The investigators observe the course of the disease among groups with and without the characteristics being studied.

In Chapter 2, we used example of birth-control pill use and strokes and learned that the type of assignment performed in case-control and cohort studies is called observed assignment. This term implies that the researcher selects individuals, who are called SUBJECTS, to include in study and control groups from those who do and do not have the characteristics under investigation.

The goal in creating study and control groups is to select subjects for each of these groups who are as similar as possible, except for the presence or absence of the characteristic being investigated. Sometimes this goal is not achieved in a particular study because of a flawed method of observed assignment that creates a *selection bias*.

Selection Bias

Few terms are less clearly understood or more loosely used than the word *bias*. Bias is not the same as prejudice. It does not imply a prejudgment before the facts are known. Bias occurs when investigators unintentionally introduce factors into the investigation that influence the results or outcome of the study. Differences between the study and control groups result in a selection bias if these specific differences affect the outcome or results under investigation. The elements of selection bias are illustrated in the following hypothetical study:[1]

> A case-control study of premenopausal breast cancer compared the past use of birth-control pills among 500 women who have breast cancer to the past use of the pill among 500 age-matched women admitted to the hospital for hypertension or dia-

[1]In reviewing this hypothetical case and others in this book, the reader should assume that all omitted portions of the study were properly performed.

betes. Investigators found that 40% of the women with breast cancer had used birth-control pills during the preceding 5 years, whereas only 5% of those with diabetes or hypertension in the control group had used the pill. The authors concluded that a strong association existed between the use of birth-control pills and the development of premenopausal breast cancer.

To determine whether a selection bias may have existed when patients were assigned to the control group, we must first ask whether the women in the control group were similar to the women in the study group except that they did not have breast cancer. The answer is no, because the women in the control group were quite different from the women in the study group because they had been admitted to the hospital for diabetes or hypertension. One must then ask whether this unique characteristic (diabetes or hypertension) was likely to have affected the results under investigation, that is, use of birth-control pills.

The answer is yes. Because birth-control pills are widely known to increase blood pressure and blood sugar, clinicians generally do not prescribe birth-control pills to women with hypertension or diabetes. Thus, the unique health characteristics of these women in the control group contributed to a lower-than-expected use of birth-control pills. This investigation's method of assignment, therefore, created the potential for a selection bias.

Thus, selection bias can occur whenever the study and control groups differ from each other by a factor that is likely to affect the results. In other words, selection bias occurs when the groups differ in a way that makes a difference in the results. Selection bias can also occur in a cohort study as illustrated in the following example:

> The effect of cigarette smoking on the development of myocardial infarctions was studied by selecting 10,000 middle-aged cigarette smokers and 10,000 middle-aged non–cigarette-smoking pipe smokers. Both groups were observed for 10 years. The investigators found that the cigarette smokers had a rate of new myocardial infarction of 4 per 100 over 10 years, whereas the non–cigarette-smoking pipe smokers had a rate of new myocardial infarction of 7 per 100 over 10 years. The results were statistically significant. The investigators concluded that cigarette smokers have a lower risk of myocardial infarctions than non–cigarette-smoking pipe smokers.

Despite the statistical significance of this difference, the conclusion conflicts with the results of many other studies. Let us see if selection bias could have contributed to this.

In analyzing this study, one must recognize two generally accepted facts: Men comprise the vast majority of pipe smokers, *and* middle-aged men have a much higher rate of myocardial infarction than do middle-aged women.

With these facts in mind, the first question is whether the study and control groups differ. The answer is yes, because men constitute the vast majority of pipe smokers, whereas more women smoke cigarettes than pipes. To establish the potential for a selection bias, we must also ask whether this difference could affect the outcome being measured. Again, the answer is yes. Men have a higher risk of myocardial infarction. Thus, both elements of selection bias are present. The study and control groups differ with regard to a particular factor that could affect the results.

Confounding Variable

Even when a study is properly designed so that selection bias is unlikely, RANDOM ERROR due to chance alone may produce study and control groups that differ according to certain characteristics that might affect the results of the investigation. When these differences in characteristics affect outcome, we refer to them as CONFOUNDING VARIABLES. Thus, a selection bias is a special type of confounding variable, which results from bias in the way the study or the control group subjects are selected. Remember, even in the absence of selection bias, differences in study and control group characteristics can result by random error. It is important to compare the study and the control group subjects to determine whether they differ in ways that are likely to affect the results of the investigation even when there is no evidence of selection bias.

Most research articles include a table, usually the first table in the article, that identifies the characteristics that the investigators know about the study and control groups. This allows the researcher and the reader to compare the groups to determine whether large or important differences have been identified. These differences may be the result of bias or chance. In either situation, they need to be recognized and subsequently taken into account or adjusted for as part of the analysis.[2]

Matching and Pairing

One method for circumventing the problem of selection bias is to match individuals who are similar with respect to characteristics that might affect the study's results. For instance, if age is related to the probability of being a member of either group, and if age is also related to the outcome being measured, then the investigator may match for age. For instance, for every 65-year-old in the control group, investigators could choose one 65-year-old for the study group and similarly with 30-year-olds, 40-year-olds, and so on. If properly performed, the result of matching guarantees that the distribution of ages in each group is the same.

Matching is not limited to making the groups uniform for age. It may be used for any characteristic related to the probability of experiencing the outcome under study. For example, if one were planning a cohort study addressing the relationship between birth-control pills and breast cancer, family history of premenopausal breast cancer would be an important characteristic to consider for matching in the study's design.

One disadvantage of matching groups is that the investigators cannot study the effect that the "matching characteristic" has on the outcome being measured. For instance, if they match for age and family history of premenopausal breast cancer, they lose the ability to study how age or family history affect the development of breast cancer. Furthermore, they lose the ability to study factors that are closely associated with the matched factor. Such pitfalls of matching are illustrated in the following example:

> One hundred patients with adult-onset diabetes were compared with 100 nondiabetic adults to study factors associated with adult-onset diabetes. The groups were matched to ensure a similar weight distribution in the two groups. The authors also found that the total calories consumed in each of the two groups was nearly identical and concluded that the number of calories consumed was not related to the possibility of developing adult-onset diabetes.

[2]Note that the reader can evaluate only those characteristics the investigator identifies, usually in tabular form. Thus the reader should ask whether there are additional characteristics that would have been important to compare. The investigators can only adjust for difference that they identify. However, randomization especially when the sample size is large, is capable of taking into account differences the investigator does not recognize.

The authors of the study, having matched the patients by weight, then attempted to study the differences in calories consumed. Because there is a high level of association between weight and calories consumed, it is not surprising that the authors found no difference in consumption of calories between the two groups matched for weight. When this type of error occurs, in which it is impossible to investigate the influence of some factor that is closely related to another used to match groups, it is called OVERMATCHING.

The type of matching used in the diabetes example is called GROUP MATCHING. Group matching seeks an equal distribution of matched characteristics in each group. A second type of matching is known as PAIRING (*i.e.,* when one study and one control group are included in an investigation). Pairing involves identifying one individual in the study group who can be compared with one individual in the control group. Pairing of individuals is a very effective way to avoid selection bias.

Despite the advantages, pairing has a distinct disadvantage. It may often be a problem to identify a control group subject who possesses all the same characteristics as the study subject to be paired. This problem can sometimes be circumvented by using a study subject as his or her own control. This may be done by comparing the results in an individual's treated and untreated eye in what is called a CROSS-OVER STUDY. In a cross-over study the same individuals are compared with themselves, for instance, while on and off medication. When properly performed, cross-over studies allow an investigator to use the same individuals in the study group and control group and to then pair their results, thus keeping many factors constant. All types of pairing allow the use of powerful statistical significance tests, which increase the probability of demonstrating statistical significance for a particular size study group. Statistical significance tests used with pairing are called MATCHED TESTS.

Cross-over studies must be used with great care, however, or they can produce misleading results as the following hypothetical study illustrates:

> A study of the benefit of a new nonnarcotic medication for postoperative pain relief was performed by giving 100 patients the medication on postoperative day 1 and a placebo on day 2. For each patient, the degree of pain was measured using a well-established pain scale on day 1 and day 2. The investigators found no difference between levels of pain on and off the medication.

When evaluating a cross-over study, one must recognize the potential for an effect of time and a carry-over effect of treatment. Pain is expected to decrease with time after surgery, so it is not accurate to compare the degree of pain on day 1 with the degree of pain on day 2.

Furthermore, one must be careful to assess whether there may be a carry-over effect in which the medication from day 1 continues to be active on day 2. Thus, the absence of benefit in this cross-over trial should not imply that pain medication on day 1 after surgery is no more effective than placebo.

Matching and pairing are two methods for preventing selection bias and can be helpful techniques when properly used.

Masking

Masking or blinding attempts to remove one source of bias by preventing each study participant and the investigator from knowing whether any individual was assigned to a study or to a control group.

The term MASKING is considered a more accurate reflection of the actual process and is currently considered the technically correct term, although the term BLIND-ING is still commonly used.

When masking is successful, we can be confident that knowledge of group assignment did not influence the outcomes that were measured. Masking is not usually feasible in either case-control or cohort investigations. In case-control studies, the patients have already experienced the outcome. In cohort investigations, the patients have already experienced the factors being investigated. Thus in both case-control and cohort investigations, it is important to consider whether the knowledge regarding the assignment influenced the measurement of the outcome. We will address this question of assessment in the next chapter.

5 Assessment

To assess the results of an investigation, researchers must define the outcome or endpoint they intend to measure. The term outcome can be somewhat confusing because it has different meanings for different types of studies. Let us review what outcome means in cohort studies and randomized clinical trials. Cohort studies and randomized clinical trials begin with the assignment of a study group that possesses the characteristic under investigation and a control group that is free of this characteristic. Individuals in the study and control groups are followed forward in time to determine whether they develop a particular condition. The occurrence of the condition that is being assessed is known as the outcome. The term *end-point* is a more general term used to designate an outcome measure that terminates assessment for a particular individual.

The investigator must use a valid measure the occurrence of the outcome or end point. For instance, in the cohort study of birth-control pills and strokes, the development of strokes is the outcome or endpoint being assessed.

Case-control studies begin with persons who have already developed a certain condition (cases) and persons who have not developed the condition (controls). The investigators review the history of the individuals in both the case and the control groups to determine whether these individuals were exposed to or possessed a specific prior characteristic. In a case-control study, this prior characteristic is the result being assessed and is thus the outcome or endpoint of the study. In the same example of birth-control pills and stroke, the use of birth-control pills is the endpoint, outcome, or characteristic being assessed.

A valid measure of the outcome or endpoint ideally fulfills the following criteria:

Appropriate: It measures a phenomenon that is relevant to the study question.
Accurate: On average, it has the same numerical value as the phenomenon being investigated. That is, it is free of systematic error or bias.
Precise: It has minimum variation as a result of the effects of chance. That is, there is minimum random error.

In addition, the implementation of the measurement should not introduce additional potential biases. The implementation should be as follows:

• **Complete:** all individuals' outcomes should be assessed
• **Unaffected:** by the process of observation

Study and control groups are followed up as completely as possible and with equal intensity. Also, the process of observing the groups over time and collecting the data does not alter the measurements that are obtained.

Appropriate Measure of Outcome

To understand the importance of the appropriateness of a measure of outcome, let us first consider an example of how the use of an inappropriate measure of outcome can invalidate a study's conclusions.

> An investigator attempted to study whether users of brand A or brand B spermicide had a lower probability of developing tubal infections secondary to Chlamydia. The investigator identified 100 women using each brand of spermicide, monitored these women, and performed annual cervical cultures for Chlamydia for 5 years. The investigator found that women using brand A spermicide had 1 1/2 times as many positive cultures for Chlamydia. The investigator concluded that brand B spermicide is associated with a lower rate of tubal infections.

Chlamydia cultures from the cervix do little to establish the presence or absence of tubal infection. The study may help to establish a higher frequency of Chlamydia infection. However, if the intent is to study the relative frequency of tubal infection, the investigator has not chosen an appropriate outcome measurement or endpoint. Investigators frequently are forced to measure an outcome that is not exactly the outcome they would actually like to measure. When this occurs, it is important to establish that the phenomenon being measured is appropriate to the question being investigated.

Accurate and Precise Measures of Outcome

Next, we look at how an outcome assessment may be affected by inaccurate measurements. Information for measuring outcome may come from two basic sources:

1. The memory of study participants or the use of data from their previous records.
2. Measurements by the study investigator.

The information obtained may be inaccurate because it produces data that are always off-target in the same direction because of bias in the way the data are collected. This is called ASSESSMENT BIAS. Alternatively, data may not be precise because of variation resulting from chance in either direction. That is RANDOM ERROR.

Information obtained from the memory of study individuals is subject to two special types of assessment bias—recall bias and reporting bias. RECALL BIAS implies defects in memory, specifically defects in which one group is more likely to recall events than other groups. REPORTING BIAS occurs in a study when one group is more likely than the other to report what they remember. Consider the following example of how RECALL BIAS can occur:

> In a case-control study of the cause of spina bifida, 100 mothers of infants born with the disease and 100 mothers of infants born without the disease were studied. Among the mothers of spina bifida infants, 50% reported having had a sore throat during pregnancy versus 5% of the mothers whose infants did not develop spina bifida. The investigators concluded that they had shown an association between sore throats during pregnancy and spina bifida.

Before accepting the conclusions of the study, one must ask whether recall bias could explain its findings. One can argue that mothers who experienced the trauma of having an infant with spina bifida are likely to search their memory more intensively and to remember events not usually recalled by other women.

Thus, recall bias is more likely to occur when the subsequent events are traumatic, thereby causing subjectively remembered and frequently occurring events to be recalled, which under normal circumstances would be forgotten. We cannot be certain that recall bias affected these results, but the conditions are present in which recall bias occurs. Therefore, the result of this case-control study may be attributable, at least in part, to recall bias. The potential for recall bias casts doubts on the alleged association between sore throats and the occurrence of spina bifida.

Reporting bias as well as recall bias may operate to impair the accuracy of the outcome assessment, as illustrated in the following example:

> A case-control study of the relationship between gonorrhea and multiple sexual partners was conducted. One hundred women who were newly diagnosed with gonorrhea were compared with 100 women in the same clinic who were found to be free of gonorrhea. The women who were diagnosed with gonorrhea were informed that the serious consequences of the disease could be prevented only by locating and treating their sexual partners. Both groups of women were asked about the number of sexual partners they had during the preceding 2 months. The group of women with gonorrhea reported an average of four times as many sexual partners as the group of women without gonorrhea. The investigators concluded that on average women with gonorrhea have four times as many sexual partners as women without gonorrhea.

It can be argued that the women with gonorrhea in this study felt a greater obligation, hence less hesitation, to report their sexual partners than did the women without the disease. Reporting bias is more likely to occur when the information sought is personal or sensitive. In addition, one group is under more pressure than another to report previous events accurately.

Thus, it is possible that women with gonorrhea may simply have been more thorough in reporting their sexual partners rather than actually having had more contacts. Reporting bias in addition to recall error may impair the accuracy of assessment in case-control studies because the individuals in a case-control study are already aware of the occurrence or absence of occurrence of the outcome being studied.

When measurements are conducted or interpreted by the investigator, human factors can produce inaccuracies in measurement as a result of both assessment bias and chance. These errors can occur when two different investigators perform the same measurements (interobserver error) or when the same individual performs the measurements more than once (intraobserver error).

Assessment bias may also occur as a result of inaccurate measurement by the testing instruments in all types of studies, as illustrated in the following example:

> The gastrointestinal side effects of two nonsteroidal antiinflammatory drugs for arthritis were assessed using an upper gastrointestinal (GI) X-ray. The investigator found no evidence that either drug was associated with gastritis.

The investigator did not recognize that an upper GI X-ray is a very poor instrument for measuring gastritis. Even if a drug caused gastritis, upper GI X-ray examination would not be adequate to identify its presence.

Thus, any conclusion based on this measurement is likely to be inaccurate. When gross instrument error occurs, as in this example, the measurement of outcome also can be considered inappropriate.

Whenever the measurement of outcome depends on subjective interpretation of data, the possibility of investigator bias exists. It is possible, however, to recognize and correct for this fundamental principle of human psychology. Human beings, including investigators, see what they want to see or expect to see. This is accomplished by keeping the investigator, who makes the assessment of outcome, from knowing an individual's group assignment. Blind or masked assessment can be used in case-control and cohort studies as well as in randomized clinical trials. Failure to use blind or masked assessment can lead to the following type of bias:

> In a study of the use of nonsteroidal antiinflammatory drugs (NSAIDs), the investigators, who were the patients' attending physicians, questioned all patients to determine whether one of the NSAIDs was associated with more symptoms compatible with gastritis. After questioning all patients about their symptoms, they determined that there was no difference in the occurrence of gastritis. They reported that the two drugs produced the same frequency of occurrence of gastritis symptoms.

In this study, the investigators making the assessment of outcome were aware of what the patients were receiving; thus, they were not masked. In addition, they were assessing the patients' subjective symptoms such as nausea, stomach pain, or indigestion in deciding whether gastritis was present. This is the setting in which masking is most critical. Even if the patients were unaware of which medication they were taking, the investigators' assessment may be biased. If the assessment conformed with their own hypothesis, their results are especially open to question. This does not imply fraud, only the natural tendency of human beings to see what they expect or want to see. The investigators' conclusions may be true, but their less-than-perfect techniques make it difficult or impossible to accept their conclusion.

Thus, masking in the process of assessment is important to eliminate this source of assessment bias.

Complete and Unaffected by Observation

Whenever follow-up of patients is incomplete, the possibility exists that those not included in the final assessment had a different frequency of the outcome than those included. The following example illustrates an error resulting from incomplete assessment:

> A cohort study of human immunodeficiency virus (HIV)-positive patients compared the natural history of the disease among asymptomatic patients with a CD4 count of 100 to 200 compared with a group of asymptomatic HIV-positive patients with a CD4 count of 200 to 400. The investigators were able to follow up with 50% of those with the lower CD4 counts and 60% of those with the higher CD4 counts. The investigators found no difference between the groups and concluded that the CD4 count is not a risk factor for developing acquired immunodeficiency syndrome (AIDS).

It can be argued that in this investigation, some of the patients who could not be followed up with were not available because they were dead. If this were the case, the results of the study might have been dramatically altered with complete follow-up. Incomplete follow-up can distort the conclusions of an investigation.

Incomplete follow-up does not necessarily mean the patients were lost to follow-up as in the previous example. They may have been monitored with unequal intensity, as the next example illustrates:

> A cohort study of the side effects of birth-control pills was conducted by comparing 1,000 young women taking the pill with 1,000 young women using other forms of birth control. Data were collected from the records of their private physicians over a

1-year period. Pill-users were scheduled for three follow-up visits during the year; other women were asked to return if they had problems. Among users of the pill, 75 women reported having headaches, 90 reported fatigue, and 60 reported depression. Among non–pill-users, 25 patients reported having headaches, 30 reported fatigue, and 20 reported depression. The average pill-user made three visits to her physician during the year versus one visit for the non–pill-user. The investigator concluded that use of the pill is associated with increased frequency of headaches, fatigue, and depression.

The problem of unequal intensity of observation of the two groups may have invalidated the results. The fact that pill-users made three times as many visits to their physician may account for the more frequent recordings of headaches, fatigue, and depression. With more thorough observation, commonly occurring subjective symptoms are more likely to be recorded.

Even if a study's end-point meets the difficult criteria of appropriate, accurate, precise, and complete assessment, one more area of concern exists. Investigators intend to measure events as they would have occurred had no one been watching. Unfortunately, the very process of conducting a study may involve the introduction of an observer into the events being measured. Thus, the reviewer must determine whether the process of observation altered the outcome. An example follows:

A cohort study was conducted of the relationship between obesity and menstrual regularity. One thousand obese women with menstrual irregularities who had joined a diet group were compared with 1,000 obese women with the same pattern of menstrual irregularities who were not enrolled in a diet group. The women were compared to evaluate the effects of weight loss on menstrual irregularities. Those in the diet group had exactly the same frequency of return to regular menstrual cycles as the nondiet group controls.

It is possible that the nondiet-group patients lost weight just like the diet-group patients because they were being observed as part of the study. Whenever it is possible for subjects to switch groups or alter their behavior, the effects of observation may affect an investigation. This is most likely to occur when the individuals in the control group are aware of the adverse consequences of their current behavior and feel pressured to change because they are being observed. This can occur only in a cohort study or in a randomized clinical trial that is begun before any of the participants have developed the outcome.

6 Analysis

In this chapter we take a look at the three key questions of analysis:

- **Estimation:** What is the magnitude or strength of the association or relationship observed in the investigation?
- **Inference:** How have the investigators performed statistical significance testing to draw inferences or conclusions regarding large populations based on the data from samples of the populations included in the investigation?
- **Adjustment:** How have the investigators accounted for potential confounding variables or differences between the groups that may affect the results?

Strength of Relationship: Estimation

When measuring the strength of a relationship using data from samples, we are attempting to use that information to estimate the strength of the relationship within a larger group called a population. Thus, biostatisticians often refer to any measurement of the strength of a relationship as an ESTIMATE or POINT ESTIMATE. The data from the samples are said to estimate the population's EFFECT SIZE, which is the magnitude or size of the association or the difference in the population. First, we will look at the basic measure of the strength of an association that is most frequently used in cohort studies. Then we turn to the basic measure used in case-control studies. Remember, by ASSOCIATION we mean that a factor, often called a RISK FACTOR, occurs together with a disease more frequently than expected by chance alone. Notice that association does not necessarily imply a cause and effect relationship, which we examine in more detail in Chapter 7.

Let us assume that we are studying the association between birth-control pills and thrombophlebitis. We want to measure the strength of the association to determine how the use of birth-control pills affects the risk for thrombophlebitis. Therefore, we must first clarify the concept of risk.

RISK measures the probability of developing a condition over a specified period of time. Risk equals the number of individuals who develop the condition divided by the total number of individuals who were possible candidates to develop the condition at the beginning of the period. In assessing the 10-year risk of developing thrombophlebitis, we would divide the number of women taking birth-control pills who developed thrombophlebitis over a 10-year period by the total number of women in the study group who were taking birth-control pills but did not have thrombophlebitis at the beginning of the study period.

A further calculation is necessary to measure the relative degree of association between thrombophlebitis for women who are on birth-control pills compared with women who are not on birth-control pills. One such measure is known as RELATIVE RISK. Relative risk measures the probability of thrombophlebitis if birth-control pills are used divided by the probability if birth-control pills are not used. It is defined as follows:

$$\text{Relative risk} = \frac{\text{Probability of developing thrombophlebitis}}{\text{Probability of developing thrombophlebitis}}$$

generally,

$$\text{Relative risk} = \frac{\text{Probability of the outcome if the risk factor is present}}{\text{Probability of the outcome if the risk factor is absent}}$$

Let us illustrate how the risk and relative risk are calculated using a hypothetical example:

> For 10 years, an investigator monitored 1,000 young women taking birth-control pills and 1,000 young women who were nonusers. He found that 30 of the women on birth-control pills developed thrombophlebitis over the 10-year period, whereas only three of the nonusers developed thrombophlebitis over the same time period. He presented his data using what is called a 2×2 table.

	Thrombophlebitis	No Thrombophlebitis	
Birth-control pills	a = 30	b = 970	a + b = 1,000
No birth-control pills	c = 3	d = 997	c + d = 1,000

The 10-year risk of developing thrombophlebitis on birth-control pills equals the number of women on the pill who develop thrombophlebitis divided by the total number of women on the pill. Thus, the risk of developing thrombophlebitis for women on birth-control pills is equal to:

$$\frac{a}{a + b} = \frac{30}{1,000} = 0.03$$

Likewise, the 10-year risk of developing thrombophlebitis for women not on the pill equals the number of women not on the pill who develop thrombophlebitis divided by the total number of women not on the pill. Thus, the risk of developing thrombophlebitis for women not on the pill is equal to:

$$\frac{c}{c + d} = \frac{3}{1,000} = 0.003$$

The relative risk equals the ratio of these two risks:

$$\text{Relative risk} = \frac{a / a + b}{c / c + d} = \frac{0.03}{0.003} = 10$$

A relative risk of 1 implies that the use of birth-control pills does not increase the risk of thrombophlebitis. This relative risk of 10 implies that, on the average, women on the pill have a risk of thrombophlebitis 10 times that of women not on the pill.[1]

---

[1]Relative risks may also be presented with the group at lower risk in the numerator. These two forms of the relative risks are merely the reciprocal of each other. Thus, the risk of thrombophlebitis for those not taking birth-control pills divided by the risk for those taking birth-control pills would be 0.003/0.03 = 0.1 or 1/10.

Now let us look at how we measure the strength of association for case-control studies by looking at a study of the association between birth-control pills and thrombophlebitis.

An investigator selected 100 young women with thrombophlebitis and 100 young women without thrombophlebitis. She carefully obtained the history of prior use of birth-control pills. She found that 90 of the 100 women with thrombophlebitis were using birth-control pills compared with 45 of the women without thrombophlebitis. She represented her data using the following 2×2 table.

	Thrombophlebitis	No Thrombophlebitis
Birth control pills	a = 90	b = 45
No birth-control pills	c = 10	d = 55
	a + c = 100	b + d = 100

Notice that in case-control studies the investigator can choose the total number of patients in each group (with and without thrombophlebitis). She could have chosen to select 200 patients with thrombophlebitis and 100 patients without thrombophlebitis or a number of other combinations.

Thus, the actual numbers in each vertical column can be altered at will by the investigator. In other words, in a case-control study the number of individuals who have and do not have the disease does not necessarily reflect the natural frequency of the disease. It is, therefore, improper to add the boxes in the case-control 2×2 table horizontally (as we did in the preceding cohort study). In a case-control study this would allow the investigator to manipulate the size of the resulting measurement.

Unfortunately, without numbers outside the boxes of the 2×2 table it is not possible to calculate relative risk as we did for the cohort study. However, often a good approximation of relative risk exists for case-control studies, which turns out to be very useful for statistical analysis. This approximation of relative risk is known as the ODDS RATIO.

First, what do we mean by odds, and how does that differ from probability or risk? Risk is a probability in which the numerator contains the number of times the event such as thrombophlebitis occurs over a specified period of time. The denominator of a risk or probability contains the number of times the event could have occurred. Odds, like probability, contain the number of times the event occurred in the numerator. However, in the denominator, odds contain only the number of times the event did not occur. The difference between odds and probability may be appreciated by thinking of the chance of drawing an ace from a deck of 52 cards. The probability of drawing an ace is the number of times an ace will be drawn divided by the total number of cards or 4 of 52 or 1 of 13. Odds, on the other hand, are the number of times an ace will be drawn divided by the number of times it will not be drawn or 4 to 48 or 1 to 12. Thus, the odds are slightly different from the probability, but when the event or the disease under study is rare, the odds are a good approximation of the risk or probability.

The odds ratio measures the odds of having the risk factor if the condition is present divided by the odds of having the risk factor if the condition is not present. The odds of being on the pill if thrombophlebitis is present are equal to:

$$\frac{a}{c} = \frac{90}{10} = 9$$

Likewise, the odds of being on the pill for women who do not develop thrombophlebitis are measured by dividing the number of women who do not have thrombophlebitis and are using the pill by the number of women who do not develop thrombophlebitis and are not on the pill. Thus, the odds of being on the pill if thrombophlebitis is not present are equal to:

$$\frac{b}{d} = \frac{45}{55} = 0.82$$

Like the calculation of relative risk, one can develop a measure of the relative odds of being on the pill if thrombophlebitis is present versus being on the pill if thrombophlebitis is not present. This measure of the strength of association is known as the *odds ratio*. Thus,

$$\text{Odds ratio} = \frac{\text{Odds of being on the pill if thrombophlebitis is present}}{\text{Odds of being on the pill if thrombophlebitis is not present}} = \frac{a/c}{b/d} = \frac{ad}{cb} = \frac{9}{0.82} = 11$$

An odds ratio of 1, parallel with our interpretation of relative risk, implies the odds are the same for being on the pill if thrombophlebitis is present as they are for being on the pill if thrombophlebitis is absent. Our odds ratio of 11 means that the odds of being on birth-control pills are increased 11-fold for women with thrombophlebitis.

The odds ratio is the basic measure of the degree of association for case-control studies. It is in and of itself a useful and valid measure of the strength of the association. In addition, as long as the disease (thrombophlebitis) is rare, the odds ratio is equal to approximately the same value as the relative risk.

It is possible to look at the odds ratio in reverse as one would do in a cohort study and come up with the same result. For instance,

$$\text{Odds ratio} = \frac{\text{Odds of developing thrombophlebitis if pill is used}}{\text{Odds of developing thrombophlebitis if pill is not used}}$$

The odds ratio then equals:

$$\frac{a/b}{c/d} = \frac{ad}{cb} = 11$$

Notice that this is the same formula for the odds ratio as the one shown previously. This convenient property allows one to calculate an odds ratio from a cohort or randomized clinical trial instead of calculating the relative risk. This makes it easier to compare the results of a case-control study with those of a cohort study or randomized clinical trial.

Thus, relative risks and odds ratios are the fundamental measures we use to quantitate the strength of an association between a risk factor and a disease. A special type of odds ratio (or relative risk) is calculated when pairing is used to conduct an investigation. Remember, there are two basic approaches to dealing with potential confounding variables. Investigators can match or pair as part of the assignment process and they can adjust as part of the analysis. When the type of matching known as pairing is used to ensure identical distribution of potential confounding variables between study and control groups, a special type of odds ratio should be used to estimate the strength of the association.

As an example, let us suppose that each pair includes one study group patient with thrombophlebitis and one control group patient without thrombophlebitis. The odds ratio then compares the odds of using and not using birth-control pills by comparing one half of the pair with thrombophlebitis to the half without thrombophlebitis.

Assume that a study of birth-control pills and thrombophlebitis postoperatively was conducted using 100 pairs of patients with thrombophlebitis and controls without thrombophlebitis. The cases and controls were paired so that each member of the pair was the same age and parity. The results of a paired case-control study are then presented using the following 2×2 table:[2]

	Controls using birth-control pills	Controls not using birth-control pills
Cases using birth-control pills	30	50
Cases not using birth-control pills	5	15

The odds ratio in a paired case-control study uses only the pairs in which the exposure (*e.g.*, the use of birth-control pills) is different between the case and the control members of a pair. The pairs in which the cases with thrombophlebitis and the controls without thrombophlebitis differ in their use of birth-control pills are known as DISCORDANT PAIRS.

The odds ratio is calculated using discordant pairs as follows:

$$\frac{\text{Number of pairs with cases using birth control pills and controls not using birth-control pills}}{\text{Number of pairs with controls using birth control pills and cases not using birth-control pills}} = \frac{50}{5} = 10$$

This odds ratio is interpreted the same way as an odds ratio calculated from unpaired studies.[3]

Alternative measurements from samples are used for estimation with other types of data. Determining which measurements to use is discussed in Part V, Selecting a Statistic.

Inference: Statistical Significance Testing

Most investigations are conducted on only a sample or subset of a larger group of individuals who could have been included in the study. Researchers, therefore, are frequently confronted with the question of whether they would achieve similar results if the entire population was included in the study or whether chance selection may have produced unusual results in their particular sample.

---

[2]The table for a paired case-control study tells us about what happens to a pair instead of what happens to each person. Thus, the frequencies in this paired 2×2 table add up to 100 (the number of pairs) instead of 200 (the number of persons in the study).

[3]Pairing, however, has an advantage of greater statistical power. That is, everything else being equal, statistical significance can be established using smaller numbers of study and control group patients.

Unfortunately, there is no direct method for answering this question. Instead, investigators are forced to test their study hypothesis using a circuitous method of proof by elimination. This method is known as statistical significance testing.

Statistical significance testing, in its most common form, quantitates the probability of obtaining the observed data or a more extreme result if no differences between groups exist in the larger population. Statistical significance testing assumes that individuals used in an investigation are representative or randomly selected from a larger group or population. This use of the term RANDOM is confusing because statistical significance testing is used in studies in which the individuals are not randomly selected. This apparent contradiction can be reconciled if one assumes that the larger population consists of all individuals with the same characteristics as those required for entry in the study. Thus, statistical significance tests actually address questions about larger populations made up of individuals just like those used in the investigation. Statistical significance testing aims to draw conclusions or inferences about a population by studying samples of that population. Therefore, biostatisticians often refer to statistical significance testing as INFERENCE.

Statistical Significance Testing Procedures

Statistical significance testing or hypothesis testing assumes that only two types of relationships exist. Either differences between groups within the study population exist or they do not exist. When we conduct statistical significance tests on study data, we assume at the beginning that no such differences exist in the population. The role of statistical significance testing is to evaluate the results obtained from the samples to determine whether these results would be so unusual, if no difference exists in the larger population, that, in fact, we can conclude: a difference does exist in the large population. Notice that the issue is whether any difference exists. Statistical significance testing itself says nothing about the size or importance of the potential difference.

Statistical significance testing begins with a STUDY HYPOTHESIS stating that a difference exists in the larger population. In performing statistical significance tests, it is assumed initially that the study hypothesis is false, and a NULL HYPOTHESIS is formulated stating that no difference exists in the larger population. Statistical methods then are used to calculate the probability of obtaining the observed results in the study sample, or more extreme results, if no difference actually exists in the larger population.

When only a small probability exists that the observed results would occur in samples if the null hypothesis were true, then investigators can reject the contention that the null hypothesis is true, that is they can reject the null hypothesis. In rejecting the null hypothesis, the investigators accept, by elimination, the existence of their only other alternative—the existence of a difference between groups in the larger population. Biostatisticians often refer to the study hypothesis as the ALTERNATIVE HYPOTHESIS because it is the alternative to the null hypothesis.

The specific steps in statistical significance testing are as follows:

1. State hypothesis
2. Formulate null hypothesis
3. Decide statistical significance cutoff level
4. Collect data

5. Apply statistical significance test
6. Reject or fail to reject the null hypothesis:

STATE HYPOTHESIS

Before collecting the data, the investigators state a study hypothesis that a difference exists between the study group and the control group in the larger population.

FORMULATE NULL HYPOTHESIS

The investigators then assume that no true difference exists between the study group and the control group in the larger population.

DECIDE STATISTICAL SIGNIFICANCE CUTOFF LEVEL

The investigators determine what level of probability will be considered small enough to reject the null hypothesis. In the vast majority of health research studies, a 5% chance or less of occurrence is considered unlikely enough to allow the investigators to reject the null hypothesis. However, we are generally left with some possibility that chance alone has produced an unusual set of data. Thus, a null hypothesis, which is in fact true, will be rejected in favor of the study hypothesis as much as 5% of the time.[4]

COLLECT DATA

The data may be collected using study designs such as a case-control, cohort, or randomized clinical trial.

APPLY STATISTICAL SIGNIFICANCE TEST

If differences between the study and control groups exist, the investigators determine the probability that these differences would occur if no true difference exists in the larger population from which both the study and control group individuals in the samples have been selected. This probability is known as the P VALUE.

In other words, they calculate the probability that the observed data or more extreme data would occur if the null hypothesis of no difference were true. To do so, the investigators must choose from a variety of statistical significance tests. Because each type of test is appropriate to a specific type of data, investigators must take care to choose the proper test, as we discuss in Part V, Selecting a Statistic.

To understand how a statistical significance test uses *P* values, let's consider an example that uses small numbers to allow easy calculation.

Assume that an investigator wants to study the question: "Are there an equal number of males and females born in the United States?" The investigator first hypothesizes that more males than females are born in the United States; a null hypothesis that an

---

[4]Investigators also need to decide whether to use a one-tailed or two-tailed statistical significance test. A TWO-TAILED test implies that the investigator is willing to accept data that deviate in either direction from the null hypothesis. A ONE-TAILED test implies that the investigator is only willing to accept data that deviate in the direction of the study hypothesis. We will assume a two-tailed test unless otherwise indicated.

equal number of males and females are born in the United States is then formulated. Then, the investigator decides the statistical significance cutoff level, which is usually set at 5% or P = 0.05. Next, the investigator samples four birth certificates and finds that there are four males and zero females in the sample of births.

Let us now calculate the probability of obtaining four males and zero females if the null hypothesis of equal numbers of males and females is true:

Probability of one male	0.50 or 50%
Probability of two males in a row	0.25 or 25%
Probability of three males in a row	0.125 or 12.5%
Probability of four males in a row	0.0625 or 6.25%

Thus, there is a 6.25% chance of obtaining four males in a row even if an equal number of males and females are born in the United States.[5] Thus, the P value equals 0.0625.

A simple form of statistical significance test such as this one can yield the probability of producing the observed data, assuming that the null hypothesis is true. Most statistical significance tests yield similar types of results. They measure the probability of obtaining the observed data or more extreme data if no true difference between groups actually exists in the larger population.

REJECT OR FAIL TO REJECT THE NULL HYPOTHESIS

Having determined the probability that the results could have occurred by chance if no true differences exist in the larger population, the investigators proceed to reject or fail to reject the null hypothesis. If the probability of the results occurring by chance is less than or equal to 0.05, investigators can reject the null hypothesis.

Thus, the probability is small that chance alone could produce the differences in outcome if the null hypothesis is true. By elimination, they accept the study hypothesis that a true difference exists in the outcome between study and control groups in the larger population.

What if the probability of occurrence by chance is greater than 0.05, as in the preceding example? The investigators then are unable to reject the null hypothesis. This does not mean that the null hypothesis, that no true difference exists in the larger population, is true. It merely indicates that the probability of obtaining the observed results, if the null hypothesis were true, is too great to reject the null hypothesis or accept by elimination the study hypothesis. When the P value is greater than 0.05 we say that the investigation has failed to reject the null hypothesis. The burden of proof, therefore, is on the investigators to show that the data obtained in the samples are unlikely before rejecting the null hypothesis in favor of the study hypothesis. The following example shows how the significance testing procedure operates in practice.

An investigator wanted to test the hypothesis that there is a difference in the frequency of mouth cancer among pipe-smokers and non–pipe-smokers. She formulated a null hypothesis stating that mouth cancer occurs with no greater frequency among pipe-smokers than among non–pipe-smokers. She then decided that she would reject the null hypothesis if she obtained data that would occur only 5% or less of the time

[5]For ease of interpretation, a one-tailed statistical significance test has been used. The births have been assumed to be independent of each other in calculating probabilities.

if the null hypothesis was true. She next collected data from a sample of the general population of pipe-smokers and non–pipe-smokers. Using the proper statistical significance test, she found that if no difference existed between pipe-smoking and mouth cancer in the general population, then data as extreme or more extreme than her data would be observed by chance only 3% of the time. She now concluded that because her data were quite unlikely to occur if there were no difference between pipe-smoking and mouth cancer, she would reject the null hypothesis. The investigator thus accepted by elimination the study hypothesis that a difference in the frequency of mouth cancer exists between pipe-smokers and non–pipe-smokers in the general population.

When a statistically significant difference between groups is obtained, we say there is an ASSOCIATION between the group and the characteristic being studied. That is, there is an association between pipe-smoking and mouth cancer. The two occur together more frequently than is expected by chance alone. Remember that we have defined small as a 5% chance or less that the observed results would have occurred if no true difference exists in the larger population.

The 5% figure may be too large if important decisions depend on the results. The 5% figure is based on some convenient statistical properties; however, it is not a magic number. It is possible to define small as 1%, 0.1%, or any other probability. Remember, however, that no matter what level is chosen, there will always be some probability of rejecting the null hypothesis when no true difference exists in the larger population. Statistical significance tests can measure this probability, but they cannot eliminate it.

Table 6.1 reviews and summarizes the steps for performing a statistical significance test.

Errors in Statistical Significance Testing

Several types of errors commonly occur in using statistical significance tests:
- Failure to state the hypothesis before conducting the study
- Failure to interpret the results of statistical significance tests correctly by not considering the TYPE I ERROR
- Failure to interpret the results of statistical significance tests correctly by not considering the TYPE II ERROR

Table 6.1. *How a statistical significance test works*

State hypothesis	Develop the study question: A difference exists between groups in a population
Formulate null hypothesis	Reverse the hypothesis: No difference exists between groups in the population
Decide significance cutoff level	5% unless otherwise indicated and justified
Collect data	Determine whether a difference between groups exists in the data collected from samples of the larger population
Apply statistical significance test	Determine the probability of obtaining the observed data or more extreme data if the null hypothesis were true (i.e., choose and apply the correct statistical significance test)
Reject or fail to reject the null hypothesis	Reject the null hypothesis and accept by elimination the study hypothesis if the statistical significance cutoff level is reached; fail to reject the null hypothesis if the observed data have more than a 5% probability of occurring by chance if there is no difference between groups in the larger population

The following example illustrates the consequences of failing to state the hypothesis before conducting the study:

> An investigator randomly selected 100 individuals known to have essential hypertension and 100 individuals known to be free of hypertension. He compared them according to a list of 100 variables to determine how the two groups differed. Of the 100 variables studied, two were found to be statistically significant at the 0.05 level using standard statistical methods: (1) Hypertensives generally have more letters in their last name than nonhypertensives, and (2) hypertensives generally are born during the first 3 ½ days of the week, whereas nonhypertensives are usually born during the latter 3 ½ days of the week. The author concluded that, although these differences had not been foreseen, longer names and birth during the first half of the week are different between groups with and without essential hypertension.

This example illustrates the importance of stating the hypothesis beforehand. Whenever a large number of variables are tested one at a time, it is likely by chance alone that some of them will be statistically significant variables. It can be misleading to apply the usual levels of statistical significance unless the hypothesis has been stated before collecting and analyzing the data. If differences are looked for without formulating a study hypothesis or only after collecting and analyzing the data, much stricter criteria should be applied than the usual 5% probability.

When a single hypothesis is not stated, a suggested rule of thumb for the reader of the health literature is to divide the observed P value by the number of variables being tested for statistical significance. The resulting P value can then be used to reject or fail to reject the null hypothesis. For instance, imagine that a study tested five variables in each of two groups without stating a study hypothesis. To reach a P value of 0.05 for any one variable, that variable must have a P value equal to:

$$\frac{0.05}{\text{Number of variables}} = \frac{0.05}{5} = 0.01$$

This P value of 0.01 should be interpreted just like a P value of 0.05 if one study hypothesis was stated before beginning the study.[6,7]

Type I Errors

Some errors are inherent in the method of statistical significance testing. A fundamental concept of statistical significance testing is the possibility that a null hypothesis will be falsely rejected and a study hypothesis will be falsely accepted by elimination. This is known as a Type I error.

[6]If there are more than two groups, the equation is the desired Type I error divided by the number of comparisons. This method is a useful approximation for small numbers of variables. As the number of variables increases much above 5, the required P value tends to be too small before statistical significance can be declared. This approach reduces the statistical power of a study to demonstrate statistical significance for any one variable. Thus, many biostatisticians argue it is better to use the multivariable method, which will be discussed in Part V, Selecting a Statistic.

[7]Remember that statistical significance testing or hypothesis testing is a method of drawing inferences in a world in which we must decide between the study and the null hypothesis based only on the data within the study. It is possible, however, to look at inference as a process that incorporates some probability that the hypothesis is true. In this process, the investigator must estimate this probability before the study begins. This might be done on the basis of the results of previous studies or other medical knowledge. When this prior probability is obtained, statistical methods are available to estimate the probability that the hypothesis is true after the results of the study are obtained. This BAYESIAN PROCESS is parallel to the use of diagnostic testing, which we discuss in Part II, Testing a Test. An advantage of the Bayesian approach is that P values need not be adjusted to account for the number of variables.

In traditional statistical significance testing, there is as much as a 5% chance of incorrectly accepting by elimination a study hypothesis even when no true difference exists in the larger population from which the study samples were obtained. This level, usually 5%, of Type I error allowed in a design of an investigation is known as the ALPHA LEVEL. Statistical significance testing does not eliminate uncertainty. Careful readers of studies are, therefore, able to appreciate the degree of doubt that exists and can decide for themselves whether they are willing to tolerate or act with that degree of uncertainty.

In some circumstances, an alpha level of 0.05 may be more than one is willing to tolerate; in other circumstances one may tolerate even more than 5% uncertainty. For instance, before introducing a new method of water purification in a community with a low frequency of water-borne disease, one might not accept the new method if there is 5% probability that the new method would fail to eliminate water-borne disease. On the other hand, in a community where water is a major source of disease transmission, one might tolerate a higher probability that the new method would fail to eliminate water-borne disease, especially if no other method is available. Let us see how failure to appreciate the possibility of a Type I error can lead to misinterpreted study results.

> The author of a review article evaluated 20 well-conducted studies that examined the relationship between breastfeeding and breast cancer. Nineteen of the studies found no difference in the frequency of breast cancer between breastfeeding and formula-feeding. One study found a difference in which the breastfeeding group had an increase in breast cancer. The results were statistically significant at the 0.05 level. The author of the review article concluded that, because a study existed suggesting that breastfeeding is associated with an increased risk of breast cancer, breastfeeding should be discouraged.

When 20 well-conducted studies are performed to test a study hypothesis that is not true for the larger population, a substantial possibility exists that one of the studies may show an association at the 0.05 level simply by chance. Remember the meaning of statistical significance at the 0.05 level: It implies that the results have a 5% probability, or a chance of 1 in 20, of occurring by chance alone when no difference exists in the larger population.

Thus, 1 study in 20 that shows a difference should not be interpreted as evidence for a difference in the larger population. It is important to keep in mind the possibility that no difference may exist even when statistically significant results have been demonstrated. If the only study showing a relationship had been adopted without further questioning, breastfeeding might have been discouraged without considering its cancer prevention benefits.

Type II Errors

A TYPE II error says that failure to reject the null hypothesis does not necessarily mean that no true difference exists in the larger population. Remember that statistical significance testing directly addresses only the null hypothesis. The process of statistical significance testing allows one to reject or fail to reject that null hypothesis. It does not allow one to prove a null hypothesis. Failure to reject a null hypothesis merely implies that the evidence is not strong enough to reject the assumption that no difference exists in the larger population.

A Type II error occurs when we are prevented from demonstrating a statistically significant difference even when a difference actually exists in the larger population. This happens when chance produces an unusual set of data that fail to show a difference, even though one actually exists in the larger population. This type of error is parallel to a Type I error, indicating that chance has played a role. A particular study may come up with an unusual outcome that could occur only a small percentage of the time. It does not imply that mistakes were made in design or implementation of the study; it merely demonstrates that, despite the best efforts and intentions, statistical methods can lead us to incorrect conclusions by the luck of the draw. This potential is inherent in statistical concepts.

Efforts to perform statistical significance testing always carry with them the probability of error.

Investigators may make the problem far worse by using too few individuals in a study. The fewer the number of individuals included in a study, the greater the chance of obtaining an unusual sample. Therefore, when using small samples, we need to see greater differences between our samples before we are ready to reject the null hypothesis. If we require larger differences to reject the null hypothesis, we have a greater chance of failing to reject a null hypothesis that actually should be rejected. Thus, the chance of making a Type II error increases as the number of observations in the sample decreases.

Statistical techniques are available for estimating the probability that a study of a particular size could establish a statistically significant difference if a specified difference actually exists in the larger population. These techniques measure the STATISTICAL POWER of the study. The statistical power of a study is its probability of demonstrating statistical significance. Thus, statistical power equals one minus the Type II error. In many studies the probability is quite large that one will fail to show a statistically significant difference when a true difference actually exists. No arbitrary number indicates how great a Type II error one should tolerate. However, well-designed studies often aim for a Type II error between 10% and 20%. Without actually stating it, investigators who use relatively small samples may be accepting a 30%, 40%, or even greater probability that they will fail to demonstrate a statistically significant difference when a true difference exists in the larger population. The size of the Type II error incorporated with the design of an investigation is known as the BETA LEVEL. Table 6.2 summarizes and compares Type I and II errors.

The following example shows the effect of sample size on the ability to demonstrate statistically significant differences between groups:

> A study of the adverse effects of cigarettes on health was undertaken by monitoring 100 cigarette smokers and 100 nonsmokers for 20 years. During the 20 years, five smokers developed lung cancer, whereas none of the nonsmokers were afflicted. During the same time, ten smokers and nine nonsmokers developed myocardial infarction. The results for lung cancer were statistically significant, but the results for myocardial infarction were not. The authors concluded that a difference in lung cancer frequency between smokers and nonsmokers had been supported, and a difference between cigarette smokers and nonsmokers with regard to the frequency of myocardial infarction had been refuted.

When differences between groups are very great, as they are between smokers and nonsmokers in relation to lung cancer, only a relatively small sample may be required

Table 6.2. *Inherent errors of statistical significance testing*

Variable	Type I Error	Type II Error
Definition	Rejection of null hypothesis when no true difference exists in the larger population	Failure to reject null hypothesis when a true difference exists in the larger population
Cause	Random error	Random error made worse by a too small sample size
Likelihood of occurrence	Setting of statistical significance cutoff level will indicate how large an error will be tolerated (usually up to 5%)	Statistical techniques can estimate occurrence from the size of the groups (probability of error may be quite large if the numbers are small)

to demonstrate statistical significance. When the true differences are smaller, it requires greater numbers to demonstrate a statistically significant difference.

This study would not refute a difference between cigarette smokers and non-smokers with regard to the frequency of myocardial infarction. It is very likely that the number of individuals included were too few to give the study enough statistical power to demonstrate the statistical significance of a difference even though other studies suggest that a difference exists in the general population. A study with limited statistical power to demonstrate a difference also has limited power to refute a difference.

Confidence Intervals

We noted that statistical significance testing does not provide information about the strength of an observed association. It is attractive to use a method that provides a summary measure (often called a POINT ESTIMATE) of the strength of an association and that also permits us to take chance into account using a statistical significance test.

The calculation of CONFIDENCE INTERVALS is such a method. These combine information from samples about the strength of an association with information about the effects of chance on the likelihood of obtaining the observed results. It is possible to calculate the confidence interval for any percentage confidence from 0 to 100. However, the 95% confidence interval is the most commonly used. It allows us to be 95% confident that the larger population's difference or ratio value lies within the confidence interval.

Confidence intervals are often calculated for odds ratios and relative risks. The calculation of these intervals is complex. The reader of the literature, however, may see an expression such as 10 (8,12), which expresses the observed odds ratio (lower confidence limit, upper confidence limit).

The term CONFIDENCE LIMIT is used to indicate the upper or lower extent of a confidence interval. The above expression usually tells us the observed odds ratio and the confidence limits for the 95% confidence interval. Other confidence intervals may be used, but they should be specifically indicated.

Imagine a study in which the odds ratio for birth-control pills and thrombo-phlebitis was 10 (8,12). How would you interpret this confidence interval?

The 10 indicates the odds ratio observed in the sample. The confidence interval on this odds ratio allows us to say with 95% confidence that the odds ratio in the larger population is between 8 and 12. Because the lower confidence limit is 8, far greater than 1, this allows us to be quite confident that a substantial odds ratio is present not only in our sample, but in the larger population from which our sample was obtained.

These expressions of confidence limits, in addition to providing additional information on estimates, have another advantage for the health literature reader: They allow us to perform hypothesis testing or inference and to rapidly draw conclusions about the statistical significance of the observed data. When using 95% confidence intervals, we can quickly conclude whether or not the observed data are statistically significant with a *P* value less than or equal to 0.05.

This calculation is particularly straightforward for odds ratios and relative risks. For these, 1 represents the point at which the odds or risk of disease are the same, whether or not the risk factor is present. Thus, an odds ratio of 1 is actually an expression of the null hypothesis which says the odds of disease are the same whether the risk factor is present or absent.

Thus, if the 95% confidence interval around the observed odds ratio does not extend beyond 1, we can conclude that the odds ratio is statistically significant with a *P* value less than or equal to 0.05. The same principles are true for relative risks. Let us look at a series of odds ratios and 95% confidence intervals:

A. 4 (0.9, 7.1)
B. 4 (2, 6)
C. 8 (1, 15)
D. 8 (6, 10)

The number to the left of the parenthesis is the odds ratio, which is obtained from the data in the investigation. The numbers within the parentheses are the upper and lower limits of the 95% confidence interval. The 95% confidence limits on odds ratios in B and D do not include 1. In C they include 1 but do not extend beyond 1.

Thus, B, C, and D are statistically significant with a *P* value less than or equal to 0.05. A is not statistically significant because one of its confidence limits extends beyond 1. Thus, when the observed odds ratio (or relative risk) is greater than 1 (*e.g.*, 4 or 8), we need to look at the lower confidence limit to see whether it extends below 1.[8]

In example A, the 95% confidence interval for the odds ratio extends below 1. This leaves us with enough uncertainty regarding birth-control pills and an actual reduced risk of thrombophlebitis that we cannot declare statistical significance. In examples B, C, and D, we can have 95% or more confidence that birth-control pills are associated with an increase in the probability of thrombophlebitis, and thus we can declare statistical significance.

---

[8]When the observed odds ratio is less than 1 (e.g., 0.8), we need to look at the upper 95% confidence limit to see whether it extends above 1. When the 95% confidence interval extends beyond 1 from either direction, the results are not statistically significant. By tradition, when the 95% confidence interval reaches, but does not extend beyond 1, the results are considered statistically significant. Thus, a *P* value of .05 is considered statistically significant.

As a reader of the literature, you will increasingly find the observed value and the confidence limits included in the analysis section. This is helpful because it allows you to gain a gestalt or a feel for the data. It allows you to draw your own conclusion about the importance of the size or strength of the observed point estimate. Finally, if you want to convert to the traditional statistical significance testing format for hypothesis testing, you can often make an approximate calculation to determine whether the results are statistically significant with a *P* value of 0.05 or less.

Adjustment: Reducing the Effect of Confounding Variables

As we discussed in Chapter 4, confounding variables can result from either random error or bias. Chance may produce random error. Unlike bias, the effect of chance is unpredictable. It may either favor or oppose the study hypothesis in a way that cannot be predicted beforehand.

Bias, on the other hand, implies a systematic effect on the data in one particular direction that predictably favors or opposes the study hypothesis. Bias results from the way the patients were assigned or assessed.

Bias and chance may each produce differences between study and control groups, resulting in study and control groups that differ in ways that can affect the outcome of the study.

In Chapter 4, we also noted that the investigator is obligated to compare the characteristics of individuals in the study group with those in the control group to determine whether they differ in any way. If the groups differ, even without being statistically significant, the investigator must consider whether these differences could have affected the results. Characteristics that differ between groups and that may affect the results of the study are potential confounding variables. These potential confounding variables may result either from selection bias or from differences between the study and control groups produced by random error. If a potential confounding variable is detected, the investigator is obligated to consider this in the analysis using a process we call ADJUSTMENT OF DATA.[9]

In performing an adjustment, the investigator may separate into groups those who possessed specific levels of the confounding variable. Groups with the same level of confounding variable are then compared to see whether an association between exposure and disease exists. For instance, if gender is a potential confounding variable, the investigator might subdivide the study and the control groups into men and women and then compare study versus control group men and study versus control group women to determine whether differences exist when the groups of the same gender are compared. Statistical techniques known as MULTI-VARIABLE METHODS are available for adjusting one or more variables at a time, as we discuss in Part V, Selecting a Statistic. Failure to recognize and adjust for a confounding variable can result in serious errors, as illustrated in the following example:

> An investigator studied the relationship between coffee consumption and lung cancer by monitoring 500 heavy coffee drinkers and 500 coffee abstainers for 10 years. In this cohort study, the risk for lung cancer in heavy coffee drinkers was 10 times

---

[9]Many biostatisticians encourage the use of adjustment, even when the differences are small or the importance of differences is not apparent, because of the possibility of interactions between variables.

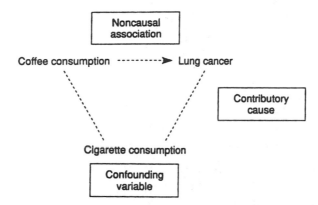

Figure 6.1. Relationship among contributory cause, confounding variable, and noncausal association. By tradition, when the confidence interval reaches but does not extend beyond 1, the results are considered statistically significant. That is, a *P* value of 0.05 is considered statistically significant.

> that of coffee abstainers. The author concluded that coffee, along with cigarettes, was established as a risk factor in the development of lung cancer.

Cigarette smoking may be considered a confounding variable in this study if it is assumed that cigarette smoking is associated with coffee drinking, or in other words, if coffee drinkers are more likely than coffee abstainers to smoke cigarettes. Cigarettes are also associated with lung cancer.

Thus, cigarettes are a potential confounding variable related to outcome, lung cancer, and coffee consumption. Figure 6.1 depicts the relationship between coffee drinking, cigarette smoking, and lung cancer. If cigarette smoking is a confounding variable, then an adjustment for cigarettes must be made as part of the analysis when studying the relationship between coffee consumption and lung cancer.

In adjusting for cigarette smoking, the investigator could divide coffee drinkers into cigarette smokers and nonsmokers and do the same with the coffee abstainers. The investigator would then compare nonsmoking coffee drinkers with nonsmoking coffee abstainers to determine whether the relationship between coffee drinking and lung cancer still holds true. Only after determining that taking into account cigarette smoking does not eliminate the relationship between coffee drinking and lung cancer can the author conclude that coffee drinking is associated with the development of lung cancer.

7 Interpretation

Contributory Cause

Can cigarettes cause cancer?
Can cholesterol cause coronary artery disease?
Can a new treatment cure cancer?
Can chemicals cause congenital defects?

Practitioners are constantly confronted with controversies about cause and effect. Thus, the reader of the health literature must have an understanding of the concept of causation used by investigators.

INTERPRETATION addresses what the results of a study mean for the participants in that study. It covers questions about cause-and-effect relationships.

One question of interpretation may be: *Is a characteristic or risk factor a contributory cause of a disease?*

Alternatively, the investigation may ask: *Does a particular treatment or other intervention prevent the disease or improve the outcome (i.e., does it have efficacy)?*

In Chapter 2, we introduced a definition of cause and effect termed *contributory cause*. This same definition is used to establish efficacy. To definitively establish the existence of a contributory cause, all three of the following criteria must be fulfilled:

- **Association:** Does the investigation establish a substantial and statistically significant association which provides convincing evidence that the cause occurs more frequently together with the effect than expected by chance alone?
- **Prior association:** Does the investigation establish that the cause precedes the effect?
- **Altering the cause alters the effect:** Does the investigation establish that altering or modifying the frequency or severity of the cause alters the frequency or severity of the disease or other effect?

Association

Establishing the first criterion of contributory cause, association, requires that we examine the magnitude and the statistical significance of the relationship established in the analysis. Usually, to establish the existence of an association, we expect a large or substantial as well as statistically significant association.

Remember, statistical significance testing is designed to help us assess the role of chance when we observe a difference or an association in an investigation. As mentioned in earlier chapters, statistical significance testing or inference tells us very little about the size of a difference or the strength of an association, that is the role of estimation. Thus, it is important to ask not only whether a difference or association is statistically significant, but whether it is large or substantial enough to be clinically useful. The world is full of myriad differences between individuals and between groups. Many of these, however, are not great enough to allow us to usefully separate individuals into groups for purposes of disease prevention, diagnosis, and therapy.[1]

As we have seen, when the sample size of a study is small, the possibility of a Type II error can be very great. Remember, a Type II error is the probability of failing to demonstrate statistical significance when a true difference or association exists. Conversely, when the sample size is quite large, it is possible to obtain a statistically significant difference or association even when the difference or association is too small or too weak to be clinically useful, as in the following example:

> Investigators monitored 100,000 middle-age men for 10 years to determine which factors were associated with coronary artery disease. They hypothesized beforehand that uric acid might be a factor in predicting the disease. The investigators found that men who developed coronary artery disease had a uric acid measure of 7.8 mg/dL, whereas men who did not develop the disease had an average uric acid measure of 7.7 mg/dL. The difference was statistically significant with a P value of 0.05. The authors concluded that, because a statistically significant difference had been found, the results would be clinically useful.

Because the difference in this study is statistically significant, it is most likely real in the larger population. However, it is so small that it probably is not clinically important. The large number of men being observed allowed investigators to obtain a statistically significant result for a very small difference between groups.

However, the small size of the difference makes it unlikely that uric acid measurements could be clinically useful in predicting who will develop coronary artery disease. The small difference does not help the clinician to differentiate those who will develop coronary artery disease from those who will not. In fact, when the test is performed in the clinical laboratory, this small difference is probably less than the size of the laboratory error in measuring uric acid.

Prior Association and Cause—Effect Link

To establish the second and third criteria, we must rely on more than statistical analysis. It may appear simple to establish that a cause precedes a disease, but let us look at two hypothetical studies in which the authors may have been fooled into believing that they had established cause preceding effect.

> Two investigators conducted a case-control study to determine whether antacids were taken by patients with myocardial infarction (MI) the week preceding an MI. They were looking for causes of the condition. MI patients were compared with patients admitted for elective surgery. The authors found that the MI patients were 10 times more likely to have taken antacids as the controls during the week preceding admission. The authors concluded that taking antacids is associated with subsequent MIs.

The authors believed that they established not only the first criterion of causation (an association at the individual level) but also the second criterion (that the cause precedes the effect).

---

[1]It is sometimes necessary to distinguish between statistically significant, substantial, and clinically important differences. At times, statistically significant and large or substantial differences between groups are not useful for decision making. We may decide medically or socially to treat individuals the same regardless of large differences in factors such as intelligence, height, or age.

But did they? If individuals have angina before MIs, they may misinterpret the pain and try to alleviate it by self-medicating with antacids. Therefore, the medication is taken to treat the disease and does not truly precede the disease. This study failed to establish that the cause precedes the effect because it did not clarify whether the disease led the patients to take the medication or whether the medication precipitated the disease. This example illustrates the potential difficulty encountered in separating cause and effect in case-control studies. Case-control studies, however, are often capable of providing convincing evidence that the cause precedes the effect. This occurs when there is good documentation of previous characteristics that are not affected by knowledge of occurrence of the disease.

Cohort studies often have an advantage in establishing that the possible cause occurs before the effect. The following example, however, illustrates that even in cohort studies, we may have difficulty determining whether this is true.

> A group of 1,000 patients who had stopped smoking cigarettes within the last year were compared with 1,000 current cigarette smokers matched for total pack-years of smoking. The two groups were monitored for 6 months to determine with what frequency they developed lung cancer. The study showed that 5% of the study group who had stopped smoking cigarettes developed lung cancer as opposed to only 0.1% of the currently smoking controls. The authors concluded that to stop cigarette smoking was associated with the subsequent development of lung cancer. Therefore, they advised current smokers to continue smoking.

The cessation of cigarette smoking appears to occur before the development of lung cancer, but what if smokers stop smoking because of symptoms produced by lung cancer?

If this was true, then lung cancer stops smoking and not vice versa. Thus, one must be careful in accepting that the hypothesized cause precedes the effect. The ability of cohort studies to establish that the cause precedes the effect is enhanced when the time lapse between cause and effect relative to the natural history of the disease is longer than in this example. Short time intervals still leave open the possibility that the presumed cause has been influenced by the presumed effect instead of the reverse.

Even if one has firmly established that the possible cause precedes the effect, to completely fulfill the criteria for contributory cause, it is necessary to establish that altering the cause alters the probability of the effect. This criterion can be established by performing an intervention study in which the investigator alters the cause and determines whether this subsequently contributes to altering the probability of the effect. Ideally, this criterion is fulfilled by performing a randomized clinical trial, as we discuss in Chapter 9.

It is important to recognize that contributory cause is an empirical definition. It does not require an understanding of the intermediate mechanism by which the contributory cause triggers the effect. Historically, numerous instances have occurred in which actions based on a demonstration of contributory cause reduced disease despite the absence of a scientific understanding of how the result actually occurred. Puerperal fever was controlled through handwashing before the bacterial agents were recognized. Malaria was controlled by swamp clearance before its mosquito transmission was recognized. Scurvy was prevented by citrus fruit before the British ever heard of vitamin C. Once we understand more about the direct mechanisms that produce disease, we are able to distinguish between indirect and direct contributory causes.[2]

Investigators must be careful to assess that any change they have observed is not associated with other unmeasured changes that are the real contributory cause. This pitfall is illustrated by the following example:

> In a poor rural region where the diet was very low in protein, diarrhea was widespread. The effect of increased protein was studied in a randomized clinical trial by using modern agricultural methods to introduce high-protein crops in the study group area. Subsequent follow-up revealed a 70% reduction in the incidence of diarrhea in the study areas and little change in the other areas. The authors concluded that a high-protein diet prevents diarrhea.

It is likely that the introduction of modern agriculture was associated with numerous other changes in water supply and sanitation that may have prompted the reduced incidence of diarrhea. Thus, care must be taken to ensure that the characteristic selected as the cause is truly the factor that brought about the effect.

In other words, the investigator and the reader must be careful that the cause has truly preceded the effect and that the presumed alteration in the effect has not been produced by other changes that are actually causal. When contributory cause cannot be definitively established, we may still need to make our best judgments about the existence of a cause-and-effect relationship. For this situation a series of ANCILLARY, ADJUNCT, or SUPPORTIVE CRITERIA for contributory cause have been developed. These include the following:

1. **Strength of association.** This indicates the strength of the association between the risk factor and the disease as measured, for example, by the size of the relative risk.
2. **Consistency of association.** Consistency is present when investigations performed in different settings on different types of patients produce similar results.
3. **Biological plausibility.** The biological plausibility of the relationship is evaluated on the basis of clinical or basic science principles.

   Biological plausibility implies that a known biological mechanism is capable of explaining the relationship between the cause and the effect. For instance, hypertension is a biologically plausible contributory cause of strokes, coronary artery disease, and renal disease because the mechanism for damage is known and the type of damage is consistent with that mechanism. On the other hand, data suggesting a relationship between hypertension and cancer would not be biologically plausible, at least on the basis of current knowledge.

   Biological plausibility also implies that the timing and magnitude of the cause are compatible with the occurrence of the effect. For instance, we assume that severe, long-standing hypertension is more likely to be a contributory cause of congestive heart failure or renal disease than mild hypertension of short duration.

---

[2]What we call a direct cause of disease depends on the current state of knowledge and understanding of disease mechanism. Thus, over time, many direct causes may come to be regarded as indirect causes. In addition, it is important to distinguish these terms from the legal concept of proximal cause. PROXIMAL CAUSE refers to actions that could prevent a particular outcome and should not be confused with the definition of causation used here.

4. A dose-response relationship. A dose-response relationship implies that changes in levels of exposure to the risk factor are associated with changes in the frequency of disease in a consistent direction.

Data that support each of these criteria help bolster the argument that a factor is actually a contributory cause. When these criteria are fulfilled, it reduces the likelihood that the observed association is due to chance or bias. The criteria, however, do not prove the existence of a contributory cause.

In addition, none of these four criteria for establishing contributory cause are essential. A risk factor with a modest but real association may in fact be one of a series of contributory causes for a disease. Consistency is not essential because it is possible for a risk factor to operate in one community but not in another. This may occur because of the existence in one community of other prerequisite conditions. Biological plausibility assumes that we understand the relevant biological processes. Finally, a dose-response relationship, although frequent in biological relationships, is not required for a cause-and-effect relationship, as illustrated in the next study example:

> An investigator conducted a cohort study of the association between radiation and thyroid cancer. He found that low-dose radiation had a relative risk of 5 of being associated with thyroid cancer. However, he found that at moderate levels of radiation, the relative risk was 10 but at high levels, it was 1. The investigator concluded that radiation could not cause thyroid cancer because no dose-response relationship of more cancer with more radiation was demonstrated.

The relative risk of 10 is an impressive association between radiation and thyroid cancer. This should not be dismissed merely because the relative risk is diminished at higher doses. It is possible that low-dose and moderate-dose radiation contributes to thyroid cancer, whereas large doses of radiation actually kill cells and thus do not contribute to thyroid cancer.

For many biological relationships, a little exposure may have little measurable effect. At higher doses, the effect may increase rapidly with increases in dose. At still higher doses, there may be little increase in effect. Thus, the presence of a dose-response relationship may depend on which part of the curve is being studied.

These ancillary, adjunct, or supportive criteria for judging contributory cause are just that: They do not in and of themselves settle the issue. If present, they may, however, help support the argument for contributory cause. An appreciation of these criteria helps in understanding the controversy and the limitations of the data.

Other Concepts of Causation

The concept of contributory cause has been very useful in studying disease causation. Contributory cause, however, is not the only concept of causation that has been used in clinical medicine. In the 19th century, Robert Koch developed a series of conditions that must be met before a microorganism can be considered the cause of a disease. The conditions, known as KOCH'S POSTULATES, include a requirement that the organism is always found with the disease. This condition is often called NECESSARY CAUSE.

Necessary cause goes beyond the requirements we have outlined for establishing contributory cause. Historically, this was very useful in the study of infectious disease when a single agent was responsible for a single disease. However, if the concept of necessary cause is applied to the study of chronic diseases, it is nearly impossible to prove a causal relationship. For instance, even though cigarettes have been well established as a contributory cause of lung cancer, cigarette smoking is not a necessary condition for developing lung cancer; not everyone with lung cancer has smoked cigarettes.

Under the rules of strict logic, causation also requires a second condition known as SUFFICIENT CAUSE. This condition says that if the cause is present, the disease will also be present. In our cigarette and lung cancer example, sufficient cause would imply that if cigarette smoking is present, lung cancer will always follow.

Even in the area of infectious disease cause and effect may not be straightforward; for instance, mononucleosis is a well-established clinical illness for which the Epstein-Barré virus has been shown to be a contributory cause. However, other viruses such as cytomegalovirus also have been shown to cause mononucleosis. In addition, evidence may show that Epstein-Barré has been present in a patient without ever causing mononucleosis, or it may manifest itself by being a contributory cause of other diseases, such as Burkitt's lymphoma. Thus, despite the fact that the Epstein-Barré virus has been established as a contributory cause of mononucleosis, it is neither a necessary nor a sufficient cause of this syndrome. If we require necessary and sufficient cause before concluding that a cause-and-effect relationship exists, we will be able to document very few, if any, cause-and-effect relationships in clinical medicine or public health. The next example illustrates the consequences of applying the necessary cause of formal logic to health studies:

> In a study of the risk factors for coronary artery disease, investigators identified 100 individuals from a population of 10,000 MI patients who experienced MIs despite normal blood pressure, normal LDL and HDL cholesterol, regular exercise, no smoking, and no family history of coronary artery disease. The authors concluded that they had demonstrated hypertension, high LDH and low HDL cholesterol, lack of exercise, smoking, and family history were not the causes of coronary artery disease because not every MI patient possessed a risk factor.

The authors of this study were using the concept of necessary cause as a concept of causation. Instead of necessary cause, however, let us assume that all these factors had been shown to fulfill the criteria for contributory cause of coronary artery disease. Contributory cause, unlike necessary cause, does not require that everyone who is free of the cause will be free of the effect. The failure of known contributory causes to be present in all cases of disease emphasizes the limitations of our current knowledge about all the contributory causes of coronary artery disease. It illustrates our current state of ignorance; if all the contributory causes were known, then everyone with disease would possess at least one such factor.

Thus, even when a contributory cause has been established, it will not necessarily be present in each and every case.

In summary, contributory cause is a useful definition of causation. It requires a demonstration that: the cause and the effect occur together in an individual more often than expected by chance alone; the presumed cause precedes the effect; and altering the cause alters the effect in some individuals. It does not require that all people who are free of the contributory cause will be free of the effect. It does not require that all people who possess the contributory cause will develop the effect.

In other words, a contributory cause may be neither necessary nor sufficient, but it must be contributory. Its presence must increase the probability of the occurrence of disease and its reduction must reduce the probability of the disease.

In addition to contributory cause or efficacy, the interpretation of health research studies may involve issues of safety or harm. At times, interpretation also addresses the results for subgroups within the study sample. We will examine these elements of interpretation in subsequent chapters.[3]

[3]The concept of contributory cause is very useful because it is directly linked to the demonstration that interventions may alter the outcome. It should not be concluded that a contributory cause that has been demonstrated is the only contributory cause or that the intervention that has been investigated is necessarily the best possible or even the best available intervention. Multiple factors may be demonstrated to be contributory causes and multiple interventions may alter the cause and thereby alter the effect. The demonstration of specific contributory causes may camouflage the larger social determinants of cause-and-effect relationships, such as poverty, pollution, or climate change.

8 Extrapolation

In the preceding chapters, we illustrated the errors that can be made in assigning patients to study and control groups, assessing a study outcome, and analyzing and interpreting study results. Having completed this process, the investigator next asks what this all means for individuals not included in the study and for situations not directly addressed by the study. In conducting extrapolation, the reader must ask how the investigators applied the results to:

- Individuals, groups, or populations who are similar to those in the investigation
- Situations that go beyond the range of the study data
- Populations that differ from those in the investigation

This is not the investigators' job alone. In fact, they are not in the best position to perform extrapolation. The investigators often want their study results to have the broadest possible implications. In addition, they cannot know the characteristics of the individuals to whom the reader may apply the results. Thus, the reader needs to be the expert on extrapolation.

Let us start by seeing how we can use the outcome data of a study to extrapolate to similar individuals, similar groups at risk, and similar communities composed of individuals with and without the factors that have been studied. We will then explore extrapolation beyond the data and to different populations.

Extrapolation to Similar Individuals, Groups, or Populations

One way we may be interested in extrapolating study results is to assess their overall meaning for an individual who is similar to the average individual included in the investigation. In doing this, we assume that the study's finding is as applicable to other very similar individuals who possess the risk factor being studied as it was for the individuals who were actually included in the investigation.

Many case-control and cohort studies estimate the odds ratios or relative risk associated with the development of the disease if a risk factor is present compared with when it is not present. Odds ratios and relative risks tell us the strength of the relationship between the risk factor and the disease. If a cause-and-effect relationship is present and the effect of the risk factor is completely reversible, the relative risks tell us important information regarding the individual patient. On average, a relative risk of 10 means the individual patient has a 10 times higher risk of developing the disease over a specified period of time if the risk factor is present than he or she does if the risk factor is not present.[1]

[1] How well estimates of relative risk apply to an individual is actually determined by how similar the individuals included in the study are to the individual to whom we wish to apply the results. Application of results to an individual assumes that the study sample is composed entirely of persons exactly like that individual. It is not enough that only some persons like that individual are included in the study sample.

Relative risks do not, however, tell us the absolute magnitude of the risk or the probability of developing the disease if the risk factor is present compared with when it is not present. A relative risk of 10 may indicate an increase in risk from 1 per 1,000,000 for those without the risk factor to 1 per 100,000 for those with the risk factor. Alternatively, a relative risk of 10 may indicate an increase in risk from 1 per 100 for those without the risk factor to 1 per 10 among those with the risk factor. Thus, despite the same relative risk, the absolute risk for individuals can be very different.

Failure to understand the concept of absolute risk can lead to the following type of extrapolation error:

> A patient has read that the relative risk of death from leukemia is increased four times with use of a new chemotherapy for Stage 3 breast cancer; the relative risk of dying from Stage 3 breast cancer without chemotherapy is 3. She therefore argues that the chemotherapy is not worth the risk.

The risk of dying from Stage 3 breast cancer, however, is far greater than the risk of death from future leukemia. The infrequent and later occurrence of leukemia means that even in the presence of a risk factor that increases the risk fourfold, the absolute risk of dying from leukemia is still very small compared with the very high risk of dying from breast cancer.

Thus, the absolute risks strongly favor the benefits of treatment despite the small probability of harm. The patient in this example has failed to understand the important difference between relative risk and absolute risk. Thus, it is desirable to have information on both the relative risk and absolute risk when extrapolating the results of a study to a particular individual or when comparing one risk to another.

When extrapolating to individuals, it is essential to appreciate that the data from an investigation address issues of averages. An investigation may include individuals who have a wide range of risk factor values, such as a diastolic blood pressure from 90 to 130 mmHg. The extrapolation, however, should address the average value (*i.e.*, the individual with a diastolic blood pressure of 110 mmHg). For instance, extrapolating results to individuals with a diastolic blood pressure of 90 mmHg can dramatically increase the number of individuals to whom the results apply, even if there is no evidence that the benefit results from treating individuals with a diastolic blood pressure of 90 mmHg. This is especially true if the range is wide and there are very few individuals in the investigation with values at the lower end of the range. Failure to focus on the average can lead to the following extrapolation error:

> An investigation was conducted on a new medication that lowers cholesterol. Patients whose only risk factor for coronary artery disease was a low-density lipoprotein level of 120 to 180 mg/dL were included in the investigation. These levels reflect the range of values for more than 50% of the adult population in the United States. Five hundred individuals were included in the study and in the control group including five individuals with a low-density lipoprotein level between 120 and 125 mg/dL. The average low-density lipoprotein was 150 mg/dL. The investigation demonstrated a clinically important and statistically significant reduction in coronary artery disease among the study group compared to the control group. The investigators concluded that all adults in the United States with low-density lipoprotein levels between 120 and 180 mg/dL should be considered candidates for the new treatment.

The investigators imply that more than half of all American adults should be considered for this new treatment. They drew this conclusion because they focused on the full range of values (120–180 mg/dL) included in the investigation rather than the average of 150 mg/dL. This was especially dangerous since there were so few individuals included with low-density lipoprotein levels near the lower end of the range.

If they had concluded that adult Americans with a low-density lipoprotein level of 150 mg/dL or above should be considered for treatment, their conclusion would have been a direct extrapolation from the results to people who are similar to those included in the investigation. Extending the conclusions to 120 mg/dl would dramatically increase the number of individuals considered for treatment based on data from a small number of similar individuals.

Thus, when extrapolating the results of an investigation to similar individuals, this should generally be limited to the average individual in the investigation.

At-Risk Groups

Relative risk and absolute risk are often used to make estimates about individual patients. Sometimes, however, we are more interested in the impact that a risk factor may have on groups of individuals with the risk factor or on a community of individuals with and without the risk factor.

When assessing the impact of a risk factor on a group of individuals, we use a concept known as ATTRIBUTABLE RISK PERCENTAGE.[2] Calculation of attributable risk percentage does not require the existence of a cause-and-effect relationship. However, when a contributory cause exists, attributable risk percentage tells us the percentage of a disease that may potentially be eliminated from individuals who have the risk factor if the effects of that risk factor can be completely removed.[3]

Attributable risk percentage is defined as follows:

$$\frac{\text{Probability of disease if risk factor present} - \text{Probability of disease if risk factor absent}}{\text{Probability of disease if risk factor present}} \times 100\%$$

Attributable risk percentage can be more easily calculated from relative risk using the following formula when the relative risk is greater than 1:[4]

$$\text{Attributable risk percentage} = \frac{\text{Relative Risk} - 1}{\text{Relative Risk}} \times 100\%$$

[2]Attributable risk percentage has also been called attributable fraction (exposed), etiologic fraction (exposed), attributable proportion (exposed), percentage risk reduction, and protective efficacy rate.

[3]This interpretation of attributable risk percentage requires that the effects of the risk factor can be immediately and completely removed.

[4]A relative risk less than 1 can be converted and expressed as a relative risk greater than 1 by using the reciprocal, *i.e.*, a relative risk of 0.5 can also be expressed as a relative risk of 2. However, using the reciprocal of a relative risk less than 1 alters the meaning since the factor in the numerator is now the factor that increases the risk. It is confusing to compare relative risks greater than 1 with relative risks less than one since relative risks greater than 1 do not have an upper limit while relative risks less than 1 cannot be less than 0. Thus there are advantages of expressing all relative risks as greater than 1.

The following uses this formula to convert relative risk to attributable risk percentage:

Relative risk	Attributable risk percentage
1	0
2	50%
4	75%
10	90%
20	95%

Notice that even a relative risk of 2 may be associated with as much as a 50% reduction in the disease among those with the risk factor.

Failure to understand this concept may lead to the following extrapolation error:

> A large, well-designed cohort study was conducted on men who exercised regularly versus men, matched for risk factors for coronary artery disease, who did not exercise regularly. The study found that those who did not exercise regularly had a relative risk of 1.5 of developing coronary artery disease. The investigators concluded that even if this was true, the relative risk was too small to be of any practical importance.

Despite the fact that the relative risk is only 1.5, notice that it converts into a substantial attributable risk percentage:

$$\text{Attributable risk percentage} = \frac{1.5 - 1}{1.5} \times 100\% = 33\%$$

This means that among men who do not exercise regularly, one third of their risk of coronary artery disease could be eliminated if the effect of their lack of exercise could be eliminated. This may affect a large number of individuals because coronary artery disease is a frequently occurring disease and lack of regular exercise is a frequently occurring risk factor.

An alternative way of expressing this information, which is applicable to cohort studies and controlled clinical trials, is known as the NUMBER NEEDED TO TREAT. The number needed to treat indicates how many patients similar to the study patient must be treated, as the average study group patient was, to obtain one less bad outcome or one more good outcome. It is calculated as follows:

$$\text{Number needed to treat} = \frac{1}{\substack{\text{Probability of the}\\\text{adverse outcome}\\\text{in the control group}} - \substack{\text{Probability of the}\\\text{adverse outcome in}\\\text{the study group}}}$$

Thus, if an investigation demonstrated a reduction of coronary artery disease over 5 years from 20 per 1,000 in the control group to 10 per 1,000 in the study group, the number needed to treat for 5 years to produce one less case of coronary artery disease would be calculated as follows:

$$\text{Number needed to treat} = \frac{1}{20/1{,}000 - 10/1{,}000}$$
$$= \frac{1}{10/1{,}000}$$
$$= 100$$

The number needed to treat may be less than 0. Negative numbers indicate that the control group patients, on average, had a better outcome. Thus, a negative number needed to treat indicates how many patients must be treated to produce an additional bad outcome.

The number needed to treat often provides a more useful way to discuss or apply research data than do the other summary statistics such as the relative risk of 2, or even the absolute risk of 20 per 1,000 versus 10 per 1,000.

Community or Population

When extrapolating the results of a study to a community or population of individuals with and without a risk factor, we need to use another measure of risk known as the POPULATION ATTRIBUTABLE RISK PERCENTAGE (PAR).[5]

The population attributable risk percentage tells us the percentage of the risk in a population that is associated with the exposure to a risk factor, and may potentially be eliminated.[6] To calculate the PAR percentage, we must know more than the relative risk (expressed as greater than 1). It requires that we know or be able to estimate the proportion of individuals in the population who possess the risk factor. If we know the relative risk and the proportion of individuals in the population with the risk factor (b), we can calculate population attributable risk percentage using the following formula:

$$\text{Population attributable risk percentage (PAR\%)} = \frac{\text{b (Relative risk} - 1)}{\text{b (Relative risk} - 1) + 1} \times 100\%$$

This formula allows us to relate relative risk, proportion of the population with the risk factor (b), and population attributable risk percentage as follows:

Relative risk	b	PAR% (Approximate)
2	0.01	1%
4	0.01	3%
10	0.01	8%
20	0.01	16%
2	0.10	9%
4	0.10	23%
10	0.10	46%
20	0.10	65%
2	0.50	33%
4	0.50	60%
10	0.50	82%
20	0.50	90%
2	1.00	50%
4	1.00	75%
10	1.00	90%
20	1.00	95%

[5]Population attributable risk percentage has also been called attributable fraction (population), attributable proportion (population), and etiologic fraction (population).

[6]This interpretation of PAR percentage requires that a cause-and-effect relationship is present and that the consequences of the cause are immediately and completely reversible.

Notice that if the risk factor is uncommon in the population (*e.g.*, 1%), the relative risk must be substantial before the population attributable risk percentage becomes impressive. On the other hand, if the risk factor is common (*e.g.*, 0.50 or 50%), even a small relative risk means the potential community impact may be substantial. When the prevalence of the risk factor is 1 or 100% (*i.e.*, when everyone has the risk factor), notice that the population attributable risk percentage equals the attributable risk percentage. This is expected because attributable risk percentage uses a study group of individuals who all have the risk factor.

Failure to understand the concept of population attributable risk percentage can lead to the following extrapolation error:

> Investigators report that a hereditary form of high cholesterol known as type III hyperlipidemia occurs in 1 per 100,000 Americans. They also report that those with type III hyperlipidemia have a relative risk of 20 for developing coronary artery disease. The authors concluded that a cure for type III hyperlipidemia would have a substantial impact on the national problem of coronary artery disease.

Using the data and our formula for population attributable risk percentage, we find that elimination of coronary artery disease secondary to type III hyperlipidemia produces a population attributable risk percentage of about one fiftieth of 1%. Thus, the fact that type III hyperlipidemia is so rare a risk factor means that eliminating its impact cannot be expected to have a substantial impact on the overall occurrence of coronary artery disease.

Extrapolation Beyond the Range of the Data

Extrapolation to new situations or different types of individuals is even more difficult and is often the most challenging step when reading research. It is difficult because the investigator and the reviewers are usually not able to adequately address the issues of interest to a particular reader. It is up to you, the reader. The investigator does not know your community or your patients. Despite the difficulty with extrapolating research data, it is impossible to be a health practitioner without extrapolation from the research. Often, we must go beyond the data on the basis of reasonable assumptions. If one is unwilling to do any extrapolation, then one is limited to applying research results to individuals who are nearly identical to those in a study.

Despite the necessity of extrapolation, it is important to recognize the types of errors that can occur if extrapolation is not carefully performed. When extrapolating to different groups or different situations, two basic types of errors can occur—those due to extrapolations beyond the data, and those that occur as a result of the difference between the study population and the TARGET POPULATION, which is the group about which we wish to apply the results.

In research studies, individuals are usually exposed to the factors thought to be associated with the outcome for only a limited amount of time at a limited range of exposure. The investigators may be studying a factor such as hypertension that results in a stroke, or a therapeutic agent such as an antibiotic that is associated with curing an infection. In either case, the interpretation must be limited to the range and duration of hypertension experienced by the subjects or the dosage and duration of the antibiotic used in the study. When the investigators draw conclusions that extrapolate beyond the duration and range experienced by the study subjects, they frequently are making unwarranted assumptions. They may assume that longer exposure continues to produce the same effect experienced by the study subjects. The following example illustrates a potential error resulting from extrapolating beyond the range of the data:

> A new antihypertensive agent was tested on 100 patients with hard-to-control hypertension. In all 100 patients with hard-to-control hypertension, the agent lowered diastolic blood pressure from 120 to 110 mmHg at dosages of 1 mg/kg and from 110 to 100 mmHg at dosages of 2 mg/kg. The authors concluded that this agent would be able to lower diastolic blood pressure from 100 to 90 mmHg at doses of 3 mg/kg.

It is possible that clinical evidence would document the new agent's efficacy at 3 mg/kg. Such documentation, however, awaits empirical evidence. Many antihypertensive agents have been shown to reach maximum effectiveness at a certain dosage and do not increase their effectiveness at higher dosages. To conclude that higher dosages produce greater effects without experimental evidence is to make a linear or straight-line extrapolation beyond the range of the data.

Another type of error associated with extrapolation beyond the range of the data concerns potential side effects experienced at increased exposure, as illustrated by the following hypothetical example:

> A 1-year study of the effects of administering daily unopposed estrogen to 100 menopausal women found that the drug relieved hot flashes and reduced the rate of osteoporosis as opposed to age-matched women given placebos who experienced no symptom relief. The authors found no adverse effects from the estrogens and concluded that estrogens are safe and effective. Therefore, they recommended that unopposed estrogens be administered long term to women, beginning at the onset of menopause.

The authors have extrapolated the data on using unopposed estrogens from a 1-year period of follow-up to long-term administration. No evidence shows that if 1 year of administration is safe, so is long-term, continuous administration of unopposed estrogen. It is not likely that any long-term adverse effects would show up in a 1-year study. Thus, the authors have made potentially dangerous extrapolations by going beyond the range of their data.

Linear extrapolation may sometimes be necessary in clinical and public health practice, but we must recognize that linear extrapolation has taken place so we can be on the lookout for new data that may undermine the assumptions and thus challenge the conclusion obtained by linear extrapolation.

Extrapolation to Different Populations

When extrapolating to a target population, it is important to consider how that group differs from the one sampled in the investigation. The following scenario illustrates how differences between countries, for instance, can complicate extrapolation from one country to another:

> In a study involving Japan and the United States, 20% of the Japanese participants were found to have hypertension and 60% smoked cigarettes, both known contributory causes of coronary artery disease in the United States. Among US participants, 10% had hypertension and 30% smoked cigarettes. Studies in Japan did not demonstrate an association between hypertension or cigarettes and coronary artery disease, whereas similar studies in the United States demonstrated a statistically significant association. The authors concluded that hypertension and cigarette smoking must protect the Japanese from myocardial infarctions.

The authors have extrapolated from one culture to a very different culture. Other explanations for the observed data are possible. If US participants frequently possess another risk factor, such as high LDL cholesterol which is rare in Japan, this factor may override cigarette smoking and hypertension and help to produce the high rate of myocardial infarctions in the US population.

Extrapolation within countries can also be difficult when differences exist between the group that was investigated and the target group to which one wants to apply the findings, as illustrated in the next example:

> A study of the preventive effect of treating borderline tuberculosis (TB) skin tests (6–10 mm) with a year of isoniazid was conducted among Alaskan Native Americans. The population had a frequency of borderline skin tests of 2 per 1,000. The study was conducted by giving isoniazid to 200 Alaskan Native Americans with borderline skin tests and placebos to 200 others with the same borderline condition. Twenty cases of active TB occurred among the placebo patients and only one among the patients given isoniazid. The results were statistically significant at the 0.05 level. A health official from the state of Virginia, where borderline skin tests occur in 300 per 1,000 skin tests, was impressed with these results. He advocated that all patients in Virginia who had borderline skin tests be treated with isoniazid for 1 year.

In extrapolating to the population of Virginia, the health official assumed that borderline skin tests mean the same thing for Alaskan Native Americans as for Virginians. Other data suggest, however, that many borderline skin tests in Virginia are not due to TB exposure. They are frequently caused by an atypical mycobacteria that carries a much more benign prognosis and does not reliably respond to isoniazid. By not appreciating this new factor in the residents of Virginia, the health official may be submitting many individuals to useless and potentially harmful therapy.

Extrapolation of study results is always a difficult but extremely important part of reading the health research literature. Extrapolation involves first asking what the results mean for people like the average individual included in the investigation. Thus, one must begin by looking closely at the types of patients and settings in which the investigation was conducted. This enables the reader to consider what the results mean for similar at-risk groups and finally communities or populations of individuals with and without the characteristics under study.

Often, the reader wants to go one step further and extend the extrapolation to individuals and situations that are different from those in the study. This extrapolation beyond the data must take into account the differences between the types of individuals included in the investigation and the target group. Recognizing the assumptions we make in extrapolation forces us to keep our eyes open for new information that challenges these assumptions and potentially invalidates our conclusions.

We have now examined how to apply the uniform framework that is applicable to the three basic study designs: case-control, cohort, and randomized clinical trial. Now, we turn our attention to applying this framework to the special characteristics of randomized clinical trials or controlled clinical trials and then nonconcurrent cohort studies or database studies. Finally, we will use the uniform framework to examine efforts to combine data from studies, which is known as *meta-analysis.*

9 Randomized Clinical Trials

Randomized clinical trials are now widely considered the gold standard by which we judge the benefits of therapy. The US Food and Drug Administration (FDA) requires them for drug approval; the National Institutes of Health (NIH) rewards them with funding; the journals encourage them by publication; and increasingly, practitioners read them and apply their results. When feasible and ethical, randomized clinical trials are a standard part of health research. Thus, it is critically important to appreciate what these trials can tell us, what can go wrong, and what questions they cannot address.

In this chapter, we follow the uniform framework to discuss the elements of study design, assignment, assessment, analysis, interpretation, and extrapolation in randomized clinical trials. Features that differ between randomized clinical trials and case-control and cohort studies are emphasized.

Study Design

Randomized clinical trials often aim to demonstrate all three criteria of contributory cause. When applied to a treatment, the term EFFICACY is used instead of CONTRIBUTORY CAUSE.[1] EFFICACY means that in the study group being investigated, the therapy reduces the probability of experiencing the adverse outcome. Efficacy, however, needs to be distinguished from effectiveness. EFFECTIVENESS implies that the therapy works under usual conditions of practice as opposed to the conditions of an investigation. Our goal usually is to use randomized clinical trials to determine whether the therapy works when given according to a defined dosage schedule, by a defined route of administration, and to a defined type of patient.[2]

Randomized clinical trials are not suitable for the initial investigation of a new treatment. When used as part of the drug approval process, randomized clinical trials are traditionally referred to as PHASE III TRIALS. As defined by the FDA, PHASE I TRIALS refer to the initial efforts to administer the treatment to human beings. They aim to establish a dosage regimen and to evaluate the potential toxicities. They provide only a preliminary look at the potential efficacy of the therapy. Phase I trials aim to establish the indications and regimen for administering the new therapy and to determine whether the new therapy warrants further study. PHASE II studies are usually small-scale controlled or uncontrolled trials that aim to establish whether full-scale randomized clinical trials should be conducted.

---

[1] A technique that removes a contributory cause has *efficacy*. However, a technique that removes an indirect contributory cause may still have efficacy even after the state of knowledge has allowed us to define a more direct contributory cause.

[2] It is possible to perform a randomized clinical trial to assess the effectiveness of therapy by using a representative sample of the types of patients to be treated with the therapy and the usual methods that are being used clinically.

Ideally, a randomized clinical, or phase III, trial should be performed after the indications and the regimen are agreed on but before the therapy has been widely integrated into clinical care. The FDA, for instance, has traditionally required two independently conducted randomized clinical trials before reviewing a drug for approval.[3] For new drugs that do not have market approval, this is relatively automatic. However, for many procedures and drugs that have been previously marketed, the treatment may have been widely used before randomized clinical trials could be implemented. This is a problem because once the treatment has been widely used, physicians and often patients have developed firm ideas about the value of the therapy. In that case, they may not believe it is ethical to enter into a randomized clinical trial or to continue participation if they discover that the patient has been assigned to the control group.

Once the time is considered right for a randomized clinical trial, the next study design question is whether it is feasible to perform one. To answer this, the investigator must define the question being asked in a randomized clinical trial.

Most randomized clinical trials aim to determine whether the new or experimental therapy results in a better outcome than placebo or standard therapy. To determine whether a trial is feasible, investigators need to estimate the necessary sample size. They must estimate how many patients are required to have a reasonable chance of demonstrating a statistically significant difference between the new therapy and the placebo or standard therapy.

The required sample size depends on the following factors:[4]

1. **Size of the Type I error that the investigators will tolerate.** This is the probability of demonstrating a statistically significant difference in samples when no true difference exists between treatments in the larger population. The alpha level for the Type I error is usually set at 5%.
2. **Size of the Type II error that the investigators will tolerate.** This is the probability of failing to demonstrate a statistically significant difference in samples when a true difference of a selected magnitude actually exists between treatments. Most investigators should aim for no more than a 20% Type II error, which is also referred to as an 80% statistical power. The statistical power plus the Type II error add up to 100%. The 80% power implies 80% probability of being able to demonstrate a statistically significant difference between the samples if a true difference exists in the larger populations.
3. **Percentage of individuals in the control group who are expected to experience the adverse outcome (death or development of disease) under study.** Often this can be estimated from previous studies.
4. **Improvement in outcome within the study group that the investigators seek to demonstrate as statistically significant.** Despite the desire to demonstrate statistical significance for even small real changes, the investigators need to decide the minimum size of a difference that would be considered clinically important. The smaller this difference between study group and control group therapy that one expects, the larger the sample size required.[5]

[3] The FDA's procedures are undergoing rapid change, with a goal of selectively introducing new treatments into practice earlier.

[4] This is all the information that is required for an either/or variable. When calculating sample size for variables with multiple possible outcomes, one must also estimate the standard deviation of the variable.

[5] The frequency of the outcome under investigation may be estimated from past studies, especially for the control group. It is often more difficult to estimate the expected frequency in the study group. Overly optimistic estimates of the results of the new therapy will result in sample size estimates that are too small to demonstrate statistical significance.

Let us take a look at the way these factors affect the required sample size. Table 9.1 provides general guidelines for sample size for different levels of these factors.

Table 9.1 assumes one study group and one control group of equal size. It also assumes that the investigators are interested in the study results whether the results are in the direction of the study treatment or in the opposite direction. Statisticians refer to statistical significance tests that consider data favoring deviations from the null hypothesis in either direction as TWO-TAILED TESTS. Table 9.1 also assumes a Type I error of 5%.

Let us take a look at the meaning of these numbers for different types of studies:

> Imagine that we wish to conduct a randomized clinical trial on a treatment designed to reduce the 1-year risk of death from adenocarcinoma of the ovary. Assume that the 1-year risk of death using standard therapy is 40%. In this study, we hope to reduce the 1-year risk of death to 20% using a new treatment. We believe, however, that the treatment could possibly increase the risk of death. If we are willing to tolerate a 20% probability of failing to obtain statistically significant results, even if a true difference of this magnitude exists in the larger populations, how many patients are required in the study and also in the control groups?

To answer this question, we can use Table 9.1 as follows:

Locate the 20% probability of an adverse outcome in the study group on the horizontal axis.

Next, locate the 40% probability of an adverse outcome in the control group on the vertical axis. These intersect at 117, 90, and 49. The correct number is the one that lines up with the 20% Type II error. The answer is 90.

Thus, 90 women with advanced adenocarcinoma in the study group and 90 in the control group are needed to have a 20% probability of failing to demonstrate statistical significance if the true 1-year risk of death is actually 40% using the standard treatment and 20% using the new therapy. Notice that the sample size required for a Type II error of 10% is 117. Thus, a compromise sample size of about 100 in each group would be reasonable for this study.

Table 9.1. *Sample Size Requirement for Controlled Clinical Trials*[a]

Adverse Outcome in the Control Group	Type II Error	Probability of Adverse Outcome in the Study Group			
		1%	5%	10%	20%
	10%	3,696	851	207	72
2%	20%	2,511	652	161	56
	50%	1,327	351	90	38
	10%	154	619	—	285
10%	20%	120	473	—	218
	50%	69	251	—	117
	10%	62	112	285	—
20%	20%	49	87	218	—
	50%	29	49	117	—
	10%	25	33	48	117
40%	20%	20	26	37	90
	50%	12	16	22	49
	10%	13	16	20	34
60%	20%	11	13	16	27
	50%		78	10	16

[a] All sample sizes obtained from this table assume a 5% Type I error.

A sample size of 100 is an approximate estimate of the number of individuals needed in each group when the probability of an adverse outcome is substantial and the investigators hope to be able to reduce it in half with the new treatment while keeping the size of the Type II error less than 20%.

Now let us contrast this situation with one in which the probability of an adverse outcome is much lower even without intervention:

> An investigator wishes to study the effect of a new treatment on the probability of neonatal sepsis secondary to delayed presentation of premature rupture of the membranes. We assume that the probability of neonatal sepsis using standard treatment is 10%, and the study group therapy aims to reduce the probability of neonatal sepsis to 5%, although it is possible that the new therapy will increase the risk of death. The investigator is willing to tolerate a 10% probability of failing to demonstrate a statistically significant difference.

Using the chart as before, we located 619, 473, and 251. Thus, we see that 619 individuals are needed for the study group and 619 individuals are needed for the control group to ensure a 10% probability of making a Type II error. If we were willing to tolerate a 20% probability of failing to demonstrate a statistically significant difference, if a difference actually exists in the larger population, 473 individuals would be required in each group. The approximate number required is 500 individuals in both the study and the control groups to be able to demonstrate statistical significance when the true difference between adverse outcomes in the larger population is only 10% versus 5%.

The neonatal sepsis example is typical of the problems we study in clinical practice. It demonstrates why large sample sizes are required in most randomized clinical trials before they are likely to demonstrate statistical significance. Thus, it is not usually feasible to investigate small improvements in therapy using a randomized clinical trial.

Let us go one step further and see what happens to the required sample size when a randomized clinical trial is performed on a preventive intervention in which the adverse outcome is uncommon even in the absence of prevention:

> Imagine that a new drug for preventing adverse outcomes of pregnancy in women with hypertension before pregnancy aims to reduce the probability of adverse pregnancy outcomes from 2% to 1%, although the new therapy could possibly increase the risk of adverse outcomes. The investigators are willing to tolerate a 20% probability of failing to demonstrate a statistically significant difference.

From Table 9.1, we can see that at least 2,511 individuals are required in each group. These enormous numbers point out the difficulty in performing randomized clinical trials when one wishes to apply preventive therapy, especially when the risk of adverse outcomes is already quite low.[6]

Even when a randomized clinical trial is feasible, it may not be ethical to perform one. These trials are not considered ethical if they require individuals to submit to substantial risks without a realistic expectation of a substantial benefit. In

---

[6] These sample sizes are designed for the PRIMARY END-POINT, which should be an end-point expected to occur relatively frequently and to be biologically important. However, it may not be the most important end-point of interest. For instance, in a study of coronary artery disease, a myocardial infarction may be a primary end-point. Other end-points that have even more clinical importance but occur less frequently, such as disability or death, are often measured as SECONDARY END-POINTS. In general, primary but not secondary end-points are used for calculating sample size.

general, investigations that use a placebo when standard therapy has been shown to have efficacy are not considered ethical. A randomized clinical trial may be conducted using standard therapy in the control group, but this may require an increase in the sample size. Thus, despite the advantages of randomized trials in defining the efficacy of a therapy, they are not always feasible or ethical.

Assignment

Participants in a randomized clinical trial are not usually selected at random from a larger population. Usually, they are volunteers who meet a series of inclusion and exclusion criteria defined by the investigators.

Participants must provide informed consent that includes an explanation of the known harms and available alternatives. Participants have the right to withdraw from the study at any time for any reason; however, they do not have a right to know their treatment group assignment while in the study and may not be eligible to receive compensation through the investigation for adverse side effects of therapy.

Individuals entered into randomized clinical trials are often a relatively homogeneous group because they share inclusion and exclusion criteria. They are not usually representative of all those with the disease or all those for whom the therapy is intended (*i.e.,* the target population). In addition, they often do not have the type of complicating factors encountered in practice. That is, they usually do not have multiple disease and multiple simultaneous therapies, and they usually do not have compromised ability to metabolize drugs as a result of renal or hepatic disease. Thus, it is important to distinguish between the study population and the target population.

In addition, some exclusion criteria may be based on evidence that the patient will follow the treatment protocol. Investigators may follow patients before entering them into a study to determine whether they meet the entry and exclusion criteria and also to determine their likely compliance with the protocol. Investigators may use what is called a RUN-IN PERIOD of prestudy therapy to exclude patients who do not take prescribed medication, do not return for follow-up, or demonstrate other evidence that they are not likely to follow the study protocol. Because this is an increasingly frequent procedure, it is important to recognize that randomized clinical trials often use patients who are especially likely to adhere to treatment.

The randomization of patients to study and control groups is the hallmark of randomized clinical trials. Randomization implies that any one individual has a predetermined probability of being assigned to each particular study and control group. This may mean an equal probability of being assigned to one study and one control group or different probabilities of being assigned to each of several study and control groups.

Randomization is a powerful tool for eliminating selection bias in the assignment of individuals to study and control groups. In large studies, it helps to reduce the possibility that the effects of treatment are due to the type of individuals receiving the study and control therapy. It is important to distinguish between randomization, which is an essential part of a randomized clinical trial, and random sampling, which is not usually a part of a randomized clinical trial. RANDOM SAMPLING implies that the individuals who are selected for a study are selected by chance from a larger group or population. Thus, random sampling is a method aimed at obtaining a representative sample (*i.e.,* one that, on average, reflects the characteristics of a larger group).

Randomization, on the other hand, says nothing about the characteristics of a larger population from which the individuals in the investigation are obtained. It refers to the mechanism by which individuals are assigned to study and control groups once they are eligible for and volunteer for the study. The following hypothetical study illustrates the difference between random sampling and randomization:

> An investigator wishes to assess the benefit of a new drug known as Surf-ez. Surf-ez is designed to help improve surfing ability. To assess the value of Surf-ez, the investigator performs a randomized clinical trial among a group of volunteer championship surfers in Hawaii. After randomizing half the group to Surf-ez and half the group to a placebo, the investigators measure the surfing ability of all surfers using a standard scoring system. The scorers do not know whether a particular surfer used Surf-ez or placebo. Those taking Surf-ez have a statistically significant and substantial improvement compared with the placebo group. On the basis of the study results, the authors recommend Surf-ez as a learning aid for all surfers.

By using randomization, this randomized clinical trial has demonstrated the efficacy of Surf-ez among these championship surfers. Because its study and control groups were hardly a random sample of surfers, however, we must be very careful in drawing conclusions or extrapolating about the effects of Surf-ez as a learning aid for all surfers.[7]

Randomization does not eliminate the possibility that study and control groups will differ according to factors that affect prognosis (confounding variables). Known prognostic factors must still be measured and are often found to be different in study and control groups as a result of chance alone, especially in small studies. If substantial differences between groups exist, these must be taken into account through an adjustment process as part of the analysis.[8] Many characteristics affecting prognosis, however, are not known. In larger studies randomization tends to balance the multitude of characteristics that could possibly be related to outcome, even those that are unknown to the investigator. Without randomization, the investigator would need to take into account all known and potential differences between groups. Because it is difficult, if not impossible, to consider everything, randomization helps balance the groups, especially for large studies.

Assessment

Masking study subjects and investigators is an important part of the assignment of patients in a randomized clinical trial. SINGLE MASKING implies that the patient is unaware of which therapy is being received; DOUBLE MASKING implies that neither the patient nor the investigator is aware of the group assignment. The impact of not masking, however, occurs in the assessment process.

Errors in assessing the outcome or end-point of a randomized clinical trial may occur when the patient or the individual making the assessment is aware of which

---

[7] Care must be taken even in extrapolating to championship surfers because we have not randomly sampled all championship surfers. This limitation occurs in most randomized clinical trials, which select their patients from a particular hospital or clinical site.

[8] Many biostatisticians would recommend using a multivariable analysis technique such as regression analysis even when no substantial difference exists between groups. Multivariable analysis then permits adjustment for interaction. Interaction occurs, for instance, when both groups contain an identical age and sex distribution, but one group contains predominantly young women and the other contains predominantly young men. Multivariable analysis then allows one to separate out the interacting effects of age and sex.

treatment is being administered. This is especially likely when the outcome or end-point being measured is subjective or may be influenced by knowledge of the treatment group, as illustrated in the following hypothetical study:

> A randomized clinical trial of a new breast-cancer surgery compared the degree of arm edema and arm strength among patients receiving the new procedure versus the traditional procedure. The patients were aware of which procedure they underwent. Arm edema and arm strength were the end-points assessed by the patients and surgeons. The study found that those receiving the new procedure had less arm edema and more arm strength than those undergoing the traditional mastectomy.

In this study, the fact that the patients and the surgeons who performed the procedure and assessed the outcome all knew which patients received which procedure may have affected the objectivity of the way strength and edema were measured and reported. This effect may have been minimized but not totally eliminated if arm strength and edema were assessed with a standardized scoring system by individuals who did not know which patients received which therapy. This system of masked assessment and objective scoring would not remove the impact of patients and surgeons knowing which surgery was obtained. It is still possible that patients receiving the new procedure worked harder and actually increased their strength and reduced their edema. This could occur, for instance, if the surgeon performing the new surgery stressed postoperative exercises or provided more physical therapy for those receiving the new therapy.

In practice, masking is often impractical or unsuccessful. Surgical therapy cannot easily be masked. The taste or side effects of medications are often a giveaway to the patient or clinician. The need to titrate a dose to achieve a desired effect often makes it more difficult to mask the clinician and in some cases the patient. Strict adherence to masking helps to ensure the objectivity of the assessment process. It helps to remove the possibility that differences in compliance, follow-through, and assessment of outcome will be affected by awareness of the treatment received.

Even when objective assessment, excellent compliance, and complete follow-up can be ensured, masking is still desirable because it helps control for the placebo effect. The placebo effect is a powerful biological process that can bring about a wide variety of objective as well as subjective biological effects. The placebo effect extends far beyond pain control. A substantial percentage of patients who believe they are receiving effective therapy obtain objective therapeutic benefits. When effective masking is not a part of a randomized clinical trial, it leaves open the possibility that the observed benefit in the study subject is actually the result of the placebo therapy.

Thus, when masking is not feasible, doubt about the accuracy of the outcome measures usually persists. This uncertainty can be reduced but not eliminated by using objective measures of end-points, careful monitoring of compliance, and complete follow-up of patients.

An assessment of outcome requires measures of outcome that are appropriate, precise and accurate, complete, and unaffected by the process of observation. The requirements are as important in a randomized clinical trial as in a case-control and cohort study, as we discussed in Chapter 5.

In randomized clinical trials, investigators often wish to use outcome measures or end-points that occur in a short period of time rather than waiting for more clinically important but longer-term outcomes, such as death or blindness. Increasingly, changes in laboratory tests are substituted for clinical end-points. These are often called SURROGATE ENDPOINTS *or* SURROGATE MARKERS. Surrogate markers can be very useful if the test is an early indicator of subsequent outcome. If that is not the situation, however, the surrogate marker can be an inappropriate measure of outcome, as suggested in the following scenario:

> Researchers note that individuals with severe coronary artery disease often have multiple premature ventricular contractions and experience sudden death, often believed to be caused by arrhythmias. They note that a new drug may be able to reduce premature ventricular contractions. Thus, they conduct a randomized clinical trial that demonstrates the new drug has efficacy in reducing the frequency of premature ventricular contraction in patients with severe coronary artery disease. Later evidence indicates that those with severe coronary artery disease taking the drug have an increased frequency of death compared with similar untreated patients.

The investigator has assumed that reducing the frequency of premature ventricular contraction in the short run is strongly associated with a better outcome in the longer run. This may not always be the situation, as has been demonstrated with treatment for premature ventricular contractions in this type of setting. The fact that treatment seems like a logical method for reducing deaths caused by arrhythmia may have allowed investigators to accept a surrogate end-point assuming, without evidence, that it would be strongly associated with the end-point of interest, which was death in this case.

An additional problem can occur when individuals are lost to follow-up before the study is completed. Even moderate loss to follow-up can be disastrous for a study if those lost move to a pleasant climate because of failing health, drop out because of drug toxicity, or fail to return because of the burdens of complying with one of the treatment protocols.

Well-conducted studies take elaborate precautions to minimize the loss to follow-up. In some cases, follow-up may be completed by a telephone or mail questionnaire. A search of death records should be conducted in an effort to find participants who cannot be located. When outcome data cannot be obtained, resulting in loss to follow-up despite these precautions, it is important to determine, as much as possible, the initial characteristics of patients subsequently lost to follow-up. This is done in an attempt to determine whether those lost are likely to be different from those who remain. If those lost to follow-up have an especially poor prognosis, little may be gained by analyzing the data regarding only those who remain, as suggested by the following hypothetical study:

> In a study of the effects of a new alcohol treatment program, 100 patients were randomized to the new program, and 100 patients were randomized to conventional treatment. The investigators visited the homes of all patients at 9 PM on a Saturday and drew blood from all available patients to measure alcohol levels. Of the new treatment group, 30 patients were at home, and one third of these had alcohol in their blood. Among the conventionally treated patients, 33 were at home, and two thirds of these had alcohol in their blood. The results were statistically significant, and the investigators concluded that the new treatment reduced alcohol consumption.

Whenever more than a small loss to follow-up occurs, it is important to ask what happened to those lost participants. In this study, if those lost to follow-up were out drinking, the results based on those at home would be especially misleading. This is important even if loss to follow-up occurs equally in study and control groups.

One method for dealing with loss to follow-up is to assume the worst regarding the lost participants. For instance, the investigator could assume that the participants not at home were out drinking. It is then possible to redo the analysis and compare the outcome in the study and control groups to determine whether the differences are still statistically significant. When the loss to follow-up is great, this procedure usually indicates no substantial or statistically significant difference between the study and control groups. However, for smaller loss to follow-up, a statistically significant difference may remain. When statistically significant differences between groups remain after assuming the worst case for those lost to follow-up, the reader can be quite confident that loss to follow-up does not explain the observed differences.

In an ideal randomized clinical trial, all individuals would be treated according to the study protocol and monitored over time. Their outcome would be assessed from their time of entry until the end of the study. In reality, assessment is rarely so perfect or complete. Patients often receive treatment that deviates from the predefined protocol. Investigators often label these individuals as PROTOCOL DEVIANTS. In addition, some patients are usually lost to follow-up before the end of the study. Deviating from the protocol, as opposed to loss to follow-up, implies that data on subsequent outcomes were obtained.

Analysis

Analysis problems can arise in randomized clinical trials as a result of protocol deviants. Let us see how this might occur by looking at the following hypothetical study:

> In a randomized clinical trial of surgery versus angioplasty for single-vessel coronary artery disease, 100 patients were randomized to surgery and 100 to angioplasty. Before receiving angioplasty, 30 of the patients deviated from the protocol and had surgery.

It is likely that many of the patients who deviated from the protocol and underwent surgery were the ones doing poorly. If that is the situation, then eliminating those who deviated from the protocol from the analysis would leave us with a group of individuals doing especially well.

Because of the potential bias, it is generally recommended that deviants from the study protocol remain in the investigation and be subsequently analyzed as if they had remained in the group to which they were originally randomized. This is known as *analysis according to the intention-to-treat.* By retaining the protocol deviants, the study question, however, is changed slightly. The study now asks whether initiating treatment with the study therapy produced a better outcome than initiating treatment with the standard therapy. This change may actually help to make the investigation more applicable to the real clinical questions, regarding the effectiveness of the therapy as actually used in clinical practice.[9]

Deviations from the protocol are relatively common in randomized clinical trials because it is considered unethical to prevent deviations when the attending physician believes that continued adherence is contraindicated by the patient's condition or when the patient no longer wishes to follow the recommended protocol.

---

[9] Investigators may perform additional calculations excluding those who deviate from the protocol. However, it is not considered proper methodology to use only this method.

Thus, in evaluating a randomized clinical trial, the reader should understand the degree of protocol adherence and determine how the investigators handled the data regarding those who deviated from the protocol.

Two other analysis questions face the investigator in a randomized clinical trial: when to analyze the data and how to analyze the data.

WHEN TO ANALYZE DATA

The seemingly simple question of when to analyze has provoked considerable methodologic and ethical controversy. The more times one analyzes, the more likely one is to find a point when the P value reaches the 0.05 level of statistical significance using standard statistical techniques.

When to analyze is an ethical problem because one would like to establish that a true difference exists at the earliest possible moment. This is desirable to avoid subjecting patients to less effective therapy. In addition, it is desirable that other patients receive an effective therapy at the earliest possible time.

A number of sequential statistical methods have been developed to attempt to deal with these problems. When multiple points of analysis are planned, statistical techniques are available to take into account the multiple analyses.

HOW TO ANALYZE DATA

LIFE TABLES are the most commonly used method of analysis in randomized clinical trials.[10] Life tables are a method of displaying how often and when the adverse outcomes occur.

In this discussion, the adverse effect under study is referred to as death. However, life tables can be used for other effects, such as permanent loss of vision or the occurrence of pregnancy after infertility therapy.

Let us begin by discussing why life tables are often, but not always, necessary in randomized clinical trials. Then, we will discuss the assumptions underlying their use and demonstrate how they should be interpreted.

In most randomized clinical trials, individuals are entered into the study and randomized over a period of time as they present for care. In addition, because of late entry or loss to follow-up, individuals are actually monitored for various periods of time after entry. Therefore, many of the patients included in a study are not followed for the full duration of the study.

If all individuals were monitored for the desired length of observation, the probability of death can be calculated simply as the number of those dead at the end divided by the number of those initially enrolled in the study. All individuals, however, are not usually monitored for the same length of time. Thus, life tables provide a method for using the data from those individuals who have been included in a study for only a portion of the possible study duration.[11] Thus, life tables allow the investigator to use all the data that they have so painstakingly collected.

The life-table method is built on the important assumption that those who were in the investigation for shorter periods would have had the same subsequent expe-

---

[10] Life-table methods can also be used in cohort studies.

[11] Variations of this type of life table are known as a Kaplan-Meier or Cutler-Ederer life table. Note that this type of life table assumes the end-point can occur only once. Thus, it is not appropriate for studies of diseases such as strep throat, which may recur.

rience as those who were actually followed for longer periods of time. In other words, the short-termers would have the same results as the long-termers if they were actually followed long term.

This critical assumption may not hold true if the short-termers are individuals with a better or worse prognosis than the long-termers. This can occur if the entry requirements for the investigation are relaxed during the course of a study. Let us see how this might occur by looking at the next hypothetical study:

> A new hormonal treatment designed to treat infertility secondary to severe endometriosis was compared with standard therapy in a randomized clinical trial. After initial difficulty recruiting patients and initial failures to get pregnant among the study patients, one woman in the study group became pregnant. News of her delivery became front-page news. Subsequent patients recruited for the study were found to have much less severe endometriosis, but the investigators willingly accepted those patients and combined their data with data from their original group of patients.

As this study demonstrates, entry criteria may not be maintained the same throughout the investigation. It is tempting to relax the inclusion and exclusion criteria if only severely ill patients are entered into an investigation at the beginning. As the therapy becomes better known in the community, at a particular institution, or in the literature, a tendency may occur for clinicians to refer, or patients to self-refer, the less severely ill.

In this case, the short-term study participants are likely to have less severe illness and thus have better outcomes than the long-termers. This problem can be minimized if the investigators clearly define and carefully adhere to a protocol that defines the type of patients who are eligible for the study on the basis of inclusion and exclusion criteria related to prognosis.

Loss to follow-up may also result in differences between the short-termers and the long-termers. This is likely if loss to follow-up occurs preferentially among those who are not doing well or who have adverse reactions to treatment. We have already discussed the importance of loss to follow-up and stressed the need to assess whether those lost are similar to those who remain.

Life-table data are usually presented as a SURVIVAL PLOT. This is a graph in which the percentage survival is plotted on the vertical axis, ranging from 100% at the top of the axis to 0% at the bottom. Thus, at the beginning of the investigation, both study and control groups start at the 100% mark at the top of the vertical axis.[12] The horizontal axis depicts the time of follow-up. Time is counted for each individual beginning with their entry into the study. Thus, time zero is not the time in which the investigation began.

Survival plots should also include the number of individuals who have been monitored for each time interval. These should be presented separately for the study and the control groups. Thus, a typical life table comparing the 5-year data on study and control groups might be examined graphically in a survival plot like Figure 9.1. The top row of numbers represents the number of study group subjects monitored through the corresponding length of time, and the bottom row represents

---

[12] Alternatively, a graphic presentation of life tables may display the percentage who experience the adverse effect and start at the 0% point on the bottom of the vertical axis. When assessing a desirable outcome, such as pregnancy in an infertility study, a life table may also begin at 0%, indicating no pregnancies.

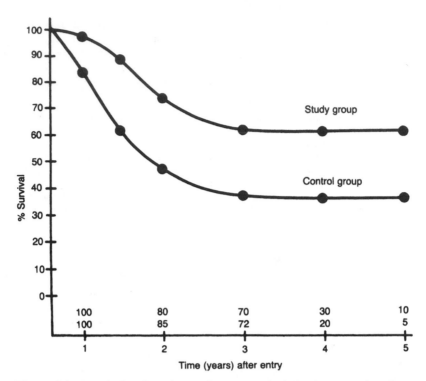

Figure 9.1. A typical study and control group survival plot demonstrating plateau effect, which typically occurs at the right end of life-table plots.

the same for control group subjects. The survival plot can be used directly to estimate the percentage death or survival at, for instance, 5 years; this probability of survival is known as the 5-year ACTUARIAL SURVIVAL. For instance, in Figure 9.1, the 5-year actuarial survival read directly from the graph is approximately 60% for the study group and 40% for the control group.

Life tables are often tested for statistical significance using the log rank or Mantel-Haenszel statistical significance tests. For these tests, the null hypothesis states that no difference exists between the overall life table results for the study and control groups. These statistical significance tests compare the observed and expected events if this null hypothesis was true. Notice that the statistical significance tests do not address the question of which treatment achieves better results at 5 years. In performing these tests, one combines data from each interval in time, using a method called WEIGHTING to take into account the number of individuals being observed during that time interval. Thus, these methods combine data from different time intervals to produce an overall statistical significance test. The combination of data from multiple intervals means that the statistical significance test asks this question:

> If no true difference exists between the overall effects of the study and control group treatments, what is the probability of obtaining the observed or more extreme results?

In other words, if a statistically significant improvement in a study group has been demonstrated on the basis of life-table data, it is very likely that a similar group of individuals receiving the therapy will experience at least some improvement compared with the control group therapy.

As we have seen, life tables can be used directly to obtain estimates of the magnitude of difference in outcome between treatments. Inference can be performed using a statistical significance test that addresses the overall differences. In addition, adjustment for potentially confounding variables may be incorporated into the life-table analysis using a technique known as COX REGRESSION *or* PROPORTIONAL HAZARD REPRESSION. Thus, life tables can address all three basic questions of statistics: estimation, inference, and adjustment.

Interpretation

Data from life tables are prone to a number of misinterpretations, as previously discussed. When displaying life-table data, it is important to display the number of individuals being monitored at each interval of time in the study and in the control groups. Usually, only a small number are monitored for the complete duration of a study. For instance, in Figure 9.1 only 10 individuals in the study group are monitored for 5 years and only 5 individuals are monitored in the control group. This is not surprising because some time is often required to start up a study, and those individuals monitored for the longest time were recruited during the first year of the study.

A 5-year probability of survival can be calculated even when only one patient has been observed for 5 years. Thus, one should not rely too greatly on the specific 1-year, 5-year, or any other probability of survival observed unless a substantial number of individuals is actually observed for the full length of the study.

In interpreting randomized clinical trial results, it is important to understand the limitations in the reliability of the estimates obtained from the life-table. Failure to recognize this uncertainty can result in the following type of misinterpretation:

> A clinician looking at the life-table curves in Figure 9.1 concluded that 5-year survival with the study treatment is 60% versus 40% for the control group. After extensive use of the same treatment on similar patients, he was surprised that the study treatment actually produced a 55% survival versus only a 50% survival among control group patients.

If the clinician had recognized that life-table curves do not reliably predict exact 5-year survival, he would not have been surprised about his subsequent experience.

Knowledge of the procedures and assumptions underlying life tables also helps in understanding their interpretation. Many survival plots have a flat or plateau phase for long time periods at the right-hand end of the plot. These may be misinterpreted as indicating a cure once an individual reaches the flat or plateau area of the survival plot. Actually, this plateau phase usually results because few individuals are monitored for the entire duration of the study. Among those few individuals who are observed for longer periods, the deaths are likely to be fewer and more widely spaced. Because the survival curve declines only with a death, a plateau is likely when fewer deaths are possible. Thus, an understanding of this PLATEAU EFFECT is important in interpreting a life table. We should not interpret the plateau as demonstrating a cure unless great numbers of patients have been observed for long periods of time.

In addition to the dangers of relying too heavily on the 5-year probability of survival derived from life-table data and of misinterpreting the plateau, it is important to fully appreciate the interpretation of a statistically significant difference between survival plots, as illustrated in the next example:

In the study depicted in Figure 9.1, a statistically significant difference occurred in outcome between the study and control groups on the basis of the 5-year follow-up. The study was subsequently extended for 1 more year, resulting in the survival plot depicted in Figure 9.2, in which the 6-year actuarial survival was identical in the study and control groups. On the basis of the 6-year data, the authors stated that the 5-year actuarial study was mistaken in drawing the conclusion that the study therapy prolonged survival.

Remember that a statistically significant difference in survival implies that patients receiving one treatment do better than patients receiving another treatment when taking into account each group's entire experience. Patients in one group may do better only early in the course, midway through, or at the end. Patients who received the better overall treatment may actually do worse early in the treatment because of surgical complications, or at a later point in time as secondary complications develop for those who survive.

Thus, when conducting a study, it is important to know enough about the natural history of a disease and the life expectancy of the individuals in the investigation to choose a meaningful time period for follow-up. Differences in outcomes are unlikely if the time period is too short, such as one that ends before the therapy is completed or can be expected to have a biologic effect.

Similarly, follow-up periods that are too long may not allow the study to demonstrate statistically significant differences if the risks of competing diseases overwhelm the shorter-term benefits. For instance, a study that assesses the 20-year outcome among 65-year-olds given a treatment for coronary artery disease might show little difference at 20 years even if differences occur at 5 and 10 years.

We have repeatedly emphasized the distinction between a statistically significant association and a cause-and-effect relationship. In randomized clinical trials,

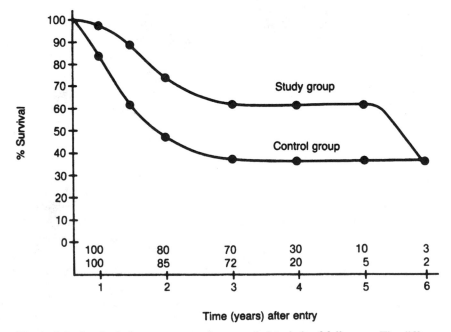

Figure 9.2. Survival plots may meet after extended periods of follow-up. The difference between the overall plots may still be statistically significant.

we use the same criteria to establish that a treatment has efficacy, meaning that it works for those in the investigation. Efficacy or a cause-and-effect relationship requires the existence of an association. Second, it requires a demonstration that the cause precedes the effect. Third, it requires that altering the cause alters the effect. One of the practical and intellectually satisfying aspects of randomized clinical trials is that they incorporate methods for helping to establish all three criteria for contributory cause and thus can establish the efficacy of a therapy as follows:

1. The investigators are able to produce study and control groups that are comparable except for the effects of the treatment being given. Thus, when substantial and statistically significant differences in outcome occur, the investigator can usually conclude that these differences are associated with the treatment itself.
2. By randomizing individuals to study and control groups at the beginning of the study, the investigators can provide strong evidence that the treatment precedes the effect and is, therefore, a prior association, fulfilling the second criterion of contributory cause.
3. By providing a treatment that alters the disease process and comparing the treatment and control groups' outcomes, the investigators can provide evidence that the treatment itself (the cause) is actually altering the outcome (the effect), thus fulfilling the third and final criterion for contributory cause.

Randomized clinical trials, therefore, can help to establish the existence of an association between treatment and outcome, can establish the existence of a prior association, and can demonstrate that altering the treatment alters the outcome. These are the three criteria necessary for establishing that the new treatment is the cause of the improved outcome. These criteria establish the efficacy of treatment. However, even after establishing that a treatment has efficacy, we need to ask what it is about the intervention that is working. The efficacy may not result from the intervention the investigator intended to study, as suggested in the following study:

> A randomized clinical trial of a new postoperative recovery program for posthysterectomy care was performed by randomizing 100 women postsurgery to a standard ward and 100 women to a special care ward equipped with experimental beds and postoperative exercise equipment and staffed by extra nurses. Women on the special care ward were discharged with an average length of stay of only 7 days compared with 12 days for women randomized to the regular ward. The results were statistically significant. The investigators concluded that the experimental beds and postoperative exercise program resulted in a substantially reduced length of stay.

This investigation established that the intervention had efficacy: It worked to produce more rapid recovery and thus to reduce length of stay. However, it is still not clear what actually worked. Before concluding that the experimental beds and postoperative exercise made the difference, do not forget that extra nurses were also required. The availability of the extra nurses may have been the cause of the early discharge rather than the beds and exercise. In an unmasked study such as this one, it is possible that the effect of observation itself helped to bring about the observed effect. Although even a well-performed randomized clinical trial may not definitively establish that the treatment caused the improvement, for practical purposes, randomized clinical trials satisfy the definition of efficacy.

The interpretation of safety data on adverse effects, side effects, or harms is an important part of randomized clinical trials, along with its emphasis on efficacy or benefits. Randomized clinical trials should display the frequency of adverse effects in both the study and the control groups. The number of individuals who experience the adverse effects in the study and control groups is usually small. Statistical significance testing is not usually performed because the statistical power is low. That is, the results would not usually be statistically significant even when they have clinical importance. Failure to appreciate this approach to adverse effects may lead to the following interpretation problem:

> A randomized clinical trial of a new hair-growth medication was conducted by randomizing 100 severely balding men to the new medicine and 100 severely balding men to placebo. Ninety percent of the men randomized to the new medication experienced substantial return of hair versus none in the placebo group. The results were statistically significant. Among the new medication group, five experienced elevated liver function tests and one acquired clinical hepatitis. Among the placebo group patients, three experienced elevated liver function tests and none acquired clinical hepatitis. The investigators concluded that the therapy had efficacy and the adverse effects may have been due to chance.

It is very tempting to dismiss the occurrence of side effects as due to chance, especially when there is no statistical significance testing and the side effect occurs in both groups. Unfortunately, this is often the situation in randomized clinical trials because of their limited size. This investigation can only provide a suggestion that the new medication is associated with liver function abnormalities. The presence of other causes for liver disease in both study and control groups must be kept in mind. In conducting this investigation, it would be very important to further investigate the cause of the elevated liver function tests to rule out other common causes, such as viral infections. In addition, the response of the liver function abnormalities to discontinuation of the treatments would provide some help in determining whether altering the potential cause alters the effect.

Demonstrating cause-and-effect relationships for adverse effects is very difficult. One approach relies on the consequences of starting and stopping treatment in a single individual. This type of investigation has been called an *n-of-1* study. In an n-of-1 study, each patient serves as his or her own control. The treatment is administered to one individual who develops a side effect such as a rash, then the therapy is discontinued and the patient is observed to see whether and when the presumed side effect resolves. The final step is to readminister the treatment to see whether the side effect occurs again.

This approach incorporates the concepts of association, prior association, and altering the cause alters the effect to help establish a cause-and-effect relationship. The potential danger to individual patients has limited the use of this technique.

Data on adverse effects are often limited to establishing the frequency of the side effect in study and control groups without expecting definitive data establishing statistical significance or contributory cause. These less definitive data, however, cannot be simply dismissed as being due to chance. Because of the small numbers, an assumption is usually made that an increase in the adverse events is caused by the study treatment. Thus, the approach to safety and efficacy is very different.

Extrapolation

Patients included in most randomized clinical trials are chosen because they are the type of patients most likely to respond to the treatment. In addition, considerations of time, geography, investigator convenience, and patient compliance are usually of paramount importance in selecting a particular group of patients for an investigation. Pregnant patients, the elderly, the very young, and those with mild disease are usually not included in randomized clinical trials unless the therapy is specifically designed for their use. In addition to these inclusion and exclusion criteria that are under the control of the investigator, other factors may lead to a unique type of patient group being entered in randomized clinical trials. Every medical center population has its own referral patterns, location, and socioeconomic patterns. A patient population referred to the Mayo Clinic may be quite different from one drawn to a local county hospital. Primary-care health maintenance organization (HMO) outpatients may be very different from the hospital subspecialty clinic outpatients. These characteristics, which may be beyond the investigator's control, can still affect the types of patients included in a way that may affect the results of the study.

The fact that the group of patients included in randomized clinical trials is different from a group of patients whom clinicians might treat with the new therapy often creates difficulty in extrapolating the conclusions to patients seen in clinical practice. If the individuals in the investigation are not representative of the intended or target population, extrapolation requires additional assumptions. This does not invalidate the result of a randomized clinical trial; however, it does mean the clinician must use care and good judgment when adopting the results to clinical practice.

Thus, despite the power and importance of randomized clinical trials, the process of extrapolation is still largely speculative. The use of convenience samples in randomized clinical trials makes it imperative that the reader examines the nature of the study institutions and the study patients before applying the study results. Clinicians should assess whether their own setting and patients are comparable to those in the study. If they are not, the differences may limit the ability to extrapolate from the study.

Patients and study centers involved in an investigation may be different from the usual clinical setting in many ways. For instance,

- Patients in an investigation are likely to be carefully followed up and very compliant. Compliance and close follow-up may be critical to the success of the therapy.
- Those in the study may have worse prognoses than the usual patients seen in clinical practice. For this reason, the side effects of the therapy may be worth the risk in the study patients, but the same may not be true for patients seen in another clinical setting.
- The study centers may have special skills, equipment, or experience that maximize the success of the new therapy. This may not be true when the therapy is used by clinicians without experience with those techniques.

Despite a clear demonstration of a successful therapy using a randomized clinical trial, clinicians must be careful to account for these types of differences in extrapolating to patients in their own practices. Randomized clinical trials are capable of assessing the efficacy or benefit of treatment performed on a carefully selected group of patients treated under the ideal conditions of an experimental study. They must be used carefully when trying to assess the effectiveness of treatment for usual clinical care. Thus, well-motivated and conscientious clinicians providing usual care with usual facilities probably cannot always match the results obtained in randomized clinical trials.

Randomized clinical trials, at their best, are capable only of assessing the benefit of treatment under current conditions. Not infrequently, however, the introduction of a new treatment can itself alter current conditions and produce secondary or dynamic effects. Clinical trials have a limited ability to assess the secondary effects of treatment. This is especially true for those effects that are more likely to occur when the therapy is widely applied in clinical practice. Consider the following study:

> A new drug called Herp-Ex was shown to have efficacy in a randomized clinical trial. It was shown to reduce the frequency of attacks when used in patients with severe recurrent herpes genitalis. It did not, however, cure the infection. The investigators were impressed with the results of the study and advocated use of Herp-Ex for all individuals with herpes genitalis.

If Herp-Ex is approved for clinical use, several effects may occur that may not have been expected on the basis of a randomized clinical trial. First, the drug would most likely be widely used, extending its use beyond the indications in the original trial. Patients with mild attacks or who present with first episodes would most likely also receive the therapy. This often occurs because once a drug is approved, clinicians have a right to prescribe it for other indications. The efficacy shown for recurrent severe attacks of herpes genitalis may not translate into effectiveness for uses that extend beyond the original indications. Second, the widespread use of Herp-Ex may result in strains of herpes that are resistant to the drug. Thus, long-term efficacy may not match the short-term results. Finally, the widespread use of Herp-Ex and short-term success may reduce the sexual precautions taken by those with recurrent herpes genitalis. Thus, over time the number of cases of herpes genitalis may actually increase despite or because of the short-term efficacy of Herp-Ex.

Randomized clinical trials are a fundamental tool for assessing the efficacy of therapy. When carefully used, they serve as a basis for extrapolations about the effectiveness of therapy in clinical practice. Randomized clinical trials, however, are not specifically designed to assess the safety of therapy.

Safety of therapy is more difficult to extrapolate than efficacy. Patients, in practice, may be on complicated treatments for multiple diseases or may have reduced renal or hepatic function, which results in exclusion from the randomized clinical trial. Thus, side effects may be more common in practice than in the randomized clinical trial. A special problem exists for rare but serious side effects. The heart of the problem stems from the large number of individuals who need to receive the treatment before rare but serious side effects are likely to be observed.

The number of exposures required to ensure a 95% probability of observing at least one episode of a rare side effect is summarized in the RULE OF THREE. According to this rule, to achieve a 95% chance of observing at least one case of penicillin anaphylaxis, which occurs on average about 1 time per 10,000, one needs to treat 30,000 individuals. If the investigator wishes to be 95% certain to observe at least one case of irreversible aplastic anemia from chloramphenicol, which occurs about 1 time per 50,000 uses, the investigator would need to treat 150,000 patients with chloramphenicol. In general terms, the rule of three states that to be 95% sure we will observe at least one case of a rare side effect, we need to treat approximately three times the number of individuals in the denominator.[13]

---

[13] These numbers assume there is no spontaneous or background incidence of these side effects. If these diseases occur from other causes, the numbers needed are even greater.

It is possible to use the rule of three in reverse to draw safety conclusions from a randomized clinical trial when there is no evidence in the investigation of rare but serious side effects. Imagine that 3,000 patients have received the new treatment and there is no evidence of a rare but serious side effect such as anaphylaxis. Then we can be 95% confident that if anaphylaxis occurs, its frequency of occurrence, on average, is no more than 1 per 1,000 uses. Most randomized clinical trials use fewer than 3,000 individuals in each group. If only 300 receive the new medication and no anaphylaxis is observed, then we can conclude with 95% confidence that if anaphylaxis occurs, its frequency of occurrence, on average, is no more than 1 per 100 uses. This may not be a very reassuring conclusion.

These numbers demonstrate that randomized clinical trials cannot be expected to detect many rare but important side effects. To deal with this dilemma, we often rely on animal testing. High doses of the drug are usually administered to a variety of animal species on the assumption that toxic, teratogenic, and carcinogenic effects of the drug will be observed in at least one of the animal species tested. This approach has been helpful but has not entirely solved the problem.

Long-term consequences of widely applied preventive treatments may be even more difficult to detect. Diethylstilbestrol (DES) was used for many years to prevent spontaneous abortions. It took decades before investigators noted greatly increased incidence of vaginal carcinoma among teenage girls whose mothers had taken DES.

It is only in clinical practice that a great number of patients are likely to receive the therapy. Therefore, in clinical practice we are likely to observe these rare but serious side effects. Alert clinicians and clinical investigators have been the mainstay of our current postmarketing surveillance. We currently have no organized systematic approach for detecting rare but serious side effects once a drug is released for clinical use. The FDA must rely on the reports received from clinicians. Thus, clinicians must remember that FDA approval should not be equated with complete safety or even with clearly defined and well-understood risks.

Randomized clinical trials are central to our current system for evaluating the efficacy of drugs and procedures. They represent a major advance. However, as practitioners reading the health literature, we must understand their strengths and limitations. We must be prepared to draw our own conclusions about the application of the results to our own patients, institution, or community. We must also recognize that randomized clinical trials can provide only limited data on the safety and effectiveness of the therapy being investigated.

10 Database Research:

Nonconcurrent Cohort Studies

The immense growth in computer capacity and the rapid acceleration of data collection in the health care system in recent years have expanded potential approaches to health research. Long-term databases collected for research or other purposes such as billing are increasingly available for research. In addition, it is now often possible for investigators to use databases collected for the primary purpose of ongoing clinical care.

Data that are collected as long-term research databases or collected in the course of health care can be used to conduct case-control studies. In addition, they can be used to conduct cohort studies. Sometimes, this type of research is called OUT-COMES research, but this name is misleading because all types of clinical studies can be used to evaluate health outcomes. More accurately, this type of cohort study done on a database is an example of what we have called a NONCONCURRENT COHORT STUDY or, less precisely, DATABASE RESEARCH.

Remember that a cohort study is defined by the fact that study and control groups are identified or observed to exist (observed assignment) before determining the study's outcome. Thus, at the time the investigators determine the observed assignment, they are not aware of the individual's end-point or outcome.

In preceding chapters, we discussed cohort studies in which individuals are observed over time to determine their outcomes. We call this a concurrent cohort study because individuals are monitored concurrently over time. In concurrent cohort studies, the treatment an individual received, or their observed assignment, is identified at the time they first receive the treatment. For example, we might observe one group of patients who underwent surgery and another group of patients who received medical treatment for recurrent otitis media in 1995. Then the individuals would be observed over time to perform the assessment. Thus, the surgical and the medical patients might be monitored until 2000 to assess their outcome.

With computerized data on patients often recorded during the course of their health care, it is now possible to conduct a second type of cohort study called a nonconcurrent cohort study. In this type of cohort study, it is not necessary to identify the treatment individuals received at one point in time and then to monitor them over time to determine the outcomes. In nonconcurrent cohort studies, the information on treatment that an individual received in 1995 can be obtained from a database in 2000. By the time a study is conducted in 2000, for instance, the assessment of outcome is already recorded in the computer database. To conduct a nonconcurrent cohort study, the investigators could proceed as follows:

> In February 2000, investigators begin a study. The investigators search the database for all patients who underwent surgery and for all patients who received medical

treatment for recurrent otitis media in 1995. Once these groups have been identified, the investigator observes their assignment to study and control groups. After performing this observed assignment, the investigators search the database to determine the outcomes that occurred after the observed assignment through January 2000.

A nonconcurrent cohort study is still a cohort study because the study and control groups are assigned before the investigators become aware of the individuals' outcomes. It is not legitimate for the investigators to obtain the outcomes until they have completed the assignment process, even though these outcomes have already occurred by the time the investigation is begun in February 2000.[1]

Figures 10.1 and 10.2 demonstrate the conduct of concurrent and nonconcurrent cohort studies. Both types of studies may be used to investigate either the cause of disease or the benefits and harms of therapy. Increasingly, however, nonconcurrent cohort studies are being used to study the outcome of therapies. Sometimes they are used to substitute for randomized clinical trials, and sometimes they are used to complement randomized clinical trials. In this chapter, we examine nonconcurrent cohort studies and contrast them with randomized clinical trials, the other common type of investigation used to evaluate therapies. We compare these types of studies in terms of their advantages and disadvantages and also examine errors that can occur in nonconcurrent cohort studies.

Study Design and Study Samples

The samples chosen for nonconcurrent cohort studies differ from randomized clinical trials in two important respects. First, randomized clinical trials are designed to include a homogeneous group of individuals who meet clearly defined inclusion and exclusion criteria. The study groups are not usually designed to reflect the target population. That is, they are not designed to reflect the entire spectrum of patients who would receive the treatment if applied in clinical practice.

Nonconcurrent cohort studies that are conducted on the basis of data from ongoing clinical care are quite different. By definition, they include those individuals who have received the treatment in clinical practice. Thus, everything else being equal, the result of a nonconcurrent cohort study is a better reflection of the result that we could expect for the average patient in clinical practice. Failure to appreciate this distinction can lead to the following type of error:

> A randomized clinical trial of nasal polyp surgery for individuals with recurrent sinusitis, aspirin allergy, and asthma demonstrated the efficacy of surgery. A nonconcurrent cohort study using a database from ongoing clinical care was also conducted. It identified all patients who had undergone the same type of nasal polyp

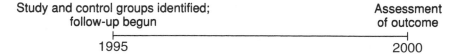

Figure 10.1. Time sequence of a concurrent cohort study.

---

[1]This type of study has also been called a RETROSPECTIVE COHORT STUDY. This term will not be used here because it often produces confusion, especially when case-control studies are referred to as retrospective studies.

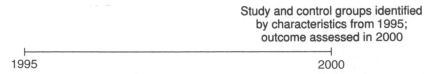

Figure 10.2. Time sequence of a nonconcurrent cohort study.

surgery and a comparable control group who had not undergone the surgery. The nonconcurrent cohort study did not demonstrate effectiveness. Reviewers of these studies relied on the randomized clinical trial exclusively because of its inherently superior study design.

The randomized clinical trial and the nonconcurrent cohort study address different questions and study different populations. Randomized clinical trials are the gold standard for determining efficacy for a specific indication. Efficacy for one clear-cut, although narrowly defined, indication for treatment such as the patient with recurrent sinusitis, aspirin allergy, and asthma may tell us very little about the outcomes the therapy produces when applied to a broader target population in clinical practice. The outcomes of a therapy on its target population in clinical practice define its effectiveness as opposed to its efficacy.

Thus, the results of a nonconcurrent cohort study, everything else being equal, may add to or complement the result of a randomized clinical trial by providing information on effectiveness in clinical practice.

Second, the number of patients included in randomized clinical trials is limited by time, money, and availability of patients. The sample sizes chosen, in fact, are often designed to be the smallest number that will provide acceptable statistical power (*i.e.*, the largest acceptable type II error, usually 10% to 20%) in addressing what is called the primary end-point. As discussed in the preceding chapter on randomized clinical trials, these numbers usually vary from less than 100 in both the study group and the control group to several thousand in each group.

The sample size in nonconcurrent cohort studies is limited mainly by the availability of patient data in the database. Thousands or even millions of patients may be included. Thus, the potential sample size for nonconcurrent cohort studies may dwarf that of randomized clinical trials. This difference in sample sizes may have important implications, as illustrated in the next example:

> A randomized clinical trial was conducted comparing removal of colon polyps versus observation. The study and control groups each included 500 patients. The investigation demonstrated a small but not statistically significant reduction in the subsequent rate of colon cancer. A nonconcurrent cohort study using 100,000 patients who had polyp removal and 100,000 patients who underwent observation demonstrates a small difference in the subsequent rate of colon cancer, but the *P* value was 0.00001 and the confidence limits were very narrow.

This type of discrepancy between the results of a randomized clinical trial and those of a nonconcurrent cohort study is expected. If the nonconcurrent cohort study is able to avoid the biases to which it is susceptible, we would expect the nonconcurrent cohort study to have a far greater statistical power. That is, it would have a much greater chance of demonstrating statistical significance if a true difference exists in the population being sampled.

Thus, for small but real differences, everything else being equal, nonconcurrent cohort studies often have a much greater probability of demonstrating statistical significance.

Assignment

When discussing nonconcurrent cohort studies and comparing them with randomized clinical trials, we have repeatedly used the phrase "everything else being equal." "Everything else" is not usually equal when we compare these two types of studies because nonconcurrent cohort studies are susceptible to a variety of potential biases. These potential biases are most dramatic in the area of assignment.

Randomized clinical trials by definition use randomization for their assignment process. The process of randomization is the hallmark of a randomized clinical trial. Remember that the process of randomization is designed to take into account not only the factors that are known to affect outcome but also those factors that have an effect on outcome we do not recognize.

In nonconcurrent cohort studies, on the basis of the results of clinical care, assignment is performed by observing the clinicians' assignment of patients to study and control groups. Clinicians try to tailor the treatment to the patient. If they are successful in doing this, they create selection biases. This occurs when clinicians assign patients with different prognoses or probability of good and bad outcomes to different treatments. In fact, we can regard the job of clinical care as one of creating biases by tailoring the treatment to the patient. The job of the clinician then is to create selection biases, and the job of the researcher is to untangle these selection biases. Selection bias created in database research has been called CASE-MIX BIAS. Let us see how this type of confounding variable may influence the results:

> A randomized clinical trial of a smoking-cessation drug demonstrated a small, statistically significant reduction in smoking among those randomized to the drug. A large, nonconcurrent cohort study identified those prescribed the drug and compared success in quitting among smokers who were prescribed the drug versus smokers who were not prescribed the drug. The investigation demonstrated a much larger reduction in smoking among those prescribed the drug.

The patients prescribed the drug in the database research may have been those who were especially motivated to stop smoking. Clinicians may have tailored their treatment by perhaps giving more intensive treatment to the patients they thought would benefit the most. This is a natural and often desirable tendency in clinical care. However, from the researcher's perspective, selecting motivated patients to receive the treatment results in a confounding variable. Those who receive the treatment are those who are especially likely to quit smoking.

Recognizing the confounding variables created by clinicians is important so they can be considered in the analysis. Unfortunately, databases often lack the data needed to measure some important variables that should ideally be taken into account in the analysis.

Randomized clinical trials are often precluded by ethical issues and practical issues. Once it is suspected that a treatment benefits patients, clinicians and patients will often be unwilling to randomize patients to receive or not to receive the treatment. Thus, a nonconcurrent cohort study may be the best available study design even when a randomized clinical trial would, in theory, be preferable.

In addition to randomized assignment, an ideal randomized clinical trial is also double-masked. That is, neither the patient nor the investigator is aware of the treatment being received. However, as mentioned in Chapter 9, double-masked studies are often either unethical, impractical, or unsuccessful. Patient masking is not possible in a nonconcurrent cohort study of a database from ongoing clinical care. In addition, the clinician who prescribes the treatment is not masked. Thus, for both randomized clinical trials and nonconcurrent cohort studies, we often need to ask what the implications are of a lack of masking. We usually need to examine how the method of assignment affects the results of the assessment process.

Assessment

The process of follow-up and assessment in well-conducted randomized clinical trials and nonconcurrent cohort studies is very different. In a randomized cohort trial, patients in the study and control groups are followed up at predetermined intervals, which are the same for the study and control groups. The same data are collected on individuals in each group at the follow-up intervals.

The process of follow-up and assessment in a nonconcurrent cohort study is very different because it occurs as part of the course of health care. Data are collected if and when the patient returns for care. This return visit may be initiated by the clinician or the patient. Thus, the frequency of data collection, the type of data, and even the accuracy of the data collected or recorded are likely to be quite different in randomized clinical trials and nonconcurrent cohort studies. These differences in follow-up may have important implications for the results obtained, as illustrated in the next example:

> A randomized clinical trial comparing surgery versus medication for benign prostate hypertrophy found that surgery produces far more retrograde ejaculation and impotence than medication. A nonconcurrent cohort study using records from ongoing medical care found no difference in these adverse effects, as recorded in the patients' charts.

Unless patients are specifically asked or tested for these side effects, they may not recognize them or report them to clinicians. Thus, in nonconcurrent cohort studies, the type of outcome measure than can be reliably used may be much more limited than in a randomized clinical trial, in which these side effects can be assessed in the same way for each group at the same time intervals.

Analysis

In randomized clinical trials, analysis is conducted using the principle of intention-to-treat. Thus, individuals are analyzed according to their assignment group even if they never received the treatment. Remember that this is done so individuals with good prognosis are not disproportionately represented among those who are left after many participants with a poorer prognosis drop out of the study.

It is possible to aim for a comparable technique in nonconcurrent cohort studies by making the assignment on the basis of the prescribed treatment and analyzing patients in their original groups on the basis of their prescribed treatment, including those who do not continue on the treatment. However, this may not be successful in database research because the only patients who appear in the database may be those who followed up on the therapy, as illustrated in the next example:

> Radiation therapy for a specific type of metastatic brain cancer was studied using a nonconcurrent cohort study. Radiation required premedication and could be started only after a month of pretreatment. The database recorded only patients who received the treatment and those who did not. Among those receiving the treatment, survival was 2 months longer on average. The results were statistically significant. The investigators concluded that the nonconcurrent cohort study had demonstrated the short-term effectiveness of radiation therapy.

The fact that the radiation therapy could not be undertaken for at least a month after it was prescribed may mean that those with the worst prognosis had already died or become too ill to receive the radiation therapy. Thus, the nonconcurrent cohort study may have examined a study group with a better prognosis than the control group, indicating the groups may not actually have been analyzed using a method analogous to the intention-to-treat method.

In randomized clinical trials, adjustment is used as a way to account for the known prognostic factors that, despite randomization, differ between the study and the control groups. Randomization itself often results in known prognostic factors being similar in the study and the control groups. In addition, randomization has the aim to produce similarity even for unknown prognostic factors. Adjustment is still used in a randomized clinical trial; however, its role is only to take into account the differences that occur despite randomization.

In a nonconcurrent cohort study, adjustment has a much larger role. It attempts to recognize and take into account all the differences between the study and control groups that may affect the outcome being measured. Adequate adjustment requires recognizing all potential confounding variables and taking them into account in the adjustment process, even though differences between groups are not substantial or statistically significant.

Interpretation

As a type of cohort study, nonconcurrent cohort studies are best designed to demonstrate that the treatment is associated with an improved outcome and that the treatment precedes the outcome. The ability to establish that the treatment alters the outcome depends on the success of the recognizing and adjusting for the potential confounding variable. This usually leaves some doubt as to the third criterion of contributory cause, or efficacy of therapy.

A special type of nonconcurrent cohort study may also help to establish that altering the cause alters the effect. This type of investigation recognizes that a change has occurred in one group over a period of time but not in another comparable group. The probability of a particular outcome before and after the change in each group is then calculated to determine whether the outcome was altered in the group that experienced the change. This type of investigation has been called a NATURAL EXPERIMENT. Let us see how a natural experiment may enable us to draw the conclusion that altering the cause alters the effect:

> Cigarettes were smoked with nearly equal frequency among male physicians and attorneys in the 1960s, and they had a similar probability of developing lung cancer. During the 1970s, a large proportion of male physicians quit smoking cigarettes,

whereas a smaller proportion of male attorneys quit smoking cigarettes. The investigators observed that both male physicians and attorneys who stopped smoking had a reduction in their probability of developing lung cancer and that the probability of developing lung cancer among male physicians in subsequent years was far lower than among male attorneys.

A randomized clinical trial of cigarette smoking would have been the ideal method for establishing that altering the cause alters the effect. This type of natural experiment is the next best method. It is often, as in this situation, the only ethical and feasible method for establishing this cause-and-effect relationship.

After analysis and interpretation are completed using all the individuals included in either a randomized clinical trial or a nonconcurrent cohort study, the investigators are often interested in examining the meaning of the results for special groups included in the study. This process is referred to as SUBGROUP ANALYSIS.[2] The large numbers of patients included in a nonconcurrent cohort study may allow the investigators to subdivide the study and control groups into smaller subgroups and examine the therapy's effectiveness for these specific groups. Because of the larger numbers, the data from the nonconcurrent cohort studies' subgroups may be more reliable than those from subgroups derived from randomized clinical trials. This may have important implications, as illustrated in the next example:

> A randomized clinical trial of one-vessel coronary artery disease demonstrated that angiography had greater efficacy, on average, than medical treatment. Subgroup analysis performed by creating groups that differed in their extent of myocardium served by the vessel, age of the patients, and gender of the patient was not able to demonstrate statistically significant differences between these groups. A large nonconcurrent cohort study demonstrated overall effectiveness of angiography but also demonstrated that this effectiveness was limited to younger men and to patients with a lesion supplying a large area of myocardium.

This type of result illustrates the principle that the larger number of patients who may be available in a nonconcurrent cohort study enables the study to better address issues among subgroups than even most well-designed, controlled clinical trials. This use of randomized clinical trials and nonconcurrent cohort studies demonstrates the potential to use the results of one type of study to supplement the results of the other.

In addition to its greater potential for investigating subgroups, a nonconcurrent cohort study may have greater potential to draw conclusions about side effects, harm, or safety. Nonconcurrent cohort studies offer two basic advantages in assessing side effects compared to randomized clinical trials. First, the large numbers make it more likely that rare but serious side effects will be recognized. These serious side effects, once they occur, are likely to be recognized and thus appear in the database. The rule of three gives us some idea of the degree of certainty that we can attach to the absence of a side effect. Remember that the rule of three suggests that if there are no cases of a side effect, we can be 95% confident that the true frequency is not greater than three divided by the number of exposures. The implications of the larger numbers often available in a nonconcurrent cohort study are illustrated in the next example:

---

[2]Subgroup analysis, in general, should only be conducted after obtaining statistically significant results using all the data. In addition they should only be conducted to examine relationships hypothesized prior to collecting the data.

In a randomized clinical trial of 300 patients receiving treatment, there were no serious side effects. In a nonconcurrent cohort study in which 3,000 patients received the treatment, there were 10 cases of a serious side effect. The authors concluded that the two studies were incompatible, and the data from the randomized clinical trial should be accepted, demonstrating that the treatment was free of serious side effects.

According to the rule of three, the data from the randomized clinical trial tells us we can be 95% confident that if there is a serious side effect of the treatment, its true frequency is no greater than 3 per 300 or 1 per 100 uses. In the larger nonconcurrent cohort study, we observed a side effect frequency of 10 per 3,000 or 1 per 300. Thus, the results of the two studies are compatible. The probability of serious side effects according to the nonconcurrent cohort study provided additional information that cannot be obtained when relying exclusively on the relatively small randomized clinical trial.

Extrapolation

Extrapolation of the results of a randomized clinical trial always requires making assumptions about the population that will receive the treatment (*i.e.*, the target population). Remember that randomized clinical trials are usually conducted using homogeneous patients who are not on multiple treatments, who do not have liver or kidney disease complicating their management, and who often do not have other diseases. In addition, special precautions may be used in randomized clinical trials to exclude patients who have special characteristics, such as those who are not likely to follow up or who are likely to become pregnant. Thus, the patients included in randomized clinical trials are often quite different than those included in nonconcurrent cohort studies on the basis of clinical practice. Therefore, the results of a randomized cohort trial and those of a nonconcurrent cohort study may look very different, even when the new therapy is administered using the same implementation procedures, as illustrated in the next example:

A randomized clinical trial of a new method of home dialysis for newly diagnosed renal failure patients demonstrated substantial improvement in outcome compared with outpatient hemodialysis. The new dialysis method was then made available using the same implementation procedures to all dialysis patients throughout the country in two stages. During the first stage, all those using the new technique were compared with all those using standard outpatient hemodialysis in a nonconcurrent cohort study. The investigators found no difference in outcome between the new home dialysis method and standard outpatient hemodialysis.

A randomized clinical trial on a small homogeneous group of new dialysis patients may show very different results compared with a nonconcurrent cohort study involving a larger number of more heterogeneous patients. For instance, patients who are accustomed to outpatient hemodialysis may have difficulty switching to the new treatment. Patients with more complications on long-standing outpatient hemodialysis may not do as well on the new therapy.

Thus, we cannot necessarily expect that the results of a randomized clinical trial and those of a nonconcurrent cohort study will be the same even when both are well designed and the therapy is administered using the same implementation procedures. It is still likely that for carefully selected patients, like those in the randomized clinical trial, the new method of home dialysis is better than the standard therapy.

As we discussed, randomized clinical trials are limited to assessing outcomes or end-points at one point in time. They actually represent a snapshot view of the therapy's effects. After they are introduced into practice, dynamic effects may occur that may alter the longer-term effectiveness of the therapy. Resistance may occur; the treatment may be used for new indications, producing more or less effectiveness; or patient behavior may change, altering the effectiveness of treatment.

Database studies may be more successful in detecting these changes in effectiveness that occur over time. The large number of patients in a database may allow the investigator to compare the outcomes that occurred when the treatment was prescribed in different years. Alternatively, the degree of effectiveness can be followed over extended periods, and an assessment can be made of the persistence of a benefit. This advantage of database studies is illustrated in the next example:

> A new high-energy treatment for kidney stones has been demonstrated in a randomized clinical trial to have efficacy in the treatment of urethral obstruction compared with surgery when patients are observed for 3 years. A nonconcurrent cohort study was performed of urethral obstruction caused by kidney stones treated with the new technique and followed for up to 10 years. The results demonstrated less efficacy for the new treatment compared with surgery. Those undergoing surgery actually did better after 3 years.

These two results may both be true. They may complement each other. This could be the case if the new treatment increases the rate of recurrence of kidney stones. The relatively short-term follow-up that is usually possible in randomized clinical trials leaves an important role for nonconcurrent cohort studies using databases obtained from ongoing clinical care in the longer-term assessment of safety and efficacy.

Remember that randomized clinical trials are the gold standard for assessing efficacy, but they have severe limitations when assessing effectiveness for the target population, when assessing the occurrence of rare but serious side effects, and when examining the longer-term results of the treatment. Nonconcurrent cohort studies can complement randomized clinical trials and compensate for some of these deficiencies.

11 Meta-Analysis

Thus far, we have examined the three basic types of investigation in the health research literature which are designed to compare study and control groups: case-control studies, cohort studies, and randomized clinical trials. Each study type can be used to address the same relationship. These investigations often provide consistent results. At times, however, studies published in the health research literature seem to conflict with one another, making it difficult to provide definitive answers to important study questions.

It is often desirable to be able to combine data obtained in a variety of investigations and to use all the information to address a study question. META-ANALYSIS is a collection of methods for combining information from single investigations in order to reach conclusions or address questions that were not possible on the basis of single investigations.

Meta-analysis aims to produce its conclusion by combining data from two or more existing investigations. Traditionally, this process of research synthesis has been the review article's role. In recent years, it has been increasingly recognized that the informal and subjective process of literature review has not always produced accurate conclusions. Let us examine one reason why this might occur.

To illustrate the principles of meta-analysis and examine its strengths and limitations, consider the following hypothetical situation:

Assume that we are interested in examining a recent innovation in the treatment of coronary artery disease known as transthoracic laser coronaryplasty (TLC). TLC is designed to treat coronary artery disease through the chest wall without using invasive techniques. The first two studies of TLC produced the following results:

Study 1

	Die	Live	Total
TLC	230	50	280
Control	530	210	740

$$\text{Relative risk} = \frac{230 \ / \ 280}{530 \ / \ 740} = \frac{0.821}{0.716} = 1.13$$

$$\text{Odd ratio} = \frac{230 \ / \ 50}{530 \ / \ 210} = \frac{4.60}{2.52} = 1.83$$

$$\text{Risk difference} = 0.716 - 0.821 = -0.105$$

$$\text{Number needed to treat} = \frac{1}{0.716 - 0.821} = -9.5$$

Study 2

	Die	Live	Total
TLC	190	405	595
Control	50	210	260

$$\text{Relative risk} = \frac{190 \, / \, 595}{50 \, / \, 260} = \frac{0.319}{0.192} = 1.66$$

$$\text{Odd ratio} = \frac{190 \, / \, 405}{50 \, / \, 210} = \frac{0.469}{0.238} = 1.97$$

$$\text{Risk difference} = 0.192 - 0.319 = -0.127$$

$$\text{Number needed to treat} = \frac{1}{0.192 - 0.319} = -7.9$$

Investigators were discouraged and feared that this new procedure would not have a bright future. Before relegating this technique to history, however, they decided to combine the results of the two studies and see what happened. Combining the data from the two studies produced the results found in the Combined Studies indicated at the bottom of this page.

Notice that the differences in outcomes now favor TLC as measured by the odds ratio, the relative risk, or the number needed to treat almost as strongly as the single studies argued against the efficacy of TLC. Thus, combining studies may produce some surprising results.

This process set into motion a widespread effort to evaluate the use of TLC in a variety of settings and for a variety of indications worldwide. Most studies focused on single-vessel coronary artery disease as assessed by new noninvasive procedures. Over the next several years, dozens of studies resulted in apparently conflicting results. Thus, it was considered important to conduct a full-scale meta-analysis evaluating the effects of TLC on single-vessel coronary artery disease.

Study Design

The process of combining information using meta-analysis can be best understood if we regard each of the studies included in the analysis as parallel to one study site in a multiple-site investigation. In a single investigation, the investigator combines the data from multiple sites to draw conclusions or interpretations. In meta-analysis, the investigator combines information from multiple studies to draw conclusions or interpretations. This parallel structure allows us to learn about meta-analysis using the studying a study uniform framework.

Combined Studies 1 and 2

	Die	Live	Total
TLC	420	455	875
Control	580	420	1,000

$$\text{Relative risk} = \frac{420 \, / \, 875}{580 \, / \, 1{,}000} = \frac{0.480}{0.580} = 0.827$$

$$\text{Odd ratio} = \frac{420 \, / \, 455}{580 \, / \, 420} = \frac{0.923}{1.381} = 0.668$$

$$\text{Risk difference} = 0.580 - 0.480 = 0.10$$

$$\text{Number needed to treat} = \frac{1}{0.580 - 0.480} = 10$$

Study Hypothesis, Study Population, and Sample Size

As with our other uses of the uniform framework, we start by defining the study question or study hypothesis. In our previous examination of studies, we emphasized the importance of defining a hypothesis before beginning an investigation. This helps us to determine appropriate individuals to include in the study and control groups.

As with our other types of investigations, we ideally begin with a study hypothesis and proceed to test that hypothesis and draw inferences. When we do this for a therapy, for instance, we may ask if that therapy works. We do this by proposing a study hypothesis that states the treatment has efficacy. We also address the question of estimation by asking how well the treatment works.

The studies that should be included in a meta-analysis depend on the purpose of the analysis. Thus, the study hypothesis of the meta-analysis helps to determine the inclusion and exclusion criteria that should initially be used in identifying relevant studies. The following example shows how the hypothesis can help to determine which studies to include:

In preparation for a meta-analysis, researchers searched the world's literature and obtained the following 25 studies of TLC for single-vessel coronary artery disease. These investigations had characteristics which allowed them to be grouped into the following types of studies:

A. Five studies of men with single-vessel disease treated initially with coronary bypass surgery versus medication versus TLC
B. Five studies of men and women treated initially with TLC versus bypass surgery
C. Five studies of men and women treated initially with TLC versus medication
D. Five studies of men treated with TLC versus medication after previous bypass surgery
E. Five studies of women treated with repeat TLC versus medication after previous TLC

If the meta-analysis is designed to test a hypothesis, then the studies to be included are chosen because they address issues relevant to the hypothesis. For instance, if the investigator wanted to test the hypothesis that men do better than women when TLC is used to treat single-vessel coronary artery disease, then study groups B and C should be used in the meta-analysis. These investigations all include comparisons of the outcomes in both men and women.

If the investigators were interested in testing the hypothesis that initial TLC is better than surgery for single-vessel coronary artery disease, then study groups A and B should be used in the meta-analysis because these groups of studies compare TLC versus surgery as the initial therapy. Alternatively, if the researcher hypothesized that medication was the best treatment for single-vessel coronary artery disease, then study groups A, C, D, and E would be used. In general, the studies that are used are determined by the study hypothesis of the meta-analysis.

Despite the many similarities between meta-analysis and single multisite investigations, there is one important difference. In original data collection research, in theory, the investigator may define the study question, then find a setting and study participants that are suited to addressing the question, and determine the desired sample size. In meta-analysis, the questions we may ask are often limited by the availability of previous studies. Thus, the study population and the sample size are largely outside the investigator's control.

To try to circumvent this problem, meta-analysis researchers often define a question or issue broadly and begin by identifying all investigations related to that issue. When this is done, the investigators are conducting an EXPLORATORY META-ANALYSIS as opposed to a HYPOTHESIS-DRIVEN META-ANALYSIS.[1]

In conducting an exploratory meta-analysis of TLC, for instance, the investigator might initially include all the studies just mentioned. Thus, the meta-analysis researcher would define the study group as consisting of those who received TLC, and the control group would consist of all the individuals receiving other therapy.

This process of using all available studies without a specific hypothesis is parallel to the process of conducting a single investigation without defining a study hypothesis. This type of exploratory meta-analysis can be useful, but must be conducted carefully and interpreted differently from hypothesis-driven meta-analyses. Despite the potential dangers of combining studies with very different characteristics, the limited number of available studies makes it important for meta-analysis to include techniques for combining very different types of studies.

Meta-analysis attempts to turn this diversity of studies into an advantage. Combining studies with different characteristics may allow us to harness the benefit of diversity. By including apples and oranges, we can ask whether it makes a difference if a fruit is an apple or an orange or whether it is enough that it is a fruit.

The approach for harnessing the benefit of diversity is discussed later. For now, we must recognize that there are actually two fundamentally different types of meta-analyses: one that is hypothesis-based and a second type called exploratory meta-analysis.

It is important to remember that the fundamental difference between meta-analysis and other types of investigations is that the data have already been collected and initially the researcher's choice is limited to including or excluding the existing study from the meta-analysis. Thus, the sample size in meta-analysis is limited by the existence of relevant studies.

Meta-analysis, like other types of investigations, usually starts by defining the question to be investigated. This question determines the types of individuals who should be included in a single investigation. Similarly, the question to be addressed by a meta-analysis determines the types of studies that should be included in the meta-analysis. Thus, in hypothesis-driven meta-analysis, the first question we need to ask is whether a particular study is relevant to the meta-analysis questions?

Assignment

Methods of Assignment

Once the study question is defined, the investigators can determine which studies to include in a meta-analysis. In meta-analysis, this selection and identification of studies to include is the assignment process, in which we ask: Have all the relevant studies been identified?

---

[1]At times, meta-analyses cannot use all the available studies because the data in some articles are not presented with enough detail to allow combination with other studies.

Identifying all relevant research is an essential step in the assignment process of a meta-analysis. It is important that the investigator describe the method used to search for research reports, including enough detail to allow subsequent investigators to obtain all the identified literature.[2] This can even include unpublished data. Doctoral dissertations, abstracts, grant reports, and registries of studies are increasingly possible to locate.

Confounding Variables Publication Bias

An extensive search for research reports as part of the assignment process in a meta-analysis is important due to the potential for a special type of selection bias known as PUBLICATION BIAS. Publication bias occurs when there is a systematic tendency to publish studies with positive results and to not publish studies that suggest no differences in outcome. Small investigations are frequently not submitted or are rejected for publication. The next example illustrates publication bias:

> After identifying the studies available through a computerized search of published articles, the TLC meta-analysis researchers identified 20 studies of the relationship between TLC and single-vessel coronary artery disease. There was a wide variation in the sample sizes of the studies and in the outcomes, as shown in Table 11.1.

One technique that can be used to assess the presence and extent of possible publication bias is known as the FUNNEL DIAGRAM. Examples of the results of the funnel approach are shown in Table 11.1 and Figure 11.1.

Table 11.1 represents the data from the initial 20 studies of TLC. The funnel diagram is based on the principle that smaller studies, by chance alone, are expected

Table 11.1. *Data from 20 studies of transthoracic laser coronaryplasty*

Study Number	Odds Ratio	Sample Size (Each Group)
1	4.0	20
2	3.0	20
3	2.0	20
4	1.0	20
5	0.5	20
6	3.5	40
7	2.5	40
8	1.5	40
9	2.5	60
10	1.5	60
11	1.0	60
12	1.5	80
13	1.0	80
14	1.5	100
15	1.0	100
16	0.5	100
17	1.5	120
18	1.0	120
19	0.5	120
20	1.0	140

[2]In performing this search, it is important to avoid double counting. Studies originally presented as abstracts, for instance, will often subsequently appear as original articles. Including the same data two or more times jeopardizes the accuracy of the results of a meta-analysis by violating the assumption that the data obtained in each of the studies are independent of the other studies.

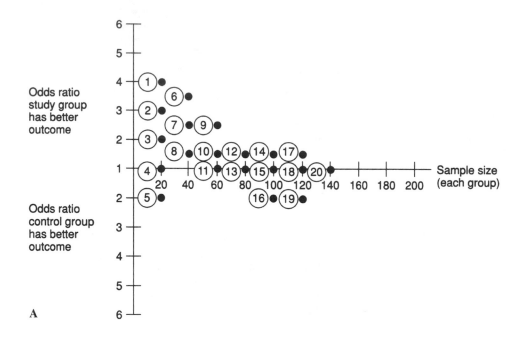

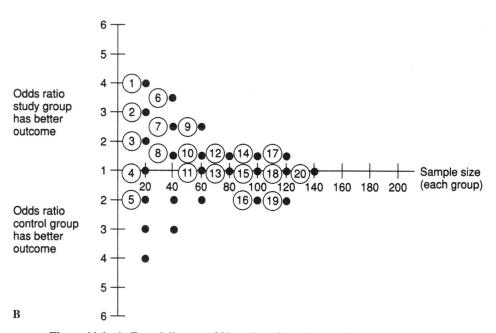

Figure 11.1. A: Funnel diagram of 20 studies of transthoracic laser coronaryplasty. **B:** Funnel diagram after adding five additional studies.

to produce results with greater variation. A funnel diagram that does not suggest the presence of publication bias should look like a funnel with larger variation in results among smaller studies. Cases in which the lower side of the funnel is incomplete, as in Figure 11.1A, suggest that some studies are missing.

Now imagine that the TLC meta-analysis researchers searched further and came up with five additional studies. After obtaining all 25 studies, they redrew their funnel diagram and obtained Figure 11.1B. From this funnel diagram, which has a more complete funnel appearance, they concluded there was no longer evidence of a publication bias and they had likely obtained all or most of the relevant studies.

Even after extensive searching, it is possible that investigations will be missed. This does not preclude proceeding with a meta-analysis. It is possible, as we will see, to take into account this potential publication bias as part of the analysis.

Another important part of the assignment process in a meta-analysis is to determine whether there are differences in the quality of studies that justify excluding low-quality studies from the meta-analysis.

There are two potential approaches to this issue. It has been argued that study types with the potential for systematic biases should be excluded for a meta-analysis. For this reason, some meta-analysis researchers have favored the exclusion of all studies except randomized clinical trials, arguing that this type of study is the least likely to produce results that have a systematic bias in one direction or the other.

If randomized clinical trials as well as other types of studies are available, however, an alternative approach is to include all types of studies at least initially. All investigations are then evaluated to determine their quality. Quality scores are usually obtained by two readers of the research report, each using the same standardized scoring system without knowledge of the other reader's score and masked to the identity of the authors. Then it is possible to compare the results of high-quality studies with those of low-quality studies to determine if the results, on average, are similar. Let us examine what might happen when we combine high-quality and low-quality studies:

> A meta-analysis of the strength of the relationship between TLC and the outcome of single-vessel coronary artery disease included all known studies, including case-control, cohort, and randomized clinical trials. The investigators had two readers score each investigation using the same standardized scoring system without knowledge of the other reader's score or the authors' identities. The outcomes on average for the low-quality studies were approximately equal to those for the high-quality studies. Thus, the investigators decided to retain all studies in their meta-analysis.

A variety of other study characteristics can potentially affect the outcome. As with single investigations, it is important that the investigator recognize these characteristics because they are potential confounding variables. The usual approach is to recognize the differences as part of the assignment process and take them into account as part of the analysis.

For instance, in the TLC studies, we should know whether some studies used only older patients, more severely ill patients, or those with other characteristics or prognostic factors that often result in a poorer outcome in coronary artery disease. In addition, we would want to know whether there were important variations in the treatment given, such as different TLC techniques or different adjunct therapy, such as duration of anticoagulation. Thus, in the assignment process in a meta-analysis, we need data on the degree of uniformity of the patients and of the procedures used.

Masking

Masking of assignment in meta-analysis has a somewhat different meaning than in other types of investigations. In one sense, the meta-analysis relies on the methods used in the individual studies, if feasible, to mask the participants and investigators as to participants in the study and control groups. In meta-analysis, masking of assignment can also be achieved by preventing the investigators from being biased by knowledge of the results, the authors, or other characteristics of an investigation when determining whether a particular investigation should be included in the meta-analysis. If masking is not feasible, more than one individual may be asked to judge whether an investigation meets the predefined criteria for inclusion in the meta-analysis.

In single investigations, whether they are case-control, cohort, or randomized clinical trials, the investigator can personally define the outcome to be studied and collect the data to assess the outcome. In meta-analysis, the researcher is usually limited to the methods used by the primary investigator for assessing the study outcome.

The meta-analysis is also limited by the extent of data presented and the statistical methods used in the original article. However, it is increasingly possible to go back and obtain all the original data. Some journals are beginning to ask investigators who submit research articles to include a complete data set from their study for later review by other investigators or for use in a meta-analysis. In the future, this may allow meta-analysis researchers to redefine the various studies' outcomes so that each investigation uses the same measurement.

Currently, the meta-analysis researcher usually must live with what is available in existing articles. Because of the differences in the definitions and measurements of outcomes in different studies, the researcher performing a meta-analysis is faced with a series of unique issues. First, the meta-analysis researcher must determine which outcome to use in comparing studies. This may pose a serious problem, as illustrated in the next example:

> In the studies of TLC, the following outcome measures were assessed. Ten studies used time until positive stress test, time until evidence of occlusion on repeat noninvasive angiography, and also time until myocardial infarction as the outcomes. Ten other studies used only time until positive stress test as their measure of outcome. Five studies used time until a positive stress test and evidence of occlusion on repeat noninvasive angiography as their measures of outcome. As a result of the different outcome measurements used, the researcher concluded that a meta-analysis could not be performed.

The need to use precise and accurate measures of outcomes do pose major issues in meta-analysis.

The researcher may be interested in an accurate and early measure of outcome, which, in this case, may be a evidence occlusion on a repeat noninvasive angiography indicating closure of the treated vessel. Despite the desirability of using this outcome measure, if it is used to assess outcome, 10 of the 25 studies would need to be excluded. Thus, the researcher performing this meta-analysis may be forced to use time until positive stress test as the measure of outcome if he wishes to include all the studies.

Even after determining that the measure of outcome will be time until positive stress test, the meta-analysis researchers' problems are not solved, as shown in the following example:

> The 25 studies define a positive stress test in several different ways. Some require greater duration and extent of stress test depression than others. The meta-analysis researcher decides to use only studies that use the same definition of a positive stress test. Unfortunately, only 12 studies can be included in the meta-analysis.

It is important to find a common end-point for a meta-analysis, but it is not essential that the end-point be defined in the same way in all the studies. This is a common problem that is not generally dealt with by excluding studies. Rather, all studies with data on follow-up stress testing are included. The results of studies that use a common definition of a positive test can then be compared with studies that use other definitions of the end-point. If the results are similar, regardless of the definition of a positive stress test, then all the studies can be combined in one analysis using their own definitions of a positive stress test. If there are substantial differences depending on the definition of a positive stress test, then separate analyses can be performed for studies that used different definitions.

Completeness and Effect of Observation

The completeness of the investigations included in a meta-analysis depends on the particular studies chosen for inclusion. The effect of observation also depends on the particular type and characteristics of the investigations that are included. Because of the large number factors that can influence the quality of the assessment process, it is tempting for the meta-analysis investigator to eliminate studies that do not meet quality standards. As we have seen, some meta-analyses are conducted using only studies that meet predefined quality standards. Other meta-analyses researchers attempt to achieve this end by including only randomized clinical trials, presuming that they constitute the preferred type of investigation. While these are accepted approaches, others argue that high- and low-quality studies should be included and that an analysis should be conducted to determine if they produce similar or different results.

Analysis

The goals of analysis in meta-analysis are the same as those in other types of clinical investigations. We are interested in the following:

- **Estimation.** Estimating effect size, that is, the strength of an association or the magnitude of a difference
- **Inference.** Performing statistical significance testing to draw inferences about the population on the basis of the data in the sample
- **Adjustment.** Adjusting for potential confounding variables to determine whether they affect the strength or statistical significance of the association or difference

The effect size in meta-analysis can be estimated using any of the estimation measures used in single studies. Most meta-analyses in the health literature use odds ratios, differences in probabilities, or number needed to treat.[3]

Unfortunately, different studies may use different measurements of effect size to present data. When the number of patients in each group and the number who experience a particular outcome in each group are reported, it is possible to convert one outcome measurement to another. At times, there are not enough data

---

[3]Measurement of a continuous dependent variable, such as weight or diastolic blood pressure, is also used in the health literature and frequently in social science and other literature. Different techniques of analysis are required for continuous dependent variables.

presented in an article to convert one estimation technique to another. Thus, it is not always possible to produce a useful estimation, even though several relevant studies are available in the literature.[4]

Even when different estimation techniques prevent calculation of an overall estimation of the relationship strength or the size of the difference, it is usually possible to perform an overall statistical significance test. As long as the type of statistical significance test used, the number of patients in each of the groups, and the P value are available, it is possible to combine the results and produce an overall statistical significance test.

When we combine a large number of studies and perform statistical significance testing, the results are often statistically significant. Remember from our previous discussion that when the number of patients is large, it is possible to demonstrate statistical significance even for small differences that have little or no clinical importance. Thus, in meta-analysis, it is especially important to distinguish between statistically significant and clinically important.

In the type of studies discussed earlier, adjustment was designed to take into account potential confounding variables, that is, differences between the study and control groups that may affect the outcome of the investigation. In meta-analysis, adjustment also has additional goals. Adjustment aims to determine whether it is legitimate to combine the results of different types of studies. It also examines the effects of including investigations with particular characteristics on the combined results. It allows us to determine whether including studies with different charac-

Table 11.2. *Studies of transthoracic laser coronaryplasty including randomized clinical trials and nonconcurrent cohort studies*

Study Number	Outcome	Study Type
1	5/100 ST 10/100 C	RCT
2	80/1,000 ST 100/1,000 C	RCT
3	25/100 ST 20/100 C	RCT
4	2/100 ST 10/100 C	RCT
5	40/1,000 ST 120/1,000 C	RCT
6	5/100 ST 20/100 C	RCT
7	10/100 ST 10/100 C	NCC
8	20/100 ST 20/100 C	NCC
9	30/1,000 ST 90/1,000 C	NCC
10	60/1,000 ST 150/1,000 C	NCC

ST, study; C, control; RCT, randomized clinical trial; NCC, nonconcurrent cohort

[4]The increasing availability of the actual data from studies may make it easier to combine data from different studies that use different estimation techniques. Odds ratios are often useful in meta-analysis, and they can be used for estimation in case-control studies, cohort studies, and randomized clinical trials.

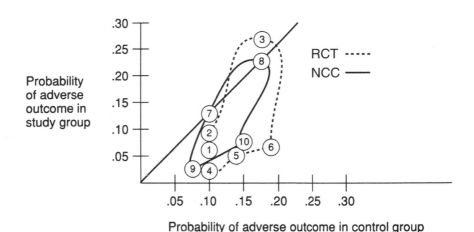

Figure 11.2. Homogeneity demonstrated by the inability to separate randomized clinical trials (RCT) from nonconcurrent cohort studies (NCC).

teristics, such as different types of patients or different approaches to treatment, affects the results. This process is what we mean by harnessing the benefits of diversity.

To combine investigations, we need to establish that the results are what we call HOMOGENEOUS. This concept is illustrated by the following example:

Assume that the randomized clinical trials and nonconcurrent cohort studies of TLC for single-vessel coronary artery disease were identified in Table 11.2 for a meta-analysis. Look at the graph in Figure 11.2, which displays these studies comparing the results of the study and control groups with respect to the common outcome measure.

Table 11.3. *Studies of transthoracic laser coronaryplasty with high and low severity of illness*

Study Number	Adverse Outcomes	Severity of Illness
1	5/100 ST 10/100 C	Low
2	80/1,000 ST 100/1,000 C	Low
3	25/100 ST 20/100 C	Low
4	2/100 ST 10/100 C	High
5	40/1,000 ST 120/1,000 C	High
6	5/100 ST 20/100 C	High
7	10/100 ST 10/100 C	Low
8	20/100 ST 20/100 C	Low
9	30/1,000 ST 90/1,000 C	High
10	60/1,000 ST 150/1,000 C	High

ST, study group; C, control group

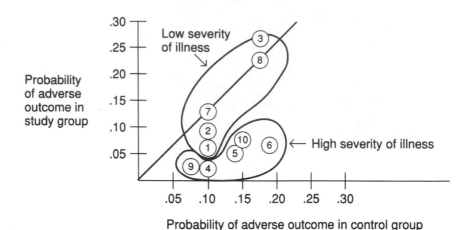

Figure 11.3. Lack of homogeneity demonstrated by the ability to separate low and high severity of illness.

The graph in Figure 11.2 that is constructed by connecting the points represented by randomized clinical trials compared with the graph for nonconcurrent cohort studies demonstrates a homogeneous effect. With a homogeneous effect, the curves formed by connecting the points overlap to a large extent. A homogeneous effect allows the meta-analysis investigator to combine the two types of studies into one analysis.

Table 11.3 and Figure 11.3, on the other hand, show that when studies including patients with more severe stenosis are compared with studies including patients with less severe stenosis, the outcome measures are not homogeneous. The curve connecting the studies including patients with a high severity of stenosis can be separated from the curve connecting studies using patients with a low severity of stenosis. Studies of more severe illness tend to have a high proportion of bad outcomes in the control group. This lack of homogeneity implies that separate analyses should be conducted, with one analysis including studies of patients with low severity of stenosis and a separate analysis including studies of patients with high severity of stenosis. The results of these meta-analyses may demonstrate that TLC is more effective for patients with a high severity of stenosis.[5]

Interpretation

Just like individual investigations are interpreted, in a meta-analysis, the investigator tries to determine whether contributory cause or efficacy has been demonstrated. As with other types of investigation, the three key questions for demonstrating contributory cause or efficacy are as follows:

- **Association.** Does the investigation establish a substantial and statistically significant association that provides convincing evidence that the cause occurs more frequently together with the effect than expected by chance alone?

[5]The degree of overlap in the graphs needed to label the effect as effect homogeneous is subjective. This is an inherent limitation of the graph technique. Statistical significance testing is also available to examine the homogeneity of studies. These statistical significance tests regard each study as the equivalent to one site in a multiple-site investigation. In general, these statistical significance tests have only a limited statistical power.

- **Prior Association.** Does the investigation establish that the cause precedes the effect?
- **Altering the cause alters the effect.** Does the investigation establish that altering or modifying the frequency or severity of the cause alters the frequency or severity of the disease or other "effect?"

In establishing associations using meta-analysis, it is important to recognize that meta-analysis aims to increase the sample's size by combining studies. This has the potential advantage of increasing the statistical power. Increases in statistical power improve the probability of demonstrating statistical significance. Thus, even small but real differences may be demonstrated to be statistically significant, although they may not have clinical importance.

The ability of a meta-analysis to establish the second and third criteria for contributory cause or efficacy depends on the type and quality of the individual investigations included. When randomized clinical trials are included, these have the potential for establishing all three criteria.

In addition, the large number of individuals included in a meta-analysis may make it possible to draw cause-and-effect conclusions about side effects and subgroups.

The greater number of individuals that may be included in a meta-analysis allows us to interpret the data on safety or harms with greater reliability. The rule of three is still a useful tool helping us to interpret the implications of the absence of an adverse effect. Thus, if a meta-analysis includes 30,000 patients and there is no evidence of anaphylaxis, we can be 95% confident that if anaphylaxis occurs, its true frequency is less than 1 per 10,000.

Once the investigators have established that there is a statistically significant association based on data from all the studies included in the meta-analysis, they can proceed to look at subgroups. The large numbers of subjects included in a meta-analysis is an advantage when examining subgroups.

For instance, if an exploratory meta-analysis of TLC used all 25 available studies, the investigator might be able to examine subgroups such as men versus women and repeat TLC versus initial TLC especially if differences between these groups were hypothesized at the beginning of the investigation. If the data were available, the investigator might also examine subgroups such as types of anticoagulation used to examine the hypothesis that this factor makes a difference. Unfortunately, data are often not presented in a way that allows the investigator to combine the subgroups from different investigations. As with other types of investigations, even when the data are available, it is important to perform a limited number of subgroup analyses on the basis of predetermined study questions.

In the process of interpretation for meta-analysis, it is important to consider removing OUTLIERS. Outliers are studies that produce results that are very different from the majority of studies. It is very tempting to merely exclude all outliers from an analysis, but this should be done only if there is very good reason. Often, in fact, additional information can be obtained by looking carefully at the outliers as part of the interpretation and asking why the results are different. This is demonstrated in the next example:

> Among the 25 studies of TLC, one demonstrated that the results of TLC were substantially worse than those associated with medication or surgery. This study was performed at the beginning of the TLC era using obsolete procedures and no anticoagulation. A second outlier demonstrated that the best results for TLC were achieved

using the newest technique at a medical center that has the largest volume and longest experience with TLC.

Here, the exceptions help to prove the rule that TLC is an effective treatment. At other times, outliers may challenge the conclusion, producing new hypotheses for further investigations. In general, outliers should not be excluded from a meta-analysis. If one outlier is excluded, the other should also be excluded. Here, examination of these two studies supports the efficacy of TLC.

When interpreting the results of a study, we need to reexamine the issue of publication bias. Publication bias is so important in meta-analysis that we often examine its potential impact as part of the interpretation. In doing so, we can estimate the number of studies that would need to be missing from the meta-analysis in order for the results to no longer be statistically significant. The investigation may calculate this number of studies assuming that the missing studies are, on average, the same size as the studies included in the meta-analysis and that the studies, on average, show no effect (*i.e.*, they have a zero difference or a ratio of 1). This number of studies is called the FAIL-SAFE-N. The following example illustrates how to interpret the fail-safe-n:

> One meta-analysis of TLC for single-vessel coronary artery disease using all 25 studies has a fail-safe-n of 100. Thus, the authors concluded that publication bias is very unlikely to affect the meta-analysis results.

It is unlikely to have 100 completed but unpublished studies that on average showed no difference between TLC and standard therapy. This degree of publication bias is unlikely to occur. Thus, we can be reasonably confident that if publication bias exists, it does not have a dramatic effect on the conclusions.

Extrapolation

To Similar Populations

Meta-analysis is designed to estimate the size of the average effect and to infer whether efficacy is likely to be real in the larger population from which the study samples were obtained. Average effect size can be very useful when making extrapolations designed for groups of individuals. These extrapolations are often called RECOMMENDATIONS and may be incorporated into practice guidelines.

However, when trying to make decisions for a particular patient, the results of meta-analysis may not be as useful as examining the results of a particularly relevant study, as demonstrated in the next example:

> A patient at the medical center with the longest experience using TLC, the newest techniques, and the largest volume is being considered for TLC. The results of the meta-analysis comparing TLC with other therapies for this type of high-risk patient indicate very little difference. However, the data from this medical center unequivocally support the use of TLC for this type of high-risk patient at this medical center.

Data available from the same institution based on similar patients are often more informative than using the average effect size obtained from a meta-analysis. Thus, despite the important role that meta-analysis can play in research and clinical care, it does not automatically produce the most useful results for a particular patient.

Beyond the Data

Issues of extrapolation are not limited to how well the therapy works. Issues of harm or safety also need consideration and require extrapolation beyond the data. The large numbers that are often included in a meta-analysis can produce more reliable extrapolation about harms or safety of therapies. The assessment of safety, however, is still limited to the duration, dosage, and types of outcomes assessed by the studies included in the meta-analysis, as illustrated in the next hypothetical example:

> The meta-analysis of TLC demonstrated efficacy of TLC for single-vessel coronary artery disease. It also demonstrated similar short-term harms compared with medication or surgery. More than a decade after the widespread use of TLC began, it was recognized that late effects on the coronary artery made it more likely to suddenly close, producing a higher incidence of late myocardial infarction.

Studies can only draw conclusions about what they measure. The ability to assess long-term consequences requires long-term follow-up. Long-term safety or effectiveness considerations are no better assessed by meta-analysis than by single studies.

Extrapolating results from a meta-analysis to practice poses the same dangerous consequences as with other types of investigations. When extrapolating to populations that are not included in the investigation, it is important to recognize and make explicit the assumptions that are being made. For instance, imagine the following situation:

> A large, well-conducted meta-analysis of TLC concluded that TLC was safe and effective and better than standard treatment for single-vessel coronary artery disease. The authors concluded that TLC should be used for treatment of coronary artery disease in two- and three-vessel disease. Subsequent studies demonstrated the superiority of TLC for single-vessel disease but found that the extensive exposure to laser treatment needed for two- and three-vessel disease was associated with side effects not previously recognized when using TLC to treat single-vessel coronary artery disease.

Whenever an extrapolation is made to new untested situations, it must be assumed that the new circumstances will not be associated with new or unexpected side effects. In this example, this assumption was not correct. Thus, regardless of the type of investigation, the reader of the health research literature must be aware of the dangers of extrapolation to new populations and situations.

Meta-analysis has gained an important role in health research. It has helped to halt continued study of issues for which there are already adequate data. It has helped us gain more accurate measures for the magnitude of effects and the degree of safety of therapies. By harnessing the benefits of diversity, meta-analysis has also helped us better understand what factors affect the outcomes of a therapy.

Despite the many advantages of meta-analysis, it requires the same type of attention to quality study design that is required for other types of research. In addition, because it relies on the existing literature, meta-analysis incorporates special techniques and is often limited in what it attempts to do and what conclusions it can draw.

The classic literature review article has been dramatically restructured by the introduction of meta-analysis. If we are to obtain the maximum amount of information from the existing literature, the principles of meta-analysis must be understood and applied.

12 Studying a Study:

Questions to Ask and Flaw-Catching-Exercises

Throughout this *Studying a Study* section, we explained how the uniform framework can be used to evaluate case-control studies, cohort studies (concurrent and nonconcurrent), randomized clinical trials, and meta-analysis. This chapter brings the pieces together by presenting checklists of key issues to address as you read each type of study in the health research literature.

Let us start by reviewing the components and key issues in the uniform framework:

1. **Study Design**
   a. Study hypothesis
   b. Study population
   c. Sample size and statistical power
2. **Assignment**
   a. Method
   b. Confounding variables
   c. Masking
3. **Assessment**
   a. Appropriate
   b. Precise and accurate
   c. Complete and unaffected by observation
4. **Analysis**
   a. Estimation
   b. Inference
   c. Adjustment/subgroups
5. **Interpretation**
   a. Association
   b. Prior association
   c. Altering the cause alters the effect
6. **Extrapolation**
   a. To similar groups
   b. Beyond the data
   c. To other populations

Application of the Uniform Framework to Case-Control Studies

Study Design

STUDY HYPOTHESIS

The study hypothesis in a case-control study generally attempts to establish that a disease or condition (such as a therapeutic success) is associated with a prior characteristic. It is possible to investigate more than one association between a disease or condition and prior characteristics but this must be done carefully, taking the multiple hypotheses into account as part of the analysis.

STUDY POPULATION

Inclusion and exclusion criteria should be specified for the study cases and for the controls. These are designed to make the cases and controls as similar as possible except for the characteristic being investigated.

SAMPLE SIZE AND STATISTICAL POWER

Case-control studies are capable of establishing associations using much smaller samples than other types of investigations. Thus, for an association of any magnitude, case-control studies have greater statistical power.

Assignment

METHOD

The cases and controls are selected by the investigator from among people who meet the inclusion and exclusion criteria. The ratio of cases to controls is under the investigator's control. Greater statistical power and similarity between cases and controls can be achieved by pairing cases and controls and subsequently analyzing them as pairs. Using multiple controls for each case is another way to increase the similarity of the cases and controls and to increase the statistical power of the study.

CONFOUNDING VARIABLES

In a case-control study, confounding variables may be due to chance or bias. Selection bias occurs in a case-control study when the cases and controls differ in ways that affect the end-point (the prior characteristic).

MASKING

Masking the study subjects and the investigators as to their assigned group is generally not possible in a case-control study because the disease being investigated has already occurred and is known to the subjects and the investigators.

Assessment

APPROPRIATE

An appropriate assessment in a case-control study measures a prior characteristic that is closely related to the study hypothesis.

PRECISE AND ACCURATE

Case-control studies are prone to recall and reporting bias as well as instrument errors.

COMPLETE AND UNAFFECTED BY OBSERVATION

A complete case-control study obtains prior data on all cases and all controls. Since a case-control study is conducted after the disease has occurred, the results are not generally affected by the process of observation.

Analysis

ESTIMATION

Odds ratios are generally the method used to estimate the magnitude of the relationship observed in a case-control investigation because an odds ratio cannot be altered by altering the number of cases relative to the number of controls. In the exceptional situation when the cases and controls are representative of a population, *i.e.*, they are population based, a relative risk can be used. Attributable risk percentages can be derived from relative risks or estimated from odds ratios. Number needed to treat cannot be obtained.

INFERENCE

The statistical significance of the odds ratio is the most common method used to perform inference for case-control studies.

ADJUSTMENT AND SUBGROUP ANALYSIS

Multiple variable analysis, such as logistic regression, may be conducted to adjust for potential confounding variables. If the case-control study is large enough, careful subgroup analyses, generally for predefined subgroups, can be performed after obtaining an overall association.

Interpretation

ASSOCIATION

Association is established by demonstrating a statistically significant and substantial odds ratio adjusted for potential confounding variables.

PRIOR ASSOCIATION

Prior association cannot be definitively established. However, if the assessment is based on objective data and the disease or condition is not likely to influence the measurement of what is being assessed, the existence of a prior association may be defended.

ALTERING CAUSE ALTERS EFFECT OR ANCILLARY CRITERIA

Case-control studies do not attempt an intervention and therefore are not capable of establishing this criterion. Case-control studies often seek to support contributory cause by examining the ancillary criteria, which are strength, consistency, biological plausibility, and dose–response relationship.

Extrapolation

TO SIMILAR GROUPS

Case-control studies may extrapolate to groups that are similar to those in the investigation. Even this type of extrapolation is dangerous, however, because case-control studies generally cannot establish contributory cause.

BEYOND THE DATA

Extrapolation beyond the data are especially dangerous with case-control studies, because these studies cannot establish all three criteria of contributory cause.

TO OTHER POPULATIONS

Extrapolation to other populations is especially dangerous in case-control studies because, again, these studies cannot establish all three criteria of contributory cause.

Application of the Uniform Framework to Cohort Studies— Concurrent and Nonconcurrent

Study Design

STUDY HYPOTHESIS

The study hypothesis in a cohort study generally attempts to establish that a characteristic or potential risk factor is associated with a subsequent outcome. It is possible for a cohort study to hypothesize more than one subsequent outcome associated with a characteristic, but that must be carefully done, taking the multiple hypotheses into account as part of the analysis.

STUDY POPULATION

Inclusion and exclusion criteria are usually set for the study and the control groups. These are designed to make the study and control groups as similar as possible except for the characteristic being investigated.

SAMPLE SIZE AND STATISTICAL POWER

Cohort investigations require much larger sample size than case-control studies to achieve the same statistical power.

Assignment

METHOD

All cohort studies identify the study and control groups prior to examining the data to assess outcome. In a concurrent cohort study, the study and control group individuals are followed over time to observe their outcome. In a nonconcurrent cohort study, the outcome has already occurred at the time the individuals are identified for the study and control groups. The investigators, however, are not aware of the outcome at the time of assignment. Once the assignment has been made, the investigators then examine the data to determine the outcome for each study and control group.

CONFOUNDING VARIABLES

In cohort studies, confounding variables may be due to chance or bias. Selection bias occurs in a cohort study when the study and control groups have different characteristics and the differences affect the outcome.

MASKING

Masking in cohort studies is generally not possible because the patients and the investigators are generally aware of the existence of the characteristic(s) under investigation.

Assessment

APPROPRIATE

An appropriate assessment in a cohort study measures an outcome that is closely related to the study hypothesis.

PRECISE AND ACCURATE

Cohort studies are less susceptible to recall and report errors if the outcome is not known to the participants at the time it is assessed. Instrument error is possible and is especially likely if the data are collected in the course of clinical care in a nonconcurrent cohort study.

COMPLETE AND UNAFFECTED BY OBSERVATION

A complete cohort study includes follow-up data on outcome for all study and control group members. Loss to follow-up is possible in cohort studies, and unequal intensity of follow-up is particularly likely in a nonconcurrent cohort study conducted as part of ongoing clinical care. The process of observation may impact the results of a concurrent cohort study.

Analysis

ESTIMATION

Relative risks are often used to estimate the magnitude of the relationship observed in a cohort study. Attributable risk, the number needed to treat, as well as life-table methods may also be used.

INFERENCE

The statistical significance of the relative risk, attributable risk, number needed to treat or statistical significance tests on the life-table survival plot may be used.

ADJUSTMENT AND SUBGROUP ANALYSES

Multiple variable analysis is performed to adjust for potential confounding variables. Subgroup analyses, generally for predefined subgroups, may be performed after obtaining an overall association. The large number of individuals who may be included in a nonconcurrent cohort study may make it feasible to conduct subgroup analysis and analysis for rare events such as side effects.

Interpretation

ASSOCIATION

In a cohort study, association is established by demonstrating the statistical significance of the results after adjusting for potential confounding variables.

PRIOR ASSOCIATION

Well-conducted cohort studies are capable of establishing the second criterion of contributory cause or efficacy, which is that the "cause" precedes the "effect."

ALTERING CAUSE ALTERS EFFECT OR ANCILLARY CRITERIA

Cohort studies are not capable of definitively establishing this criterion. However, a special type of nonconcurrent cohort study called a natural experiment may observe an intervention in one group and compare it to a comparable group in which the intervention has not occurred. The ancillary criteria may be used to defend the existence of a contributory cause.

Extrapolation

TO SIMILAR GROUPS

Cohort studies often attempt to extrapolate to groups that are similar to those in the study. Extrapolation is based on the assumption that a cause-and-effect relationship has been established. Nonconcurrent cohort studies have the potential to include large numbers of patients who receive therapy in the course of clinical care and thus have potential for extrapolation for safety as well as effectiveness.

BEYOND THE DATA

Extrapolation beyond the data assumes that a cause-and-effect relationship has been established. Extrapolation beyond the data always includes the additional assumption that the observed effect will continue when the duration or dose is extended beyond what is observed in the study.

TO OTHER POPULATIONS

Extrapolation to other populations assumes that a cause-and-effect relationship has been established in the study population. Extrapolation to other populations always includes the additional assumption that the observed effect will occur despite the different characteristics of the other population.

Application of the Uniform Framework to Randomized Clinical Trials

Study Design

STUDY HYPOTHESIS

The study hypothesis in a randomized clinical trial generally attempts to establish that an intervention such as a treatment is a contributory cause of an outcome (*i.e.*, the intervention has efficacy).

STUDY POPULATION

Inclusion and exclusion criteria are used to determine who is eligible for the study. Actual participation requires informed consent. A run-in period may be used to ensure adherence to the treatment prior to entry into the randomized clinical trial. This results in a study population that is especially likely to adhere to therapy.

SAMPLE SIZE AND STATISTICAL POWER

Randomized clinical trials require much larger sample size than case-control studies to achieve the same statistical power.

Assignment

METHOD

Once individuals meet the inclusion and exclusion criteria, provide informed consent, and are enrolled in the investigation, their study or control group assignment is achieved by randomization. Individuals have a known but not necessarily equal probability of being assigned to each of the study (treatment) or control (placebo or standard treatment) groups.

CONFOUNDING VARIABLES

Confounding variables in a randomized clinical trial may be due to chance but not to bias since randomization eliminates bias. Despite randomization, small randomized clinical trials are particularly likely to contain differences between groups that may affect the outcome.

MASKING

Masking may or may not be feasible in a randomized clinical trial.

Assessment

APPROPRIATE

Assessment of the primary end-point or outcome needs to address the study hypothesis. Surrogate end-points that occur earlier and more frequently than important clinical outcomes are often used to perform assessment. Surrogate outcomes must correlate well with eventual clinical outcome. Additional outcomes that are less frequent or generally take longer to occur are often assessed as secondary outcomes. Side effects may be regarded as a tertiary outcome.

PRECISE AND ACCURATE

Recall and report bias are not likely to occur in a randomized clinical trial; however, instrument error is possible.

COMPLETE AND UNAFFECTED BY OBSERVATION

A complete randomized clinical trial includes follow-up data on outcome for all study and control group members. Loss to follow-up is possible in randomized clinical trial, but unequal intensity of follow-up should not occur with good study design. The process of observation may impact the results of a randomized clinical trial, especially when masking is not possible or successful.

Analysis

ESTIMATION

Analysis should be conducted by intention-to-treat. Relative risk, attributable risk, number needed to treat, as well as life-table methods may also be used.

INFERENCE

The statistical significance of the relative risk, attributable risk, number needed to treat, or statistical significance tests on the life-table survival plot may be used.

ADJUSTMENT AND SUBGROUP ANALYSES

Multiple variable regression analysis is performed to adjust for potential confounding variables. If the size of the investigation is adequate, subgroup analyses, generally for predefined subgroups, may be performed after obtaining an overall association.

Interpretation

ASSOCIATION

In a randomized clinical trial, association is established by demonstrating the statistical significance of the result after adjusting for potential confounding variables. Data on secondary outcomes or end-points and data on safety are not expected to be statistically significant.

PRIOR ASSOCIATION

Well-conducted randomized clinical trials are capable of establishing the second criterion of contributory cause or efficacy, which is that the "cause" precedes the "effect."

ALTERING CAUSE ALTERS EFFECT OR ANCILLARY CRITERIA

Well-conducted randomized clinical trials are capable of establishing the third criterion of contributory cause or efficacy (*i.e.*, altering the "cause" alters the "effect"). The ancillary criteria may be used as additional evidence.

Extrapolation

TO SIMILAR GROUPS

> Randomized clinical trials often attempt to extrapolate to groups that are similar to those in the study. This extrapolation is more reliable for primary end-points than for secondary end-points or safety.

BEYOND THE DATA

> Extrapolation beyond the data assumes that a cause-and-effect relationship has been established. Extrapolation beyond the data always includes the additional assumption that the observed effect will continue when the duration or dose is extended beyond what is used in the study. One form of extrapolation beyond the data known as risk–benefit (or harm–benefit) analysis is an extrapolation beyond the data in which a particular value is placed on the potential harm and efficacy or benefit.

TO OTHER POPULATIONS

> Extrapolation to other populations assumes that a cause-and-effect relationship has been established in the study population. Extrapolation to other populations always includes the additional assumption that the observed effect will occur despite the different characteristics of the other population. Extrapolations regarding safety are particularly dangerous based on randomized clinical trials.

FLAW-CATCHING EXERCISES

The following hypothetical studies illustrate the potential errors that can occur in each component of the basic uniform framework. These flaw-catching exercises are designed to test your ability to apply the basic framework in order to study a study critically. Examples of case-control, concurrent, and nonconcurrent cohort studies and randomized clinical trials and meta-analysis are presented. A sample critique that points out important errors follows each exercise.

Case-Control Study

Flaw-Catching Exercise No. 1: Factors Associated With Congenital Heart Disease:

> A case-control study was undertaken to study the factors associated with the development of congenital heart disease (CHD). Two hundred women with first-trimester spontaneous abortions in which congenital heart abnormalities were found in the fetus on pathologic examination were used as the study group. The control group included 200 women with first-trimester induced abortions in which no congenital heart defects were found.
> An attempt was made to interview each of the 400 women within 1 month after her abortion to determine which factors in the pregnancy may have led to CHD. One hundred different variables were studied. The interviewers gained the participation of 120 of the 200 study group women who experienced spontaneous abor-

tions and 80 of the 200 control group women who underwent induced abortions. The other women refused to participate in the study.

The investigators found the following differences between women whose fetuses had CHD and those whose fetuses were not affected:

1. Women with CHD fetuses were three times more likely to have used antinausea medications during pregnancy than were women whose fetuses did not have CHD. The difference was statistically significant.
2. There was no difference in the use of tranquilizers between the study and control group.
3. Women with CHD fetuses had an average age of 23 years versus 18 years for women whose fetuses did not have CHD. The results were statistically significant.
4. The women with CHD fetuses drank an average of 3.7 cups of coffee per day, whereas women whose fetuses did not have CHD drank an average of 3.5 cups of coffee per day. The differences were statistically significant.
5. Among the other 96 variables studied, the authors found that women with CHD fetuses were twice as likely to have blond hair and be taller than 5 ft. 6 in. Both differences were statistically significant using the usual statistical methods.

The authors drew the following conclusions:

1. Antinausea medications cause CHD because they are more often used by women whose fetuses have CHD.
2. Tranquilizers are safe for use in pregnancy because they were not associated with an increased risk of CHD.
3. Because women in their 20s are more likely to have fetuses with CHD, women should be encouraged to have their children before age 20 years.
4. Because coffee drinking increases the risk of CHD, coffee drinking should be eliminated completely during pregnancy, which would largely eliminate the risk of CHD.
5. Despite the fact that no one had hypothesized height and hair color as risk factors for CHD, these were proved to be important predictors of CHD.

Critique: Exercise No. 1

STUDY DESIGN

The investigators have not clarified the aims of their study. Are they interested in specific types of CHD? Congenital heart disease consists of a variety of conditions involving valves, septum, and blood vessels. In lumping all conditions under CHD, the investigators are assuming that a common cause exists for all these conditions. In addition, the specific hypotheses being tested are not clarified in this study. The groups chosen consist of a study group that underwent spontaneous abortions and a control group that underwent voluntary induced abortions. These groups can be expected to differ in a variety of ways. It would have been preferable to choose more comparable groups of women, for instance, those who had induced abortions with and without CHD or those who had spontaneous abortions with and without CHD.

With this study design, remember that the population of women consisted only of those with abortions. This implies that the investigator must be cautious in drawing conclusions about live births. The population being studied includes only CHD that was severe enough to cause early spontaneous abortion. Although this may provide important information, the factors causing CHD severe enough to abort fetuses may be different from the factors causing CHD in full-term infants.

ASSIGNMENT

To determine whether a selection bias exists, we first consider whether the study and control group differ in some respect. Second, we assess whether these differences could have affected the results. The experiences of women having induced abortions versus those having spontaneous abortions are likely to be different in many ways. The women probably also have different attitudes about their pregnancies, which may affect their use of medications during pregnancy. Such differences between the study and control group could affect the results so that selection bias may well be present.

ASSESSMENT

The high rate of subjects lost to follow-up because they refused to participate suggests the possibility that those who were lost to follow-up had different characteristics than those who participated in the study. A high rate of loss to follow-up weakens the conclusions that can be drawn from any observed differences. Recall bias by participants is possible, particularly when a traumatic event has occurred. In addition participants were asked to recall frequently and may have subjectively remembered events, such as use of medication or coffee consumption. The retrospective reporting of medication use, for instance, may be influenced by the emotions caused by losing the fetus among those women who experienced an unexpected spontaneous abortion. The result may be a closer scrutiny of the memory, leading to a more thorough recall of medication use among those who had a spontaneous abortion.

ANALYSIS, INTERPRETATION, AND EXTRAPOLATION

The investigators' five conclusions may contain the following flaws:

1. Even if one assumes that the relationship between antinausea medications and CHD was properly derived, no cause-and-effect relationship has been shown. Case-control studies cannot definitively settle the question of which factor is the cause and which is the effect. It is possible that women with CHD fetuses have more nausea and, therefore, take more antinausea medications. Before a contributory cause is established, investigators must show that the postulated cause precedes the effect and that altering the cause alters the effect. The authors of this study have made an interpretation that is not warranted by the data.

2. The absence of a difference between groups in terms of tranquilizer use does not necessarily ensure the safety of these drugs. The samples may be too small to determine the existence of and association between tranquilizer use and CHD. The rule of three tells us that we should not expect to observe rare but serious side effects in small studies. Even if there is no association between tranquilizers and CHD, this does not ensure the absence of other adverse effects

on the fetus that make tranquilizers unsafe for use during pregnancy. The investigators have, therefore, extrapolated too far beyond the data.

3. The difference in age between the two groups of women may be related to both their abortion type and their CHD status. Thus, age may be a selection bias if women are more likely to undergo induced abortion in their teenage years rather than later in life; this relationship alone may explain the differences in age between the groups. Even if the study had shown that the risk of CHD was lower for pregnancies among teenagers, the medical and social risks of pregnancy among teenagers might outweigh this benefit. The mere presence of a statistically significant difference does not mean that a clinically important conclusion has been reached. Additional assumptions are required to make this extrapolation.

4. The difference between the average amount of coffee consumed by women with a CHD fetus compared with the amount consumed by women without a CHD fetus is statistically significant, but it is not large. A statistically significant result is one with a low probability of occurring by chance if no true differences exist in the larger populations from which the sample data were drawn. However, it is clinically unlikely that such a small reduction in coffee consumption would have a great effect on the risk of CHD. Statistical significance must be distinguished from clinical importance and from contributory cause. Coffee drinking may have an effect, but with such small differences, one must be careful not to conclude too much.

5. By testing 100 variables, it is not surprising that the authors found associations that were statistically significant by chance alone. When using many variables, one cannot use the usual level of statistical significance to reject the null hypothesis of no association. The usual 5% level assumes one hypothesis is developed before the study. Because it was not anticipated that height and hair color would be associated with CHD, these differences are likely to be the results of chance. Thus, the authors cannot safely conclude that height and hair color are risk factors for CHD.

Concurrent Cohort Study

Flaw-Catching Exercise No. 2: A Study of Screening in the Military

During their first year in the military service, 10,000 18-year-old male privates were offered the opportunity to participate in a yearly health maintenance examination that included history, physical examination, and multiple laboratory tests. The first year, 5,000 participated and 5,000 failed to participate. The 5,000 participants were selected as a study group, and the 5,000 nonparticipants were selected as a control group. The first-year participants were then offered yearly health maintenance examinations during each year of their military service.

On discharge from the military, each of the 5,000 study group members and each of the 5,000 control group members were given an extensive history, physical examination, and laboratory evaluation to determine whether the yearly health maintenance visits had made any difference in the health and lifestyle of the participants.

The investigators obtained the following information:

1. On the basis of self-reporting, participants had half the frequency of alcohol consumption as nonparticipants.

2. Participants had twice as many examinations and twice as many diagnosed ill-nesses during military service as did nonparticipants.
3. Participants had advanced an average of twice as many ranks as nonpartici-pants.
4. No statistically significant differences occurred between the groups in the rate of myocardial infarction (MI).
5. No differences were found between the groups in the frequency of development of testicular cancer or Hodgkin's disease, the two most common cancers in young men.

The authors then drew the following conclusions:

1. Yearly screening can reduce the frequency of alcoholism in the entire military by half.
2. Because participants had twice as many examinations and twice as many diag-nosed illnesses during their military service, their illnesses were diagnosed at an earlier stage in the disease process, when therapy is more beneficial.
3. Because participants had twice the military advancement of nonparticipants, the screening program must have contributed to the quality of their work.
4. Because the groups did not differ in the rate of MI, screening and intervention for coronary risk factors should not be included in a future health maintenance screening program.
5. Because testicular cancer and Hodgkin's disease occurred with equal frequency in both groups, future health maintenance examinations should not include efforts to diagnose these conditions.

Critique: Exercise No. 2

STUDY DESIGN

This is a concurrent cohort study because individual assignment is observed and mon-itored to assess outcome. The investigators have stated only a general goal of study-ing the value of the annual health maintenance examination in the military. They do not identify the target population to which they wish to apply their results. They do not state specific hypotheses or clearly identify their specific study questions.

If the investigators' goal was to study the effects of an annual health mainte-nance examination, they have not accomplished this goal because no evidence exists that first-year participants actually took part in subsequent examinations.

Furthermore, the authors' choice of a population to be investigated may not have been appropriate for the study question. The study selected young men who already had been screened for chronic illness by virtue of passing the entry physical for military service. Being a young and healthy group, they may not have been an appropriate population for testing the usefulness of health maintenance for older or higher-risk populations in which the frequency of pathologic conditions would be expected to be much higher.

ASSIGNMENT

Individuals in this study were self-selected; that is, they decided whether or not to participate. The participants, therefore, can be considered volunteers. The researchers presented no evidence to indicate that those who elected to participate differed in any way from those who elected not to participate. It is likely that participants had health habits and health risks that were different from those of the nonparticipants. These differences may well have contributed to the observed differences in the outcome. Because no baseline evaluation is available on the control group, it is not known whether or how they differed from the study group. Thus, it is not known whether the study and control group were comparable.

The individuals in both the study and control groups were self-assigned on the basis of their participation in the first year of the health maintenance examinations. Because the examinations were conducted on a yearly basis, those who initially participated may not have continued to participate.

ASSESSMENT

Without a clear hypothesis, it is not possible to determine if the assessment is appropriate. Problems with precision and accuracy as well as reporting errors are likely when confidential and subjectively remembered measures such as alcohol consumption are used. Assessment of outcome was conducted only on those who were discharged from the military; thus, it was not complete. Those who remained in the military service would not have been included. Individuals who had died during military service would not have been included among those assessed at discharge. The individuals who had died may have been the most important in terms of assessing the potential benefits gained by screening.

Individuals participating in multiple health maintenance examinations were under much more intensive observation than the nonparticipants. The unequal intensity of observation may have resulted in the greater number of illnesses diagnosed during their military service. Nonparticipants may have had the same number of conditions, without all of them resulting in a recorded diagnosis. The absence of masked assignment and masked assessment may have affected the results.

ANALYSIS, INTERPRETATION, AND EXTRAPOLATION

The five conclusions made by the investigators may contain the following flaws:

1. Participants had a lower rate of alcohol consumption than nonparticipants, perhaps due to differences between the groups before entry into the study. If heavy drinkers were less likely to participate in the health screening, then the screening would only appear to have altered the frequency of alcohol consumption. Comparative baseline data on alcohol consumption and other variables and adjustment for these differences were lacking in the analysis. Potential assessment errors draw into question the validity of the measurement of outcome. Even if none of these potential errors existed, there is no evidence in the study that the screening itself was the causative factor in producing a lower rate of alcohol consumption. Extrapolating to the military in general went well beyond the range of the data.

2. The greater intensity of observation among participants compared with nonparticipants may explain the greater number of diagnoses. This greater number does not in and of itself ensure that the diseases were detected at an earlier stage or that their treatment benefits the patients.

3. If a higher level of motivation is associated both with the participation in the study and advancement in the military, then motivation would be a confounding variable, related to both the participation status and the outcome. Without the use of randomization or adjustment for this potentially confounding variable, no conclusion can be reached about the relationship between participation status and advancement.

4. Many of the participants with an MI may have died and thus were excluded from the assessment. In addition, one would expect a very low rate of MI in a young population. Even with the great numbers included in this study, the sample may not have been large enough to observe small differences between the groups. There is no evidence that those who participated had either more recognized risk factors or more risk factors altered. Even if they had more altered risk factors, the effects of these alterations may not become apparent until years after the participants have left the military. Therefore, this study was incapable of answering the question of whether screening for risk factors for coronary artery disease alters prognosis.

5. The absence of differences in the frequency of testicular cancer and Hodgkin's disease cannot be assessed on the basis of those discharged alive. Even if the frequencies of developing these diseases were identical, they say little about the success or failure of the screening program. A cancer screening program aims to pick up disease at an early stage; it does not aim to prevent disease. Thus, the frequency of cancer cannot be used to evaluate the success or failure of a screening program. Therefore, one would expect nearly identical frequency of Hodgkin's disease and testicular carcinoma. The stage of illness at diagnosis and the prognosis for those who developed either of the conditions would be more appropriate measures for assessing the success of the screening program. No such data are presented here; thus, no interpretation can be made. In addition, even if the author's conclusions were used for males in the military, they may not be valid when extrapolated to females.

Nonconcurrent Cohort Study

Flaw-Catching Exercise No. 3: Cesarean versus Vaginal Delivery after Previous Cesarean

A large database was available to study all births that occurred after a previous cesarean section delivery. The investigators hypothesized that repeat cesarean section delivery would result in improved pregnancy outcomes. During the time period of the study, it was up to individual physicians and patients to decide whether to perform repeat cesarean section or vaginal delivery.

Of 20,000 available in the database, 10,000 repeat cesarean section deliveries were chosen. These repeat cesarean section deliveries were included because complete data were available on delivery, hospital course, and child's health and development at age 12 months. The vaginal deliveries included all 10,000 deliveries after a previous cesarean section that were available in the database even if they did not return for a developmental assessment at 12 months.

Data from study and control group deliveries were collected on parity, mother's age, and mother's socioeconomic status. Outcome measures included the Apgar score for live births, stillbirths, mother's and child's length of hospital stay, child's health and developmental status at 12 months, and mother's health outcomes.

The parity was nearly identical between the groups; however, the repeat cesarean section group had an average age of 34 years versus an average age of 28 years for the vaginal delivery group. The repeat cesarean section patients were five times more likely to be in the top half of the socioeconomic scale.

Apgar scores for the repeat cesarean section deliveries were a mean of 8 compared with a mean of 7.8 for the vaginal deliveries. There were 60 stillbirths in the repeat cesarean delivery group versus 6 in the vaginal delivery group. The length of hospital stay in the repeat cesarean section group was 5 days longer, on average, than the vaginal delivery group. The developmental indices at 12 months of children born by cesarean section were 1% better on average than children delivered vaginally. All these differences were statistically significant. There were 100 cases of thrombophlebitis and one death among the women who underwent repeat cesarean section and 10 cases of thrombophlebitis and one death among the women who delivered vaginally.

The authors drew the following conclusions:

1. Although this was not a randomized clinical trial, the large number of deliveries and the nearly identical parity ensure that the two groups were similar.
2. The relative risk is 10 and the attributable risk percentage is 90% for stillbirth among repeat cesarean section deliveries compared with vaginal deliveries. This implies that 90% of the stillbirths are caused by cesarean section delivery and could be eliminated by vaginal delivery.
3. The difference in length of stay was expected because of the need to recover from surgery and was, therefore, not a relevant finding.
4. The increase in Apgar score and developmental scores at 12 months among repeat cesarean section deliveries was caused by the repeat cesarean delivery.
5. Because the number of maternal deaths is equal in the two groups, the harms to the mothers do not need to be considered in making recommendations.
6. The authors concluded that repeat cesarean section deliveries result in better Apgar scores and improved child development at 12 months. This more than compensates for the increased thrombophlebitis and the longer length of hospital stay.

The authors recommended repeat cesarean section for all women who had previously delivered by cesarean section.

Critique: Exercise No. 3

STUDY DESIGN

This investigation is designed to be a large, nonconcurrent cohort study or database investigation. It intended to compare the results of a subsequent delivery conducted vaginally or by repeat cesarean section after a previous cesarean section delivery. The investigation is a nonconcurrent cohort study because the investigators started by identifying a study group exposed to repeat cesarean section and a control group exposed to vaginal delivery before the investigators were aware of the outcomes.

The two groups are intended to be the same except for the method of delivery. This goal is difficult to achieve in the best of circumstances in a nonconcurrent cohort study. However, the choice of method for identifying the study and control groups in this investigation has compounded this problem. The repeat cesarean section deliveries are a subgroup of all repeat cesarean section deliveries chosen because of the availability of complete data. The vaginal deliveries include all available patients. When groups selected because they have complete data are compared with groups with incomplete data, we expect to find differences in the patient characteristics which may affect the outcomes being assessed.

In addition, the process of study design requires identifying a study population by defining inclusion and exclusion criteria for study and control group patients. This may not have been fully performed in this investigation because we do not know whether patients with more than one previous cesarean section delivery were included.

ASSIGNMENT

The major problem with cohort studies is the need to recognize and address clinicians' tendency to tailor the therapy to their perceptions of what individual patients need. This often clinically beneficial tendency can create selection bias, which must be recognized and taken into account in research studies.

For instance, imagine that clinicians are willing to perform a vaginal delivery in women who have had a previous cesarean section only if the women were progressing very well in their deliveries. This would create a strong selection bias favoring the outcomes of vaginal delivery. In addition it is possible that clinicians may only be willing to perform vaginal delivery on women in their 20's. This could explain the younger age of the women undergoing vaginal deliveries. This difference between groups may produce a selection bias if women in their 20's have a better outcome of their deliveries. The difference in average age needs to be recognized and taken into account in the analysis.

The investigators do record a number of baseline patient characteristics that are useful for comparison. However, the characteristics that are not recorded may affect the results. For instance, there are no data on the duration of pregnancy before delivery by either method. It is possible that repeat cesarean section deliveries were used predominantly for premature or delayed delivery. These deliveries may be for pregnancies that were developing complications and required intervention. If this was the case, it would create a selection bias, which would greatly affect the results by making stillbirths far more likely in the repeat cesarean section group.

ASSESSMENT

The investigators did not assess the perinatal deaths that occur in either group. This may be an end-point that may reflect an important clinical outcome.

Nonconcurrent cohort studies often assess patients on the basis of data collected in the course of ongoing medical care. This leads to the potential for bias because those who return for follow-up may not be an accurate reflection of all those entered into the study. We know that the repeat cesarean section deliveries were all followed up to assess child development at 12 months, whereas the vaginal deliveries did not have complete follow-up. If those who returned for follow-up child development assessment had a worse outcome than those who failed to return, this difference could explain the small difference in results between the two groups.

The assessment process did not fully take into account adverse maternal effects of the cesarean. To the extent that thrombophlebitis represents an adverse and costly effect, for instance, the authors did not recognize its importance and acted as though the only important adverse maternal effect was death.

ANALYSIS

The investigators do not distinguish between outcomes that reflect substantial differences between the groups or the results that represent small differences. When the sample sizes are large, many small differences may be statistically significant. These differences, however, are not likely to be clinically important.

The small difference in Apgar scores or the differences in child development at 12 months, for instance, are not likely to represent a clinically important difference. The use of multiple outcome measures requires caution in interpreting the meaning of small differences. On the other hand, the large differences in numbers of still-births, length of stay, and frequency of thrombophlebitis are likely to have clinical importance. The investigators, however, did not consider the possibility that these differences were the result of confounding variables that require adjustment.

INTERPRETATION

The authors drew six conclusions about those included in the study which may contain the following flaws:

1. Similar parity and the large number of deliveries do not ensure that the two groups were similar. The failure to adjust for differences in the study and the control groups for potential confounding variables, such as age and socioeconomic status, may have altered the results.
2. The relative risk is 10 for stillbirths because there were 60 stillbirths per 10,000 deliveries in the repeat cesarean group compared with 6 per 10,000 deliveries in the vaginal delivery group. From this, the investigators correctly derived an attributable risk percentage of 90%. However, the relative risk and the attributable risk percentage can be calculated even in the absence of a cause-and-effect relationship. If repeat cesarean sections are performed when premature delivery is threatened, then stillbirths may cause repeat cesarean sections and not the other way around. Attributable risk percentages can only be used to imply the ability to remove a percentage of the bad outcome risk if contributory cause has been demonstrated (and the effect is immediately and proportionately reduced by any reduction in the cause).
3. The length of stay is a relevant outcome even if it is completely expected on the basis of the type of delivery. The costs and harms associated with the extended hospitalization are relevant to the decision whether or not to deliver by repeat cesarean section. This is true even if its impact is completely predictable.
4. It is not clear that the cesarean delivery causes the slight increase in Apgar scores or the slightly improved development score at 12 months. These may have been the result of selective follow-up, differences in socioeconomic status, or multiple outcome measures.

5. The potential harms to the mother should not be limited to death. Death is typically a rare occurrence. More frequent events such as thrombophlebitis are important outcome measures. Thrombophlebitis produces considerable morbidity and cost in addition to any deaths that may result.
6. The conclusion that the benefits of repeat cesarean section outweigh the harms assumes that both the benefits and the harms are real. There is considerable doubt concerning the benefits. Even if the investigation's outcomes are valid, this is not the only possible conclusion. The small benefits may be viewed as less important than the substantial increase in the length of stay and the probability of developing thrombophlebitis.

EXTRAPOLATION

The uncertainties about the efficacy of repeat cesarean among the women in the study make extrapolation even to other women like those included in the investigation difficult. It is especially dangerous to make recommendations for a target population of all women who have undergone previous cesarean section. Even if the data established the benefits of cesarean section, including a modest increase in Apgar score and 12-month child development, these benefits would still need to be balanced against the potential harms of greatly increased thrombophlebitis risk and extended hospital stays before recommending cesarean section deliveries for all women who had previously delivered by cesarean section.

Randomized Clinical Trial

Flaw-Catching Exercise No. 4: Blood Safe—A New Treatment to Prevent AIDS

An investigator believed he discovered an improved method for preventing human immunodeficiency virus (HIV) infection through blood transfusions. His method required treating all transfusion recipients with a new drug called Blood Safe. At the time of his discovery, the rate of HIV transmission via blood transfusions was 1 per 100,000 transfusions.

Having gained approval to study this drug in humans, the investigator set out to design a randomized clinical trial for the initial use of the drug. He designed a study in which a random sample of all blood transfusion recipients in a major metropolitan area was asked whether they wished to receive the drug within 2 weeks after their blood transfusion.

The study enrolled 1,000 study group individuals who accepted the therapy. An additional 1,000 individuals who refused Blood Safe were used as the control group. Control group individuals had received an average of 1.5 blood transfusions compared with 3 for the average individual receiving Blood Safe. The investigators were able to obtain a follow-up HIV blood test on 60% of those receiving Blood Safe and 60% of those who refused approximately 1 month after their date of receiving a blood transfusion.

Those performing the follow-up blood testing were not aware of whether the patient did or did not receive Blood Safe. The investigator found that one patient in the study group was HIV-antibody–positive within 1 month after treatment with Blood Safe. In the control group, two individuals were HIV-antibody–positive.

The investigator did not find any evidence of side effects caused by Blood Safe during the 1-month follow-up period. The investigator concluded that the study established that Blood Safe was effective and safe. He advised administration of Blood Safe to all blood transfusion recipients.

Critique: Exercise No. 4

STUDY DESIGN

The investigator intended to conduct a randomized clinical trial to test the hypothesis that Blood Safe has efficacy in preventing HIV infection via blood transfusions.

Randomized clinical trials are best suited to assessing the efficacy of a therapy once a defined dose and method of administration have been developed during initial studies on humans. They are not well suited to the initial human investigations. The absence of HIV testing before entry into the study is a major error in defining the population because we cannot be sure that the HIV-antibody–positive patient converted after their blood transfusion.

The risk of HIV from blood transfusions at the time of the study was 1 per 100,000, a very low risk. Randomized clinical trials, which aim to reduce an already low risk, require a very large number of individuals. Millions of individuals would be required to properly conduct a randomized clinical trial when the probability of occurrence of the disease, without the treatment, is 1 per 100,000. A study of this size does not have adequate statistical power. In other words, this study would not be able to demonstrate statistical significance for this therapy, even if Blood Safe were capable of substantially reducing the incidence of AIDS from blood transfusions, for instance, from 1 per 100,000 to 1 per 1,000,000.

ASSIGNMENT

The investigator identified a random sample of patients comparable to those who might receive an effective therapy. Random sampling is not a requirement of randomized clinical trials, but it does make extrapolation to those in the target or the intended population who are not included in the trial more reliable.

The investigator did not randomize patients to the study and control groups. The control group consisted of those who refused administration of Blood Safe. This is not an ideal control group, because those who refused to participate may be different from those who agreed to participate in a number of ways related to the potential for acquiring HIV infection. Randomization, as opposed to random selection, is considered a critical characteristic of a randomized clinical trial. Therefore, this study is not truly a randomized clinical trial. No attempt was made to identify potential confounding variables and no masking of assignment was attempted.

ASSESSMENT

It is important to remember that the study is actually measuring HIV status after the blood transfusion rather than conversion. This could be considered an inappropriate measure because the important issue is conversion.

Those who assessed the outcome of this study were not aware of whether the patient had received Blood Safe. This masked and objective assessment helps to prevent bias in the assessment process. The lack of masking in the assignment process, however, means that patients were aware of whether they received Blood Safe. This may have affected the precision or accuracy of assessment outcome; for instance, those who received Blood Safe believed they were protected from acquiring HIV infection.

The investigators assessed HIV-antibody status 1 month after the patients received a transfusion. This is too early to assess adequately whether an individual actually will convert to an HIV-antibody–positive status.

The large number of study and control patients who were lost to follow-up is an important assessment problem even though the percentages lost were equal in both groups. When the number of adverse outcomes is low, those lost to follow-up become especially important. They may disproportionately experience side effects or develop symptoms.

ANALYSIS

The investigator did not report statistical significance testing or confidence intervals. The investigator would not have been able to demonstrate statistical significance. This is not surprising because a single additional case of HIV infection would have made the outcome in the study and control groups equal.

The confidence interval in this study would be very wide, indicating that the results of this study are compatible with no difference or even a difference in the opposite direction.

The higher number of blood transfusions among those who received Blood Safe is a confounding variable that should be taken into account through an adjustment as part of the analysis. The number of blood transfusions is a confounding variable because it is different in the two groups and is related to the probability of developing HIV infections secondary to blood transfusions.

INTERPRETATION

The previous study design, assignment, assessment, and analysis problems mean that the study must be interpreted with great care.

The result of statistical significance testing and confidence intervals imply that this difference in HIV infections between the study and control groups could be due to chance.

The probability of developing an HIV infection from blood transfusion in the absence of administration of Blood Safe is so small that other means of acquiring the HIV infection may be much more likely. Therefore, any difference between a study group and a control group cannot automatically be attributable to Blood Safe. The difference may be due to other risk factors for AIDS or even in their HIV status before the study. No data are presented that deal with these factors, which may be far more important risk factors than blood transfusions. Thus the investigation clearly does not achieve its goal of establishing all three criteria of contributory cause through use of a well-designed randomized trial.

EXTRAPOLATION

Even if Blood Safe was shown to have efficacy in preventing transfusion-associated HIV infections, one could not draw conclusions about its effectiveness or safety from this study.

Randomized clinical trials can draw conclusions about the efficacy of therapy under the ideal conditions of an investigation. Effectiveness implies that the therapy has benefit under the usual conditions of clinical practice.

Using Blood Safe in clinical practice would imply administering Blood Safe to very large numbers of individuals. Thus, rare but serious side effects are important. Despite the absence of side effects among those who received Blood Safe in this study, rare but serious side effects may still occur. The rule of three states that if a serious side effect occurs once per 1,000 uses, then 3,000 individuals must be observed to be 95% certain of observing at least one case of the side effect. Thus, this study is too small to accurately detect rare side effects.

In extrapolating the use of a treatment from randomized clinical trials to clinical practice, one must at a minimum consider the following:

- Whether the study establishes the efficacy of therapy under ideal conditions
- If individuals in the study are similar to those who will receive therapy in clinical practice; that is, the intended or target population
- If known safety hazards or the possibility of rare but serious side effects not observed in randomized clinical trials outweigh the potential benefits
- At times, it may also be important to consider the cost of the treatment compared with other options

Meta-Analysis

Flaw-Catching Exercise No. 5: Magnesium Channel Blockers and Coronary Artery Disease

A meta-analysis was conducted to determine whether a class of medications called magnesium channel blockers used for the treatment of hypertension is associated at high dose with an increased frequency of coronary artery disease.

Studies were identified by searching for all articles published in the leading peer-reviewed journals. The authors initially sought to use only randomized clinical trials, believing that these would provide the highest quality data. Because of the inability to identify randomized clinical trials, case-control and cohort studies were used. Studies were used in the meta-analysis regardless of the specific magnesium channel blocker or the antihypertensive medication used by the control group as long as the outcome being assessed was coronary artery disease. A funnel diagram revealed an incomplete funnel with missing small negative studies.

The studies examined the frequency of coronary artery disease regardless of the definition of coronary artery disease used in the studies. Graphic and statistical methods were used to evaluate homogeneity. Separate meta-analyses were conducted only when the results of a statistical significance test indicated that there was heterogeneity. Separate meta-analyses were conducted for high-dose verses low-dose treatment. Short- and long-acting medications were separable by graphical analysis, but the differences were not statistically significant.

Overall, the meta-analysis demonstrated an odds ratio of 1.3 for coronary artery disease comparing all patients on magnesium channel blockers with those on other types of antihypertensive medications. The results were statistically significant after two outlier studies were removed. For those on high-dose treatment, the odds ratio for coronary artery disease was 1.8; it was 1.2 for low-dose treatment.

The authors drew the following conclusions:

1. This meta-analysis included all appropriate investigations.
2. The methods used to search for relevant investigations was ideal.
3. The use of coronary artery disease as assessed by each article was the only way to perform this meta-analysis.
4. As performed here, separate meta-analyses are appropriate only when statistical significance tests indicate that there is heterogeneity.
5. The fact that the results of the meta-analysis were statistically significant implies that magnesium channel blockers cause coronary artery disease.
6. This meta-analysis establishes that magnesium channel blockers should be removed from the market.

Critique: Exercise No. 5

STUDY DESIGN

This was a hypothesis-driven meta-analysis designed to test the hypothesis that magnesium channel blockers used at high dose for the treatment of hypertension are associated with coronary artery disease. In a hypothesis-driven meta-analysis, articles may be selected to meet the specific features of the hypothesis. The authors attempted to use only randomized clinical trials and exclude other types of investigations. This is a common approach but an alternative approach is to include all types of investigations as was eventually done in this investigation. When there is a question of the quality of the investigations included in a meta-analysis, it may be possible to compare the results of different types of studies.

ASSIGNMENT

This meta-analysis included only studies published in leading peer-reviewed journals. Thus, other published articles and unpublished research was excluded. Even if the authors argue that leading peer-review articles are the hallmark of quality, they should search for all relevant articles before deciding which to use. The incomplete funnel with missing small negative studies suggests the existence of publication bias.

ASSESSMENT

When there are a variety of ways to define the outcome under investigation, the authors must decide how to measure it. At times, it may be desirable to use the outcome as measured by each investigation in the meta-analysis, even if each investigation measures the outcome differently. However, it is desirable to determine if the results depend on the way the outcome is defined. Thus, it is often desirable to use more than one measure of outcome and to determine if the results are different depending on the definition used. If the results do not depend on how the outcome is measured, then it is reasonable to use an outcome measure that allows the meta-analysis to use the largest number of relevant studies. Using the measure employed by each study accomplishes this goal of increasing the number of usable studies.

ANALYSIS

Using statistical significance testing to assess homogeneity has become a common practice in meta-analysis. However, when the number of investigations is relatively small, these tests have limited statistical power to demonstrate statistical significance. Graphical measures, on the other hand, give a better sense of the relationship between the results of the investigations. When doubt exists, it is preferable to perform separate meta-analysis using homogeneous groupings of studies. For instance, in this example, it might have also been important to perform a meta-analysis separately for short-acting and long-acting magnesium channel blockers. It is permissible to perform separate analyses if there is graphical evidence that the results are heterogeneous. Differences between short-acting and long-acting magnesium channel blockers might have helped to define the nature of the relationship.

INTERPRETATION

The existence of a statistically significant association in a meta-analysis does not in and of itself establish that a clinically important relationship exists. As with any investigation, it is important to look at the magnitude of the effect and not just at whether it is statistically significant. In a meta-analysis that combines a large number of investigations, the total number of patients can be quite large. In this situation, it is often possible to demonstrate statistical significance even when the magnitude of the difference is quite small.

Outliers should be included in a meta-analysis of the overall data. Close examination of outliers as part of the interpretation is often useful in gaining new insights. The presence of a hole in the funnel diagram suggesting publication bias indicates that the interpretation should include calculation of a fail-safe-n.

The issue of interpretation is really one of contributory cause. This investigation hypothesizes that high-dose magnesium channel blockers increase the frequency of coronary artery disease. When case-control studies are used, the meta-analysis may really be looking at whether an association exists. The availability of case-control and cohort studies and the lack of availability of randomized clinical trials means it is difficult to definitively establish a cause-and-effect relationship. In this situation the ancillary criteria was useful. Thus it was desirable to examine high- and low-dose treatments to determine whether a dose–response relationship exists. The existence of a dose-response relationship provides support for but does not establish contributory cause. Thus, the evidence presented in this example may support but does not fully establish the existence of a contributory cause.

EXTRAPOLATION

The conclusion to take magnesium channel blockers off the market depends on more data than this meta-analysis contains. Assuming an association exists, assumptions must be made that relate to the relative benefits and harms. To address this, one needs to ask such questions as: Are there other equally effective alternatives? Can the harm be eliminated by limiting the dose or duration? Are there other important indications for magnesium channel blockers?

Summary

Having critiqued the flaw-catching exercises in this chapter, you may feel that there are too many errors in research to draw useful conclusions. Of course, most health research studies have far fewer errors than the hypothetical exercises presented here. However, it may help you to remember that a certain number of errors are unavoidable and that identifying errors is not the same as invalidating research.

The practice of clinical medicine and public health requires that practitioners act on probabilities; therefore, a critical reading of the health literature helps the practitioner to define these probabilities more accurately. The art of reading the literature is based on the ability to draw useful conclusions from uncertain data. Learning to detect errors not only helps the practitioner to recognize the limitations of a particular study, but also helps to temper the tendency to automatically put the newest research results immediately into practice.

Testing a Test

II

13 Introduction to Testing a Test

The process of diagnosis may be regarded as an attempt to make adequate decisions using inadequate information. The uncertainty that is inherent in diagnosis is due to the fact that diagnoses are made based on the results of tests that typically provide less than certain conclusions. Although diagnostic tests have traditionally been regarded as a way to reduce the uncertainty in diagnosis, they can only be used successfully if the clinician understands how tests decrease uncertainty about a patient's condition and also how they describe and quantitate any uncertainty that remains.

Historically, the diagnostic tools available to clinicians were largely limited to a patient history and physical examination. These are still powerful diagnostic tools. Today, however, we also have a massive array of ancillary technology, which can provide a more precise diagnosis when properly and selectively used. Learning whether and when we should apply each element of the history, physical examination, and ancillary technology constitutes the essence of diagnosis.

Today's emphasis on cost-conscious quality care requires that clinicians understand the fundamental principles of diagnostic tests: which questions they answer and which they do not, which tests increase the diagnostic precision and which merely increase the cost.

To paraphrase Will Rogers, clinicians traditionally have believed that nothing is certain except biopsy and autopsy. However, even these gold standards for diagnosis may miss the mark or be performed too late to help. Understanding the principles of specific diagnostic tests helps to define the extent of diagnostic uncertainty as well as to increase certainty when they are used appropriately. Knowing how to live with uncertainty is a central feature of good clinical judgment: The skilled clinician has learned when to perform tests to increase certainty and when to simply tolerate uncertainty.

The fundamental principle of diagnostic testing rests on the belief that individuals with disease are different from individuals without disease and that diagnostic tests can distinguish between these two groups. Diagnostic testing in an ideal world would have the following features: (1) all individuals without the disease under study have one uniform value on the test, (2) all individuals with the disease under study have a different but uniform value for the test; *thus,* (3) all test results would coincide with the results of the diseased or those of the disease-free group (Figure 13.1).

If this was the situation in reality, then one perfect test could distinguish disease from health, and the clinician's work would be merely to order the right test. The real world is not so simple. None of these three conditions is usually present. Variations exist within each of the three basic factors: the tests, the group with disease, and the disease-free group (Figure 13.2).

The assessment of diagnostic tests is largely concerned with describing the variability of these three factors and thereby quantitating the conclusions that can be reached despite or because of this variability.

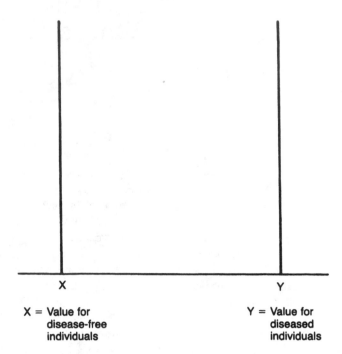

Figure 13.1. Conditions required for a perfect diagnostic test.

The accuracy and precision of tests themselves are discussed in Chapter 14. In Chapter 15, the variability of the disease-free population is reviewed and assessed using a concept known as the reference interval. In Chapters 16 and 17, the variability of the diseased population and its relationship to the disease-free population are quantitated using the concepts of sensitivity, specificity, and predictive values. These concepts are outlined and common errors in their implementation are

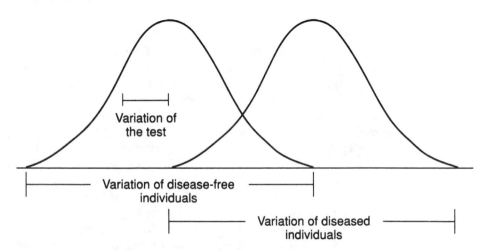

Figure 13.2. The three types of variations that affect diagnostic testing.

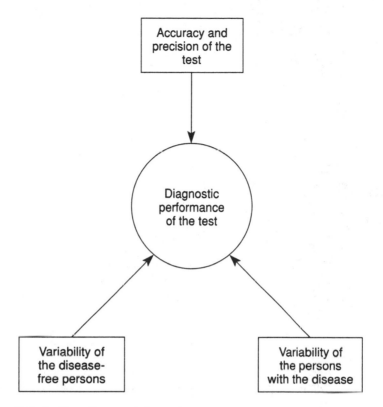

Figure 13.3. Uniform framework for testing a test.

illustrated. Chapter 18 examines how we compare tests and define their roles in practice. Chapter 19 examines the special use of screening tests and the potential strategies for combining tests. Flaw-catching exercises then provide an opportunity to apply these principles in evaluating diagnostic and screening tests.

As with critically reading research studies, it is helpful to have a generalized framework for evaluating a test. This framework is depicted in Figure 13.3, which illustrates the variability that exists in tests, in the disease-free population, and in the population with the disease. It also emphasizes that these variations must be studied and incorporated into any assessment of the diagnostic performance of a test.

14 Variability of the Test

There are two fundamental reasons for errors that result from the test itself. We can think of these as parallel to errors that occur when shooting at a target. The bull's-eye may be missed because of a tendency to shoot in one particular direction. This systematic tendency to deviate from the true value is called BIAS. The absence of bias is ACCURACY. Alternatively, error can occur because the bullets scatter in every direction from the bull's-eye. We call this scattered deviation from the true value RANDOM ERROR. The absence of random error is PRECISION.

There are three general sources of variation in test results. The subjects, the instruments, and the observers may all contribute to this variation. The ideal is accurate results that are free of bias and precise results that are free of random error. A test with completely precise and accurate results would produce identical results on repeat testing. Precise and accurate results are not always obtained or obtainable. The sources of error that produce bias or random error include the following:

- **Subject variation.** The condition of the individual subject being tested may vary from performance to performance, resulting in changes in the phenomenon being assessed.
- **Instrument variation.** Variation may occur as a result of the technical methods used to perform the test. Errors may occur because of variations when using the same testing instrument (*intrainstrument error*) or when using different instruments (*interinstrument error*).
- **Observer variation.** Variation may occur as a result of the observer who assesses the results. Errors may occur because of variations in measurement by the same observer (*intraobserver error*) or error using different observers (*interobserver error*).

To minimize subject variation, it is important that the conditions under which the subject is tested are as identical as possible. Failure to follow this precaution can result in the following type of error:

> The precision and accuracy of a test of serum cortisol levels were evaluated by selecting 100 study subjects and drawing two blood samples from each individual. The first test was obtained at 6 AM and a second at noon. The authors found that, on average, the second test results were twice the level found in the individual's first test. They concluded that the large variation indicated that the test was not precise or accurate.

Precision requires the test to be reproducible, that is, it must produce nearly the same results when conducted under the same conditions. In this example, the investigators did not repeat the test under the same conditions. Throughout the day and night, a physiologic cycle occurs in individuals' cortisol levels, in which they are lowest in the early morning. By drawing blood at 6 AM and again at noon, the investigators were testing at two different points in this cycle. Even if the test itself was completely precise and accurate, the different condition of the subjects would produce variation in the test results.

In addition to subject variation, instrument and observer variation may influence the results of a test. The apparent precision and accuracy of test results may be affected when the observer making the assessment of the results knows of the results of a previous performance of the test, as illustrated in the next example:

> An investigator studying the precision and accuracy of urinalysis asked an experienced laboratory technician to read a urinalysis sediment, to leave the slide in place, and then to repeat the reading in 5 minutes. The investigator found that the reading performed under the same conditions produced perfectly precise and accurate results.

In this example, the technician knew the results of the first test and was likely to have been influenced by the first reading when reexamining the urine 5 minutes later. Determining that a test's results are precise and accurate requires that the second measurement be performed without knowing the results of the first measurement.

Whenever an observer's assessment is needed to obtain the results of a test, there is potential for interobserver and intraobserver variations. Two radiologists frequently read the same X-ray film differently (*i.e.*, interobserver variation). An intern may interpret an electrocardiogram differently in the morning than he or she did when reading the same test performed in the middle of the night (*i.e.*, intraobserver variation). These variations do not in and of themselves destroy the usefulness of a test. They do, however, require that the clinician be alert to these sources of variation of the test results.

The variation within test results caused by subjects, instruments, and observers should be relatively small compared with variations between individuals that result from biologic factors. That is, the variation resulting from the test should be relatively small compared with variation among those who are free of the disease and among those who have the disease under investigation.

A test may be precise in that it produces the same results each time, even though these results are not accurate, as illustrated in the next example:

> A study was conducted on 100 patients undergoing surgery for navicular fractures. Each of the study patients had two X-ray films conducted on different X-ray machines and read by observers who had no knowledge of the other observer's reading. Both X-ray films were negative for navicular fracture within a week of the initial injury. The authors concluded that both the radiologists had been negligent in missing the fracture.

The consistently negative results do not ensure that the results are accurate. Tests may produce the same results even if they are not accurate. That is, they may be free of random error even though they are not free of bias. Navicular fractures are frequently not diagnosed correctly, or at all, by X-ray film at or near the time of injury. Anatomically, the fracture may be there, but the X-ray film is not usually capable of detecting its presence until evidence of healing appears. Therefore, the result do not have random error, but they do contain bias. They do not measure the fracture accurately. Therefore, it is not the negligence of the radiologist but rather the inaccuracy of the X-ray tests that causes the error in this example. Repeating the X-ray film confirms the precision of the results but not their accuracy.

A test may be quite accurate when studied in an experimental situation but may not be as accurate when used in a clinical or public health setting, as illustrated in the next sample:

In a university hospital, a study was conducted of 500 patients after a 10-day, low-fat diet. The study showed that the fat content of the stools collected over a 72-hour period successfully separated those patients with malabsorption from those without malabsorption. An identical study protocol administered to 500 outpatients failed to identify the presence of malabsorption successfully.

The performance of a test is usually initially assessed under ideal experimental conditions. The clinical or field conditions under which it is used often may be less than ideal. A 72-hour stool collection after a 10-day low-fat diet may be very difficult to collect on an outpatient basis. The fact that the outpatient data do not agree with the inpatient data may merely reflect the challenging realities of trying to collect stools on an outpatient basis.

We have now examined the general sources of variation in test results. The subjects, the instruments, and the observers may all contribute to this variation. Accurate results that are free of bias and precise results that are free of random error are ideal. A test that is precise may not be accurate, and a test that is accurate under experimental conditions may not be accurate under clinical or field conditions. These sources of variation cannot be entirely removed. However, they should be relatively small compared with the variation that results from differences among those who are free of the disease and those who have the disease under investigation. Now let us turn our attention to the variation that can occur among those who are free of the disease.

15 Reference Interval

Disease-free human populations are subject to inherent biologic variations. You need only to walk down the street to appreciate the differences among people. Individual height, weight, and color, for instance, reflect the wide, but not unlimited, variations that can occur among healthy individuals.

In a world with complete information, we would know exactly what an individual's measurement on a particular test such as hematocrit should be when they are free of a particular disease. This would enable us to compare the results of a test to the individual's expected disease-free measurement of hematocrit. In reality, we rarely know what an individual's measurement should be, so we are forced to compare one individual's level with those of other individuals who are believed to be free of the disease. To perform this comparison, we use a REFERENCE INTERVAL, which has also been called a RANGE OF NORMAL. The reference interval is built on the assumption that a particular individual should be similar to other individuals.

The reference interval is an effort to measure and quantify the variation in values that exists among individuals believed to be disease-free or at least free of the disease that the test attempts to diagnose. A reference interval can be derived for any measurement in which multiple possible numerical values exist for disease-free individuals. These include measurements of physical examination characteristics such as blood pressure, liver size, and heart rate, or laboratory values such as hematocrit, sedimentation rate, or creatinine. Although the reference interval measurements are often wide, this range of normal does not include all those who are free of disease. It intentionally leaves out 5% of the individuals who are believed to be disease-free to create a reference interval that is wide enough to include most disease-free measurements but not so wide as to include all possible numerical values. If the reference interval included the measurements on all individuals without disease, it would be too wide and would not be generally useful for separating those with disease from those who are disease-free. The reference interval is descriptive, not diagnostic. It describes disease-free individuals; it does not diagnose disease. Values outside the reference interval may be the result of biologic variation, physiologic changes unassociated with disease, or pathologic changes secondary to disease.

Developing the Reference Interval

The reference interval values may be developed as follows:

1. The investigator locates a particular group of individuals who are believed to be disease-free. This group is known as the REFERENCE SAMPLE GROUP. These individuals are frequently students, hospital employees, or other easily accessible volunteers. Usually, they are merely assumed to be disease-free, although they may undergo extensive testing to ensure they are disease-free or at least do not have the disease that the test attempts to diagnose.

2. The investigator then performs the test of interest on all the individuals in the reference sample group.

3. The investigator next plots the distribution of test measurements among this disease-free reference sample group.

4. The investigator then calculates a reference interval that includes the central 95% of the reference sample group. Strictly speaking, the reference interval includes the mean or average measurement plus or minus the measurements within two standard deviations from the mean. Unless there is a reason to do otherwise, when the spread of test results are symmetrical, the investigator generally chooses the central part of the range so that 2.5% of disease-free individuals have measurements above the reference interval and 2.5% of disease-free individuals have measurements below the reference interval.[1]

To illustrate the method for developing the reference interval, imagine that investigators have measured the heights of 100 male medical students and found numerical values that looked like those in Figure 15.1. The investigators would then choose a reference interval that includes 95 of the 100 male medical students. Unless they had a reason to do otherwise, they would use the middle part of the range so that the reference interval for this reference sample group would be from 60 to 78 inches. Individuals outside this range may not have any disease; they may simply be healthy individuals who are outside the reference interval.

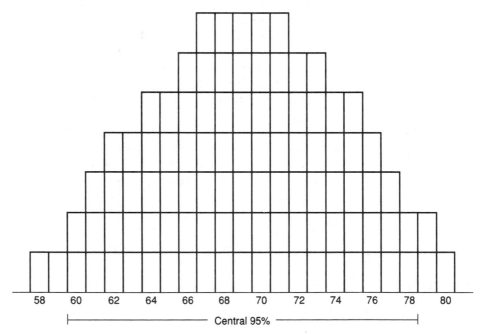

Figure 15.1. Heights of 100 male medical students used to derive a reference interval.

[1]There is often a reason to do otherwise. In addition to the issues raised in this chapter, cost considerations may influence the choice of a cutoff line for the reference interval.

Basic Principles

Let us look first at the implications of those principles for calculating the reference interval and then illustrate the errors that can result from failure to understand these implications.

1. **By definition, 5% of a group without disease will have a measurement on a particular test that lies outside the reference interval.** Thus, "abnormal" and "diseased" are by no means synonymous. The more tests that are performed, the more disease-free individuals there will be whose numerical values are outside the reference interval on at least one test. Taking this proposition to its extreme, one might conclude that a "normal" person is anyone who has not been investigated sufficiently. Despite the absurdity of this proposition, it emphasizes the importance of understanding that the definition of the reference interval or range of normal intentionally places 5% of disease-free individuals outside the reference interval. Thus, the phrase outside normal limits or outside the reference interval must not be equated with disease.

2. **Values that lie within the reference interval do not ensure that the individual is fully disease-free or specifically free of the disease being assessed.** The ability of the reference interval or range of normal on a test to discriminate diseased from disease-free individuals varies from test to test. Unless the test is perfect in ruling out disease, as few tests are, some individuals with the disease will have test measurements that lie within the reference interval.

3. **Changes within the reference interval may be pathologic.** Because the reference interval includes a wide variation in numerical values, an individual's measurement may change considerably and still be within the reference interval. For instance, the reference interval for the liver enzyme AST is 8 to 20 U/L, the range of normal serum potassium may vary from 3.5 to 5.4 mEq/L, and the reference interval for serum uric acid may vary from 2.5 to 8.0 mg/dL. It is important not only to consider whether an individual's measurement lies within the reference interval but also whether the individual's test result has changed over time. The concept of a reference interval is most useful when no historic data are available for a comparison of individual patients. When previous results are available, however, they should be taken into account.

4. **A particular individual may come from a group with an inherently different reference interval from the reference interval reported for the test.** The reference interval is calculated using a reference sample group of individuals who are believed to be disease-free. Therefore, when applying a reference interval to a particular individual, one must ascertain whether this individual has a reason to be different from the reference sample group used to calculate that reference interval. For instance, if male medical students are used to obtain a reference interval for height, this reference interval may not be applied to women or older individuals or perhaps even nonmedical students.

5. **The reference interval must not be confused with the desirable range of test results.** The reference interval is an empirical measurement of the way things are among a group of individuals currently believed to be disease-free. It is possible that large segments of the community may have test results that are higher than ideal and may be predisposed to develop a disease in the future.

6. The upper and lower limits of the reference interval can be altered for diagnostic purposes. The reference interval generally includes 95% of those who do not have a particular condition or disease. It does not require, however, that the same number of individuals who are free of the disease have test results below the reference interval as do those with test results above it. Various factors help to determine where the upper and lower limits of the reference interval should be set. Where to set the limits depends on what the practitioner desires to accomplish by using the test.[2] For instance, suppose that most of the individuals with a disease are found to have measurements nearer the upper limits of the reference interval for the test. If the investigator is willing to lower the upper limits of the reference interval, a larger proportion of those with the disease can be expected to have test results above the reference interval. Then, however, the investigator makes the trade-off of labeling a larger proportion of the disease-free population as outside the reference interval. At times, it may be worth making this trade-off, especially when it is important to detect as many individuals as possible with the disease or when the follow-up testing to clarify the situation is cheap and convenient. This trade-off is illustrated in Figure 15.2.

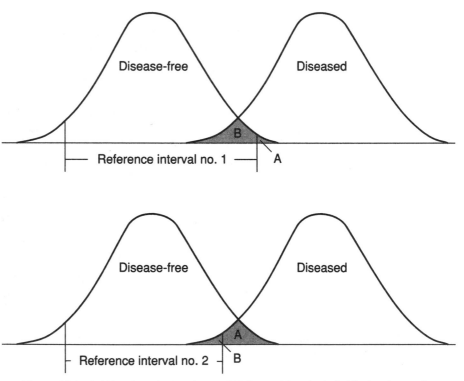

Figure 15.2. Shifting the reference interval. False positive, **A:** Individuals who are disease-free and who have values higher than the reference interval. False negative, **B:** Individuals who have disease and who have values within the reference interval.

[2]The level set for the reference interval defines the specificity of the test. This level may subsequently be adjusted to increase (or decrease) the specificity. Thus, in actual use, the reference interval has been adjusted whenever the specificity is not 95%.

By shifting the reference interval to the left as in the reference interval no. 2, note that area B becomes smaller than in the reference interval no. 1 and that area A becomes larger. In other words, a decrease in the number of those with disease who are within the reference interval (*i.e.*, false negatives) leads to an increase in the number of people without disease who are outside the reference interval (*i.e.*, false positives) and vice versa. More persons with the disease are now identified as outside the reference interval or outside normal limits by the test. At the same time, more individuals who are disease-free are classified as outside the reference interval; therefore, in reference interval no. 2, we are trading off more false-positive readings for less false-negative ones.

How many false positives and how many false negatives the health system is willing to tolerate depends on ethical, economic, and political considerations as well as testing data. Where to set the lower limits may be a critical issue if therapeutic interventions depend on where the line is drawn. Testing technology alone is inherently unable to set these reference limits or cutoff lines.[3]

Examples of Common Errors in Interpreting Reference Intervals

The following examples demonstrate errors that result from failure to apply each of the basic principles in calculating reference intervals:

> In a series of 1,000 consecutive health maintenance examinations, a series of 12 laboratory tests was done on each patient even though no abnormalities were found on a history or physical examination. Five percent of the SMA-12s were outside the reference interval, a total of 600 abnormal tests. The authors concluded that these test results fully justified doing SMA-12s on all health maintenance examinations.

Let us look at how we might interpret these test results. A reference interval, by definition, includes only 95% of those who are believed to be free of the condition. If a test is applied to 1,000 individuals who are free of a condition, 5% or 50 individuals will have test results outside the reference interval. If 12 tests are applied to 1,000 individuals without evidence of disease, then on average 5% of 12,000 tests performed will be outside the reference interval. Five percent of 12,000 equals 600 tests. Thus, even if these 1,000 individuals were completely free of disease, one could expect 600 test results that are outside the range of normal or the reference interval. These would merely reflect the method of determining the reference interval. Remember that test results outside the reference interval do not necessarily indicate disease and do not by themselves justify doing multiple laboratory tests on all health maintenance examinations.

In considering the implications of test results, it is important to realize that all levels outside the reference interval do not carry the same meaning. Numerical values well beyond the limit of the reference interval may be much more likely to be caused by disease than numerical values that are near the borderlines of the reference interval. Test results nearer the limits of the reference interval are more likely to be due to variation of the test or to biologic variation. For instance, if the upper limits of male hematocrit are 52, then a value of 60 is more likely to be associated with disease than a value of 53.

---

[3]A technique known as *receiver operator curve*, or ROC, can be used to help define the most useful cutoff line for a specific purpose. However, when setting cutoff lines, it is still necessary to determine the relative importance of obtaining false-negative and false-positive results.

> One hundred long-term alcoholics underwent AST determinations to assess liver function. Most were found to have AST results within the reference interval. The authors concluded that these alcoholics had well-functioning livers.

This example illustrates the difference between reference interval for laboratory tests and the disease-free state. The fact that these individuals had laboratory tests within the reference interval did not in and of itself establish that their livers were functioning properly because, on any one test, some individuals with the disease will be within the reference interval. The poorer the capacity of the test to diagnose disease, the more individuals there will be with a disease despite test results within the reference interval of the test.

On certain tests, individuals with a disease may not be distinguishable from disease-free individuals. Both groups may have test results mostly within the reference interval. This appears to have occurred for the AST results. The failure of the test to separate individuals with the disease from disease-free individuals indicates that the test had poor diagnostic performance in this application, and it is not useful for diagnosis of liver disease associated with long-term alcoholism. This emphasizes the distinction between being within the reference interval and disease-free.

Figures 15.3 through 15.5 illustrate three possible relationships between disease-free persons and those with the disease. Figure 15.3 illustrates a test that completely separates those with disease from those who are disease-free. The diagnostic performance of this test is perfect. Figure 15.4 illustrates the usual situation in which a test partially separates those with disease from those without disease. Figure 15.5 illustrates the situation in which a test provides no diagnostic information. Individuals with disease have the same test results as individuals without disease. In the AST example, the situation closely resembles Figure 15.5. Despite its use in identifying many liver diseases, AST determination does not appear useful for identifying the long-term effects of alcohol consumption on the liver. Thus, despite the ability to calculate a reference interval for any test, the reference interval alone does not indicate whether the test will be useful in diagnosis. Measurements for individuals with a particular disease may be identical to those of the disease-free group or vice versa, indicating that the test is not useful for diagnosing a particular disease.

> Among 1,000 asymptomatic Americans with no known renal disease and with no abnormalities showing on urinalysis, the reference interval for serum creatinine was found to be 0.7 to 1.4 mg/dL. A 70-year-old woman was admitted to the hospital with a serum creatinine of 0.8 mg/dL and was treated with gentamicin. On discharge, she

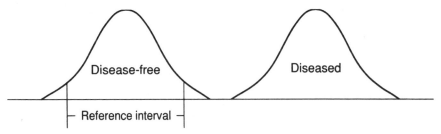

Figure 15.3. A test with complete separation of groups results in perfect diagnostic performance.

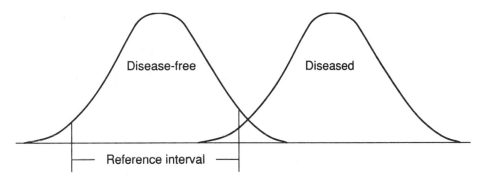

Figure 15.4. A test with partial separation of groups results in intermediate diagnostic performance.

> was found to have a creatinine value of 1.3 mg/dL. Her physician concluded that because her creatinine was within the reference interval on admission as well as on discharge, she could not have had renal damage secondary to gentamicin.

The presence of a result within the reference interval does not ensure the absence of disease. Each individual has a disease-free measurement that may be higher or lower than the average measurement for individuals without disease. In this example, the patient increased her serum creatinine over 60% but still fell within the reference interval. The change in the creatinine measurement suggests a new pathologic process occurred. It is likely that the gentamicin produced renal damage. When historic information is available, it is important to include it in evaluating a test result. Changes within the range of normal may be a sign of disease.[4]

> A group of 100 medical students was used to establish the range of normal values for granulocyte counts. The reference interval was chosen so that 95 of the 100 granulocyte counts were included in the reference interval. The reference interval for granulocyte count was determined to be 2,000 to 5,000. When asked about an elderly black man with a granulocyte count of 1,900, the authors concluded that this patient was clearly outside the reference interval and needed to be further evaluated to identify the cause of the low granulocyte count.

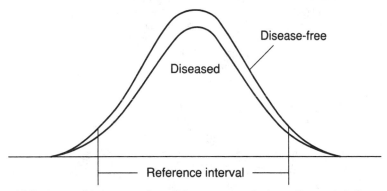

Figure 15.5. A test with no separation of the groups results in no diagnostic information.

---

[4]This example also reflects the fact that older individuals have a different creatinine reference interval than young individuals, and women have a different creatinine reference interval than men because serum creatinine reflects the quantity of muscle mass.

The reference interval is dependent on the disease-free reference sample group chosen; it is usually defined as the interval around an average value, which includes 95% of the individuals in a particular reference sample group. However, the disease-free reference sample group used for determining a reference interval may have different measurements from the group of individuals for whom we want to use the test.

It is unlikely that there are many elderly black men among the group of medical students used to establish the reference interval. In fact, black men have a different reference interval for granulocyte count than white men. Thus, the reference interval established for the medical students may not have reflected the reference interval applicable to this elderly black man. He was probably well within the reference interval for an individual of his age, race, and sex. Because elderly black men are known to have a lower reference interval for granulocyte counts, this must be taken into account when interpreting the test results.

> The central 95% of total serum cholesterol level, as determined among 100 white American men aged 30 to 60 years, was found to be 200 to 300 mg/dL. A 45-year-old white American man was determined to have a serum cholesterol of 280 mg/dL. His physician informed him that because his cholesterol was within the traditionally defined reference interval he did not have to worry about the consequences of high cholesterol.

A reference interval is calculated using data collected from a reference sample group currently believed to be disease-free. It is possible that the group used consists of many individuals whose results on the test are higher (or lower) than desirable. A result within the central 95% does not ensure that an individual will remain disease-free. American men as a group, today, may have higher than desirable cholesterol levels.

Since this is true, the patient with a cholesterol of 280 mg/dL may well suffer the consequences of high cholesterol. When research data are available strongly suggesting a range of desirable numerical values for a test, it is permissible to substitute the desirable range for the usual reference interval. This is now standard procedure for serum cholesterol.

> A study found that 90% of people with intraocular pressure greater than 25 mmHg will develop visual defects secondary to glaucoma within the next 10 years. Of those with pressures of 20 mmHg, 20% will have similar changes, whereas 1% of individuals with pressures of 15 mmHg will develop defects. The authors concluded that performance on the test could be improved by setting the upper limits of the reference interval at 15 mmHg instead of 25 mmHg because the test then could identify nearly everyone at risk for visual defects (Figure 15.6).

If 25 mmHg is the upper limit of the reference interval, then nearly everyone who will not develop glaucoma will fall within the reference interval, but a great number of individuals who will develop glaucoma will also be included within the reference interval. On the other hand, if we set the upper limit of the reference interval at 15 mmHg, very few individuals with glaucoma will fall within the reference interval, and a great number of individuals who will never develop glaucoma will fall outside the reference interval.

The ability of a test to detect disease can be increased by altering the limits for the reference interval. If the limits are extended far enough, the test will include nearly everyone with the condition. Unfortunately, this attractive solution also classifies a larger number of individuals who do not have and will not have a patho-

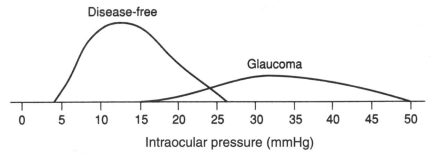

Figure 15.6. Possible distribution of intraocular pressure for people with glaucoma and those who are disease-free.

logic condition as outside the reference interval. By increasing the upper limit of the reference interval, the investigators increased the ability to detect future disease, but only by paying the price of following up on a greater number of individuals who are destined to remain disease-free. In determining where to set the upper limits, the following factors might be considered:

• Vision loss from glaucoma is largely irreversible and may develop before it is apparent to the patient.
• Treatment is generally safe but only partially effective in preventing progressive visual loss.
• Follow-up is safe and involves little harm, but follow-up of a great number of individuals is time-consuming and costly, requiring multiple repeated examinations extending over long periods of time. It also produces anxiety among those requiring follow-up.

The trade-offs then are not simply related to health. Additional social, psychologic, economic, and political considerations should all be considered in deciding where to set the cutoff line. These trade-offs indicate that false-negative results and false-positive results have different implications. The relative importance or value that we place on false-negative and false-positive results ultimately determines where we draw the line. There is often no perfect answer. The only way out of this no-win situation may be to come up with a better test, one that leaves less overlap between persons who will develop disease and those who will not.

As mentioned, creating a reference interval is an attempt to deal with the variability that exists among humans. An understanding of the usefulness and limitations of this concept is central to an understanding of diagnostic tests. The reference interval defines the numerical values found for 95% of a particular reference sample group who are believed to be disease-free individuals. The reference interval may not reflect the desirable level, and it does not take into account changes from previous test results.

The reference interval per se tells us nothing about the diagnostic usefulness of a test. Every test has a reference interval that may or may not help in distinguishing individuals with disease from those without disease. To determine the usefulness of a test for diagnosing disease, it is necessary to look at the test results for a group of individuals with a particular disease and to compare those values with the reference interval of a disease-free group, as we do in Chapter 17. Before we can do this, however, we must examine how we define those with disease.

16 Defining Disease:

The Gold Standard

Individuals with disease, like disease-free individuals, show variations in their measurements on any test. This variability among individuals with disease may result from different severities of the disease or from differences in individual responses to the disease. Despite this variability, it is essential to define a group of patients who definitely have the disease.

The test or criterion used to unequivocally define the disease is known as a GOLD STANDARD. The gold standard may be a biopsy, an angiogram, a subsequent autopsy, or any other established test. The use of a gold standard to definitively identify those with the disease in question is a necessary prerequisite to examining the diagnostic usefulness of any new or unevaluated test. In other words, the usefulness of a new test rests on its comparison with the gold standard. Thus, a new test is compared with any older and better established test to determine if it can perform as well as the traditional gold standard.

Notice that it is assumed when using the gold standard tests that it is possible to be 100% correct in making a diagnosis. In other words, the assumption is that it impossible to invent a better performing mouse trap because you cannot do better than 100%. There might be a cheaper or more convenient mouse trap but, by definition, not one that catches more mice. We can ask only whether the test measures up to the gold standard.

Despite the inherent limitation of our ability to initially evaluate a new test, time and repeated applications tell us which are the better "mouse traps." Once a new test is applied in clinical practice, for instance, it may eventually prove to be superior than the gold standard at predicting a subsequent clinical course. Over time, the new test might even be accepted as a gold standard. Often, however, a particular test that provides a definitive diagnosis is often too dangerous or is useful too late in the course of a disease to be of maximum clinical benefit. In such instances, an adequate gold standard may exist, but it is not a clinically practical test. Thus, one must be sure that the best available gold standard test is being used for the particular case. Let us see what can happen when the gold standard is less than ideal, as illustrated in the following example:

> One hundred individuals, who were admitted to a hospital with diagnostic Q waves on their electrocardiograms (ECGs) and who died within 1 hour of admission, were autopsied for evidence of myocardial infarction (MI). The autopsy was used as the gold standard for MI. Autopsy revealed evidence of MI in only 10 patients. The authors concluded that the ECG was not a useful method of making the diagnosis of an MI. They insisted on the gold standard of pathologic diagnosis.

The usefulness of all diagnostic tests is determined by comparison to a gold standard test that has previously been shown by experience to diagnose the disease under study. Autopsy diagnoses are frequently used as a gold standard against which all other tests are judged. At times, even an autopsy is a less-than-perfect measure of disease as illustrated in this example because the pathologic criteria for MI may take considerable time to develop. It is possible that the diagnostic Q waves on an ECG are a better reflection of an MI than pathologic changes at autopsy. The investigator should be sure that the gold standard selected has, in fact, been shown to be the gold standard before using it as a basis for comparison.

Unfortunately, even the best available gold standards often do not unequivocally differentiate all those with the disease from those without it. Individuals with early or mild disease may not fulfill the gold standard test criteria. When this is the situation, investigators are often tempted to include only those individuals who have clear-cut evidence of disease as measured by the gold standard. Despite the seemingly intellectual certainty that this approach provides, it may produce an investigation which includes only persons with severe or far advanced disease. This danger is illustrated in the next example:

> An investigator studied the ability of urine cytology to diagnose bladder cancer compared with unequivocal biopsy-diagnosed cases of invasive bladder cancer that fulfilled the gold standard criteria. The cytologic examination detected 95% of those with bladder cancer. However, when applied in clinical practice when patients were observed long term, urine cytology detected only 10% of those with bladder cancer.

By using cases of advanced invasive bladder cancer, the investigators have eliminated those with early or equivocal disease that are seen in clinical practice. Thus, we should not be surprised to find that the test fails to perform as well in identifying bladder cancer in clinical practice as it performed when compared to a group of individuals with a clear-cut gold standard test.

When assessing the diagnostic performance of a test, it is important to ask whether the gold standard was used to define those with the disease in question. However, it is also important to ask whether those with the disease spanned the entire spectrum of individuals who have the disease. We must recognize that at times it is impossible to satisfy both of these goals simultaneously.

Even if these conditions are fulfilled, one must appreciate that the goal of testing a test is limited to determining whether the test being studied is as good as the gold standard. The methods used do not allow us to address the possibility that the new test might be better than the gold standard.

17 Diagnostic Performance of Tests

It is now possible to measure the ability of a test to distinguish between individuals with disease and those who are disease-free. In doing so, it is important to remember the following three prerequisites for such an assessment:

1. Variability of the test: Make an assessment of the precision and accuracy of the test results. This variability should be relatively small compared with the reference interval.
2. Variability of the disease-free group: Set the limits of the reference interval for the test which will be used to determine the diagnostic performance of the test.
3. Definition of the gold standard: Identify groups of individuals who definitely have and do not have the disease as defined by the gold standard.

Sensitivity and Specificity

The traditional measures of a test's diagnostic value are its sensitivity and specificity. They measure a test's diagnostic performance compared with that of the gold standard, which by definition has a sensitivity of 100% and a specificity of 100%. Sensitivity and specificity have been chosen as measures because they are inherent characteristics of a test that should be the same when the test is applied to a group of patients in whom the disease is rare or to a group of patients in whom the disease is frequent.[1] Thus, they provide measurements of a test's diagnostic performance which should be the same regardless of the probability of disease before performing the test. The stability of a test's sensitivity and specificity allows researchers in Boston, Bombay, or Beijing to apply the same diagnostic test and interpret the results of testing despite their very different populations.

SENSITIVITY measures the proportion or percentage of people with the disease as defined by the gold standard who are correctly identified by the test. In other words, it measures how sensitive the test is in detecting the disease. It may be helpful to remember sensitivity as POSITIVE IN DISEASE (PID). SPECIFICITY measures the proportion of people without the disease who are correctly labeled free of the disease by the test. Specificity can be thought of as a NEGATIVE IN HEALTH (NIH).

Notice that sensitivity and specificity tell us only, as defined by the gold standard, the proportion or percentage of people with or without a disease who are correctly categorized. These measures do not tell us the actual number of individuals who will be correctly categorized. The actual number will also depend on the frequency of the disease in the group being tested.

Sensitivity and specificity are useful measures because they allow readers and researchers to obtain the same results when assessing a test on groups of patients

---

[1]This may not be strictly true if the proportion of early disease changes along with the frequency of disease. A test may have different sensitivity and specificity for early versus more advanced disease.

with different frequencies of the disease. Sensitivity and specificity, however, may have different numerical values when they are obtained using a group of patients with early stages of a disease compared with using a group of patients with more advanced disease.

Let us first outline the mechanism for calculating sensitivity and specificity and then outline the implications and limitations. In calculating the sensitivity and specificity of a test in comparison to the gold standard, researchers proceed in the following manner:

1. The investigators choose the gold standard to be used in defining individuals with and without the disease.
2. The investigators perform the gold standard test and identify one group of patients that the gold standard indicates has the disease and another group that the gold standard indicates does not have the disease. In implementing this criterion, it is important to know whether investigators included a representative group of individuals with and without the disease. In other words, do the individuals chosen represent a full spectrum of individuals who have the disease and who are disease-free, or do they represent only those with severe disease and those who are unequivocally disease-free? In choosing these individuals, it has become common practice to select an equal number of individuals with the disease as defined by the gold standard test and individuals who are free of the disease according to the results of gold standard test. This 50-50 split, however, is not necessary.[2]
3. Researchers must now use the test being investigated to categorize all study individuals as positive or negative. To do this for tests with results that are presented as numerical values, such as hematocrit or creatinine, they must use the reference interval. For instance, if most individuals with the disease have values above the reference interval, then investigators use the upper end of the reference interval as the cutoff point. Investigators test all individuals with the new test and classify them as positive or negative.
4. The investigators have now classified each patient as either having the disease or being disease-free according to the gold standard test, and as positive or negative by the test being evaluated. They then can calculate the number of individuals for whom the test and the gold standard test agree and the number for whom they disagree and then display their results in a 2×2 table as follows:

Test	Gold Standard Disease	Gold Standard Disease-Free
Positive	a = Number of individuals with the disease and positive: true positive	b = Number of individuals disease-free and positive: false positive
Negative	c = Number of individuals with the disease and negative: false negative	d = Number of individuals disease-free and negative: true negative
	a + c = Total number of individuals with the disease	b + d = Total number of disease-free individuals

[2]The 50-50 split provides the greatest statistical power for a given sample size.

5. Finally, investigators apply the definitions of sensitivity and specificity and calculate their values from the data in the 2×2 table.

$$\text{Sensitivity} = \frac{a}{a+c} = \begin{array}{l} \text{The proportion of those with disease,} \\ \text{according to the gold standard test, who are} \\ \text{labeled positive by the test being evaluated} \end{array}$$

$$\text{Specificity} = \frac{d}{b-d} = \begin{array}{l} \text{The proportion of those who are disease-free,} \\ \text{according to the gold standard test, who are} \\ \text{labeled negative by the test being evaluated} \end{array}$$

To illustrate this procedure using numbers, imagine that a new test is performed on 500 individuals who have the disease according to the gold standard and 500 individuals who are free of disease according to the gold standard. We can now set up the 2 × 2 table as follows:

Test	Gold Standard Disease	Gold Standard Disease-Free
Positive	a	b
Negative	c	d
	500	500

Now suppose that 400 of the 500 individuals with the disease are labeled positive by the test and that 450 of the 500 individuals who are free of the disease are labeled negative by the test. One can now fill in the 2×2 table:

Test	Gold Standard Disease	Gold Standard Disease-Free
Positive	400	50
Negative	100	450
	500	500

Sensitivity and specificity can now be calculated:

$$\text{Sensitivity} = \frac{a}{a+c} = \frac{400}{500} = 0.80 \text{ or } 80\%$$

$$\text{Specificity} = \frac{d}{b+d} = = \frac{450}{500} = 0.90 \text{ or } 90\%$$

A sensitivity of 80% and a specificity of 90% are fairly typical of many tests used clinically to diagnose disease.

Notice that the test being evaluated has been applied to a group of patients in which 500 have the disease and 500 are disease-free as defined by the gold standard. This division of 50% with the disease and 50% disease-free is the usual division chosen for study. The sensitivity and specificity obtained in the investigation would have been the same regardless of the proportion who are disease-free as determined by the gold standard. That is, if 10% of the individuals included in the investigation were positive by the gold standard and 90% were negative by the gold standard, the sensitivity and specificity would be the same as obtained in the study, *i.e.*, a sensitivity of 80% and a specificity of 90%. One way to convince yourself of the truth of this important principle is to look at how the sensitivity and specificity are calculated:

$$\text{Sensitivity} = \frac{a}{a+c} \text{ and specificity} = \frac{d}{b+d}$$

Notice that a and c, which are necessary to calculate sensitivity, are both contained in the left column of the chart. Similarly, b and d, which are necessary to calculate specificity, are both contained in the right column of the chart. Thus, the relative number of individuals in the two columns does not really matter because sensitivity and specificity each relate only to the results for patients who are within a single column. That is, sensitivity and specificity are not affected by the number of individuals with the disease compared to the number who are free of disease as defined by the gold standard.

Once the sensitivity and specificity have been calculated, it is possible to work backward and fill in the table when different numbers of individuals with the disease and disease-free individuals, as defined by the gold standard, are used. This time, assume there are 900 disease-free individuals and 100 individuals with disease. In other words, 10% of the individuals being tested have the disease. Thus, the average individual has a 10% chance of having the disease even before the test is performed.

Test	Gold Standard Disease	Gold Standard Disease-Free
Positive	a	b
Negative	c	d
	100	900

Now, let us apply the sensitivity and specificity measures as previously determined.

Sensitivity equals 80%; therefore, 80% of those with the disease will be correctly labeled as positive (80% of 100 = 80). The remaining 20% of those with the disease will be incorrectly labeled as negative (20% of 100 = 20).

Specificity equals 90%; therefore, 90% of those who are disease-free will be correctly labeled as negative (90% of 900 = 810). The remaining 10% of disease-free people will be incorrectly labeled as positive (10% of 900 = 90).

The following 2×2 table can now be constructed:

10% Probability

Test	Gold Standard Disease	Gold Standard Disease-Free
Positive	80	90 False positives
Negative	20 False negatives	810
	100	900

This is a situation in which 10% of the patients under study have the disease as defined by the gold standard; therefore, we can say that in this group of patients, the probability of having the disease is 10%.

Let us now compare this table to the one developed when sensitivity and specificity were first calculated. Because we used 500 individuals with the disease and 500 disease-free individuals, we were actually using a group of patients with a 50% probability of having the disease.

50% Probability

Test	Gold Standard Disease	Gold Standard Disease-Free
Positive	400	50 False positives
Negative	100 False negatives	450
	500	500

Notice that with our original 50% chance of having disease, 100 individuals were falsely labeled as negative and 50 were falsely labeled as positive. In the group of patients with 10% chance of having disease, however, 20 individuals were falsely labeled as negative and 90 individuals were falsely labeled as positive. The change in numbers is solely the result of the difference in relative frequency of disease or probability of disease in the two groups of patients studied (50% vs. 10%) as determined by the gold standard test. Notice that when 10% of the individuals have the disease, there are actually more positives who are disease-free (90) than positives who have the disease (80).

This may be surprising in light of the relatively high sensitivity and specificity. However, this result illustrates a principle that must be recognized in applying the concepts of sensitivity and specificity. Despite the fact that sensitivity and specificity are not directly influenced by the relative frequency or probability of the disease, the actual number of individuals who are falsely labeled positive and falsely labeled negative is often very much dependent on the probability that the disease is present.

Now let us look at an even more extreme situation in which only 1% of the group being tested has the disease as determined by the gold standard test. This is typical when we screen a group of individuals who have risk factors for a common disease but no clinical evidence of disease. This situation may be charted as below:

1% Probability

Test	Gold Standard Disease	Gold Standard Disease-Free
Positive	8	99 False positives
Negative	2 False negatives	891
	10	990

In this screening situation, we have again used the same test with 80% sensitivity and 90% specificity. This time, however, there are 8 true positives and 99 false positives; this is more than 12 false positives for every true positive.

Thus, sensitivity and specificity alone do not provide a complete indication of how useful a result will be in diagnosing a disease for a particular group of individuals. As practitioners, we need to know more than a test's sensitivity and specificity. We must be able to address the questions:

- What is the probability of disease if the test being evaluated is positive?
- What is the probability of the individual being free of the disease if the test being evaluated is negative?

Before we can answer these questions, we must consider the probability of disease before the patient receives the test. This PRETEST PROBABILITY,[3] along with the test's sensitivity and specificity, allows one to calculate measures known as the PREDICTIVE VALUES OF THE TEST.

Predictive Value of Positive and Negative Tests

As previously discussed, the major advantage of sensitivity and specificity as measures of a test is that they are not directly dependent on the relative frequency or pretest probability of the disease. This advantage is particularly useful for articles in the health research literature. Sensitivity and specificity, however, have shortcomings in answering two clinically important questions: If the test is positive, how likely is it that the individual has the disease? If the test is negative, how likely is it that the individual does not have the disease? These questions are of practical concern to clinicians because they ask about the probability of the disease being present once the results of the test are known, or the POSTTEST PROBABILITY of disease.

The measures that address these questions are known as the PREDICTIVE VALUE.

Predictive value of a positive test = Proportion of those with a positive test who have the disease

Predictive value of a negative test = Proportion of those with a negative test who do not have the disease

The pretest probability of disease may be based on the probability of disease in a group of individuals, taking into account their risk factors for the disease. For instance, the pretest probability of coronary artery disease may be estimated on the basis of age, gender, LDL cholesterol level, cigarette smoking, and other risk factors. In clinical practice, in addition to overall frequency of disease and risk factors, the patient's clinical symptoms are taken into account. Thus, the type, location, and duration of chest pain are also included when estimating the probability of coronary artery disease before interpreting test results to make a diagnosis.

PREDICTIVE VALUE means the probability of the disease being present (or absent) after obtaining the results of the test. Thus, predictive values can be thought of clinically as the posttest probability of the disease.

As a rough guide to interpreting the numbers, it may be helpful to use the following approximate pretest probabilities:

1% = Pretest probability of those with risk factors for a common disease but without any symptoms

10% = Pretest probability when a disease is unlikely but possible clinically and the clinician wishes to rule it out

[3]Pretest probability for an asymptomatic individual may be the same as prevalence, or the probability that the disease is present in the population from which the individual comes. However, if additional information on the individual is available based on history, physical or laboratory testing, these may be used, in addition to prevalence, to estimate the pretest probability of the disease.

50% = Pretest probability when there is considerable uncertainty but the clinical presentation is compatible with the disease and the clinician wants to rule the disease both in and out

90% = Pretest probability when the disease is very likely clinically but the clinician wishes to rule it in

The following 2×2 tables illustrate how to calculate the predictive values. Remember we must perform this calculation for one particular relative frequency or pretest probability of the disease at a time.

Test	Gold Standard Disease	Gold Standard Disease-Free	
Positive	a = Number of individuals with the disease and positive	b = Number of individuals disease-free and positive	a + b = Total number of positives
Negative	c = Number of individuals with the disease and negative	d = Number of individuals disease-free and negative	c + d = Total number of negatives

The following formulas are used for calculating the predictive values of a positive test and a negative test:

$$\text{Predictive value of a positive test} = \frac{a}{a+b}$$ Proportion of those with a positive test who actually have the disease (as measured by the gold standard)

$$\text{Predictive value of a negative test} = \frac{d}{c+d}$$ Proportion of those with a negative test who actually do not have the disease (as measured by the gold standard)

Let us again use our test with 80% sensitivity and 90% specificity to calculate predictive values starting with pretest probabilities of 90%, 50%, 10%, and 1%. Remember that the number of positives and negatives will be different for each pretest probability of the disease. The calculations which we perform from our 2×2 tables are an example of BAYES' THEOREM.

90% Pretest Probability

	Gold Standard Disease	Gold Standard Disease-Free	
Test positive	720	10	730
Test negative	180	90	270
	900	100	

90% Pretest Probability

Predictive value of a positive test $= \dfrac{a}{a+b} = \dfrac{720}{730} = 98.6\%$

Predictive value of a negative test $= \dfrac{d}{c+d} = \dfrac{90}{270} = 33.3\%$

Using the previous 2×2 charts, the other predictive values are as follows:

50% Pretest Probability

Predictive value of a positive test $= \dfrac{a}{a+b} = \dfrac{400}{450} = 88.9\%$

Predictive value of a negative test $= \dfrac{d}{c+d} = \dfrac{450}{550} = 81.8\%$

10% Pretest Probability

Predictive value of a positive test $= \dfrac{a}{a+b} = \dfrac{80}{170} = 47.1\%$

Predictive value of a negative test $= \dfrac{d}{c+d} = \dfrac{810}{830} = 97.6\%$

1% Pretest Probability

Predictive value of a positive test $= \dfrac{a}{a+b} = \dfrac{8}{107} = 7.5\%$

Predictive value of a negative test $= \dfrac{d}{c+d} = \dfrac{891}{893} = 99.8\%$

For a test with a sensitivity of 80% and a specificity of 90%, these data can be summarized as follows:

	Pretest Probability			
	1%	10%	50%	90%
Predictive value of a positive test	7.5%	47.1%	88.9%	98.6%
Predictive value of a negative test	99.8%	97.6%	81.8%	33.3%

These calculations of predictive values have important clinical implications. They indicate that the probability of a disease being present or absent after obtaining the results of a test depends on the best possible estimate of the probability of disease made before performing the test. When the probability of disease is moderately high before performing the test, such as 50%, even a negative test like the one used in the example leaves an 18.2% (100% − 81.8%) probability that the disease is present. When the probability of disease is relatively low before performing the test, such as 10%, even a positive test leaves a 52.9% (100% − 47.1%) probability that the disease is absent.

The situation is even worse when the same test is used as a screening test. For instance, we might be testing a group of individuals who have a risk factor for the disease but only a 1% probability of having active disease. As we can learn from our example with a 1% probability or pretest probability of disease, when we apply our test with 80% sensitivity and 90% specificity to this group of individuals, those with a positive test will still have only a 7.5% probability of having the disease. That is what a predictive value of a positive test of 7.5% means. Failure to understand the effect of pretest probability on predictive values can lead to the following error:

> A new, inexpensive test for lung cancer was evaluated by applying it to a group of 100 individuals with lung cancer and 100 individuals with no evidence of lung cancer. A positive test was shown to have a predictive value of 85%; that is, 85% of those with a positive test had lung cancer. The authors concluded that this test was well suited for screening a high risk population because 85% of those with a positive test will have lung cancer.

The predictive value of a positive test is the percentage of persons with a positive test who have the disease. That predictive value depends on the relative frequency or pretest probability of the disease in the group of individuals tested. In evaluating a test, it is often applied to individuals of whom half are known to have the disease. In this example, the test was applied to a group in which 50% of the individuals had the disease (100 with lung cancer, 100 without lung cancer). Thus, the pretest probability of the disease in the test group was 50%. The lower the pretest probability of the disease, the lower the predictive value of a positive test will be regardless of the sensitivity and specificity.[4]

In a high-risk population, even among those with a long history of smoking cigarettes, the pretest probability of lung cancer will be much lower than 50%; therefore, the predictive value of a positive test when applied to an average individual, even one with risk factors for lung cancer, will be far less than 85%. The ability of a positive test to correctly identify disease changes dramatically when the test is used on groups of individuals with different probabilities of having the disease. A positive test may have a high predictive value in one group of patients with a high pretest probability of disease; however, in another group of patients with a lower pretest probability of disease, the same positive test may have a much lower predictive value. Such a test may be useful for diagnosis in a group of patients with a high suspicion of disease, but it will be nearly useless for screening a general community with low suspicion of disease.

Until now we have been examining one test at a time and seeing how well it performs. Now let us see how we can compare the performance of tests.

---

[4]In this example, we assume that the test does not have 100% sensitivity or 100% specificity. If the sensitivity and the specificity are both 100%, the test would be as good as the gold standard, and pretest probability would not influence interpretation of the results.

18 Comparing Tests

When comparing tests to determine which is best to use, it is important to ask what we are trying to achieve. There are a number of different purposes for using tests:

1. Testing may be used to rule out disease when the probability of the disease being present is relatively low.
2. Testing may be used to rule in disease when the probability of the disease being present is relatively high.
3. Testing may be used to assess the prognosis of a disease by repeating the test to monitor for progression of the disease.
4. Testing may be used to detect disease in the absence of symptoms. We call this *screening for disease.*

A particular test may be used at different times for more than one purpose. Nonetheless, it is useful to make these distinctions because the same test may not perform well for all purposes.

When comparing tests to decide which is better to use to rule in a disease, it is common to choose the test with the greatest specificity. Likewise, when choosing a test for ruling out a disease, it is common to choose the test with the greatest sensitivity. Often, this method does identify the better test. However, there are circumstances when using the test with greatest specificity to rule in a disease and the test with the greatest sensitivity to rule out a disease is not the best choice, as demonstrated in the next example:

> A new disease, called Lemon disease, has been found to occur following a killer bee sting. The disease can cause heart disease that occurs months to years after the initial stings. Treatment instituted after early diagnosis is most effective for preventing the development of heart disease. However, treatment causes rare but serious side effects and carries substantial cost. Two tests are available for the early diagnosis of Lemon disease. Test #1 has a sensitivity of 80% and a specificity of 70%, and test #2 has a sensitivity of 85% and a specificity of 50%. After more than 10 killer bees stings, the probability of developing Lemon disease is 5%.

The following demonstrates the calculation for the predictive value of a positive test and the predictive value of a negative test when tests #1 and #2 are used and the pretest probability of Lemon disease is 5%.

Figure 18.1 displays the use of tests #1 and #2 in a situation when the probability of disease or the pretest probability is 5%. This 5% pretest probability is indicated by imagining 500 individuals with the disease and 9,500 individuals without the disease. As indicated in Figure 18.1, test #1 has the greatest predictive value of a positive result and also the greatest predictive value of a negative result. Thus, test #1 is better for ruling in and also slightly better for ruling out disease. Therefore, we cannot always choose the best test by using only specificity or only sensitivity.

	Test 1			Test 2	
	Disease (+)	Disease (–)		Disease (+)	Disease (–)
Test (+)	400	2,850	Test (+)	425	4,750
Test (–)	100	6,650	Test (–)	75	4,750
	500	9,500		500	9,500

Sensitivity = 80%   Sensitivity = 85%
Specificity = 70%   Specificity = 50 %

Predictive Values   Predictive Values

of a positive test $= \dfrac{400}{3,250} = 12.3\%$ of a positive test $= \dfrac{425}{5,175} = 8.2\%$

of a negative test $= \dfrac{6,650}{6,750} = 98.5\%$ of a negative test $= \dfrac{4,750}{4,825} = 98.4\%$

Figure 18.1. Lemon disease.

The best test to use when seeking to rule in disease and also to rule out disease can be determined by using sensitivity and specificity together.

When comparing one test to another to determine which is the better test for ruling in or for ruling out a disease, other measurements can be used to compare the tests. These are known as likelihood ratios. The likelihood ratio of a positive test tells us how well a positive test does by comparing its performance when the disease is present compared with when it is absent. Thus, the formula for the likelihood of a positive test is:

$$\frac{\text{Likelihood ratio}}{\text{of a positive test}} = \frac{\text{Probability of a positive test if the disease is present}}{\text{Probability of a positive test if the disease is absent}}$$

The likelihood ratio of a positive test is related to sensitivity and specificity as follows:

$$\frac{\text{Likelihood ratio}}{\text{of a positive test}} = \frac{\text{Sensitivity}}{100\% - \text{Specificity}}$$

Let us calculate the likelihood ratio of a positive test for the two tests for Lemon disease. For test #1, the likelihood ratio of a positive test is as follows:

$$\frac{80\%}{100\% - 70\%} = 2.66$$

For test #2, the likelihood ratio of a positive test is as follows:

$$\frac{85\%}{100\% - 50\%} = 1.7$$

The best test to use for ruling in a disease is the one with the largest likelihood ratio of a positive test. A likelihood ratio of a positive test of 1 means that a positive test does not provide any additional information for ruling in disease. That is, it does not change the pretest probability of the disease. The greater the likelihood ratio of a positive test, the more information the test provides for ruling in the disease. A perfect test with 100% sensitivity and 100% specificity has a likelihood ratio of a positive test of infinity.

The formula for the likelihood ratio of a negative test is as follows:

$$= \frac{\text{Probability of a negative test if the disease is present}}{\text{Probability of a negative test if the disease is absent}}$$

$$= \frac{100\% - \text{Sensitivity}}{\text{Specificity}}$$

Let us calculate the likelihood ratios of a negative test for the two tests for Lemon disease. For test #1, the likelihood ratio of a negative test is as follows:

$$\frac{100\% - 80\%}{70\%} = .28$$

For test #2, the likelihood ratio of a negative test is as follows:

$$\frac{100\% - 85\%}{50\%} = .30$$

The better test to use to rule out disease is the one with the smaller likelihood ratio of a negative test. A likelihood ratio of a negative test of 1 means that a negative test does not provide any additional information for ruling out a disease. That is, it does not change the pretest probability of the disease. The smaller the likelihood ratio of a negative test, the more information the test provides for ruling out the disease.[1] A perfect test with 100% sensitivity and 100% specificity has a likelihood ratio of a negative test of 0.

Using only the likelihood ratios to determine the better test to use makes an important assumption: that the consequences of a false-positive test are equal to the consequences of a false-negative test. This may not be true, as illustrated in the next example:

> After a test is performed and a positive result obtained, the patient with Lemon disease remains under observation to detect early heart disease. The disease can be successfully treated and heart disease prevented only if the heart disease is detected early. Thus, a false positive results in unnecessary observation, whereas a false negative results in irreversible heart disease. The investigators advise use of test #1, knowing it has the greater likelihood ratio of a positive test and thus is the better test to use to rule in disease.

When the value or importance of a false positive is equal to the value or importance of a false negative, the likelihood ratios alone are enough to tell us which is the better test to use to rule in and to rule out a disease. In this situation, the better test to use to rule in a disease is the one with the highest likelihood ratio of a positive test: test #1. However, in this example, a false negative seems to be more important than a false positive. Looking at the results of test #1, it has produced 100 false negatives compared with only 75 false negatives for test #2. Thus, we

[1]This relationship can be most easily appreciated by using the odds form of Bayes' theorem. Using this expression, the posttest odds of a disease are equal to the pretest odds multiplied by the likelihood ratio. Thus, here the pretest odds are 1 to 19 or 1/19. Multiplying the likelihood ratio of a positive test by 1/19 gives us the posttest odds of the disease after obtaining a positive test. Similarly, multiplying the likelihood ratio of a negative test by 1/19 gives us the posttest odds of disease after obtaining a negative test.

need to take into account the fact that false negatives are worse than false positives. In this situation, we would most likely prefer to use test #2 to rule out disease, because the smaller number of false negatives with their important consequences should more than make up for its larger number of false positives with their less severe consequences.[2]

In addition to the relative importance of false positives and false negatives, considering the best test to use also requires taking into account the safety and sometimes the cost of the tests, as illustrated in the next example:

> A new test for Lemon disease has a likelihood ratio of a positive test of 100 and a likelihood ratio of a negative test of 0.01 when used for diagnosis. Thus, it is clearly better than either of our other tests for both ruling in and ruling out Lemon disease. However, the test uses a new intravenous dye that produces severe reactions in 1% of all patients.

Even though the new test is clearly a better test, its severe adverse effect makes it unsuitable for either ruling in or ruling out Lemon disease unless the consequences of the disease are very frequent and severe.[3]

In addition to using testing to rule in and rule out a disease, testing is often used after a disease has been diagnosed. Prognosis may be evaluated by tests that assess the extent of involvement at the time of diagnosis. For instance, prognosis is often assessed by staging patients. In addition, tests may be used to monitor progression by repeatedly using the same test and comparing the results over time. The better test to use for this type of follow-up assessment may be quite different from the best test to use for ruling in or ruling out a diagnosis, as illustrated in the next example:

> A safe and inexpensive test had a likelihood ratio of a positive test of 1 and a likelihood ratio of a negative test of 1 when used for diagnosis of early Lemon disease. However, the test is found to be useful in following progression of the disease when a patient has been diagnosed using other tests. The test is repeated on a monthly basis, and the subsequent results are compared with the initial results. Despite being worthless for diagnosis when the test is used to monitor progression after treatment for Lemon disease, it is shown to rise in titer before the development of heart disease in time to adjust the dosage of treatment and prevent cardiac complications.

This test, which provides no additional information for diagnosis, is still very useful for monitoring progression of the disease. A test for monitoring progression should have very different characteristics than a test for diagnosis. It does not require a large likelihood ratio of a positive test because other tests are being used to rule in the disease. The key features of a test for monitoring progression are that it can be used repeatedly and it accurately predicts outcome. Considerations of safety are very important with these types of prognosis tests because the test must be used repeatedly. Cost may be of less concern with tests that monitor for progression because they only need to be performed on a relatively small number of patients who already have been diagnosed with the disease.[4]

---

[2]This adjustment can be done quantitatively if we can place a numerical value on the ratio of the harm of a false negative to the harm of a false positive.

[3]Cost may be the dominant consideration in testing, especially when two tests have nearly the same performance.

[4]It is possible to calculate the likelihood ratio for tests that monitor progression if progression to an adverse outcome is used as the equivalent of the presence of the disease and absence of progression to an adverse outcome is used as the equivalent of the absence of the disease.

Using the same test repeatedly on the same individuals offers a special advantage. By using the patient as his or her own comparison, we are better able to avoid many of the issues that are inherent in using a reference interval. Remember that the reference interval is actually a "necessary evil." We compare an individual to a reference sample group because we do not know the measurement that individual should have previously had on a particular test. With repeat testing, we are aware of the individual's previous measurement, and we can then define a positive test in terms of a change from their previous level. This advantage may help us to use tests that are not useful for diagnosis to observe patients and monitor progression.[5]

Thus, before knowing which is the best test to use in a particular situation, we first need to ask what we are trying to achieve. That is, are we trying to rule out a quite unlikely cause of symptoms or to rule in a quite likely cause of symptoms, or are we trying to monitor to assess progression? The criteria we use to determine the better testing strategy for each of these goals are different. We have reviewed the criteria for selecting a test to rule in disease, to rule out disease, and to monitor progression. Selecting a strategy for screening has a number of special features, as we will see in the next chapter.

[5]Test results may change over time in the same individual, even in the absence of progression of disease. Changes may be due to random variations, biologic changes over time such as aging, or diseases other than the one being assessed. If the initial measurement was unusually high, the subsequent measurement may be lower by chance alone.

19 Screening

Whether to Screen

The goal of screening for a disease is to test individuals without current symptoms of the disease, that is asymptomatic individuals, in order to detect the disease at an early stage in its natural history. Before considering screening, the following criteria should be fulfilled:

- The particular disease detected early by screening would otherwise go on to cause substantial morbidity or mortality
- Treatment is available that is more effective when used at the early stage before symptoms develop than when used after symptoms develop

The evidence in the literature that supports the ability to detect disease at an early stage often comes from studies that compare the stage of disease among individuals who were diagnosed through screening versus those whose disease was diagnosed in the usual course of health care. The probabilities of detecting disease in early stages through screening and alternatively through the usual course of health care are calculated and then compared. If there is a higher probability of detecting disease with screening, the results may suggest early detection is possible through screening.

Early detection, however, is not necessarily the same as detecting disease that will go on to cause morbidity or mortality. It is possible that the disease detected by screening may never become clinically important, as illustrated in the next example:

> A new test is able to detect thyroid cancer in 40% of all men older than 80 years. Cancers detected in these men using the new test are generally found to be microscopic foci that are at an earlier stage than thyroid cancers diagnosed during the course of usual health care. The investigators are enthusiastic about the possibility of early detection of thyroid cancer and argue that this test is likely to be useful in early detection.

The ability to detect disease early is not the same as the ability to detect cancers that are likely to go on to become clinically important. Patients may die with thyroid cancer rather than die from thyroid cancer. The goal of early detection, as mentioned, is not just to identify cancer early, but also to identify those cases that need effective therapy to prevent progression to clinically important disease.

In addition, screening should not be recommended unless a therapy is available that can alter the outcome of patients detected by screening. Thus unless there is effective therapy that has additional effectiveness when used early in the disease, there is generally no reason to conduct screening for disease.[1] The benefit of early

---

[1]At times screening may be worthwhile for other reasons. It may be worthwhile to detect infectious disease in order to prevent spread even if no effective treatment is available.

therapy is ideally demonstrated using a randomized clinical trial that randomizes patients to a screening group and a usual medical care control group.[2]

Often, however, it is not possible to perform randomized clinical trials with long-term follow-up. Thus, we often rely on studies that compare the outcome of groups that have been screened and compare their outcome with that of groups that have not been screened by conducting nonconcurrent or concurrent cohort studies. These studies may provide important data that suggest the ability of screening to successfully improve outcome.

Cohort studies of screening, however, are also susceptible to misleading results due to LEAD-TIME BIAS. This bias results from comparing the time from diagnosis to an outcome, such as death, between those diagnosed through screening and those diagnosed in the usual course of medical care. The potential for lead-time bias is illustrated in the next example:

> An X-ray screening program to detect lung cancer among smokers was performed among a group of smokers who were asked to participate. Their outcomes were compared with the outcomes of individuals in a control group whose lung cancer was diagnosed in the usual course of medical care. The study and control groups' individuals were matched for age and number of pack-years of cigarette smoking. The screened group had a greatly improved survival 1 year after their diagnosis of lung cancer compared with the 1-year survival rate after diagnosis among the unscreened control group.

Even if the treatment for lung cancer has no effect, we would expect the results for the screened group to be better. By detecting the disease earlier, screening has moved back the time of diagnosis. As illustrated in Figure 19.1, unfortunately, it has not moved forward the time of death. The increase in time between diagnosis and death may be entirely due to lead-time bias or the early detection without improved prognosis.

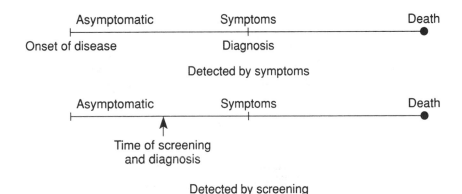

Figure 19.1. Lead-time bias in which earlier diagnosis by screening does not alter outcome.

[2]Even when using a randomized clinical trial, it is necessary to follow up those diagnosed with the disease. They should be monitored not just until they are diagnosed, but until they have had an opportunity to develop the adverse outcome we hope to prevent. That is because a randomized clinical trial that demonstrates improvement in early outcome is not always sufficient. The outcome in the screened group should remain better than groups undergoing the usual course of care even years after the disease is detected.

There is a second reason why comparing screened and unscreened populations using a cohort study to assess their outcome may not produce convincing evidence of an improved outcome among those screened. This is known as LENGTH BIAS. As illustrated in Figure 19.2, length bias occurs when there are two or more types of disease, such as slow-growing and rapidly growing cancer. When screening is performed initially, most cases that are detected will be slow growers. This is because slow growers remain in the presymptomatic stage for a longer period of time and thus constitute the majority of individuals whose cancer is detected by screening. Fast growers, on the other hand, remain in the presymptomatic stage for a shorter period of time and constitute a smaller proportion of the individuals detected by screening.[3]

Satisfying the first two criteria for recommending a disease screening demonstrates that identification and treatment of a disease at an early presymptomatic stage improves outcome. The third criterion is a feasible testing strategy, which requires us to define who should be screened, how they should be screened, and when they should be screened.

Who to Screen

In general, it is not feasible to screen everyone for a disease. It is usually necessary to identify groups of individuals who have an increased probability of having the disease in question. We usually need to rely on studies in the literature to identify risk factors, which increase the probability of having the disease. Risk factors are not necessarily a cause of the disease; they may be age, gender, or race, for instance. However, by alerting us to the increased frequency of disease, they help us to identify groups with an increased pretest probability of having the disease.

When performing screening, we are usually testing presymptomatic individuals. Thus, we cannot rely on their symptoms to help us estimate the pretest probability of disease. Instead, we need to rely on the frequency of the disease itself and the presence of risk factors to help us identify groups with adequately high pretest probabilities of disease.

Without being able to identify individuals who have one or more risk factors for the disease, we would often be starting with a very low pretest probability. In Chap-

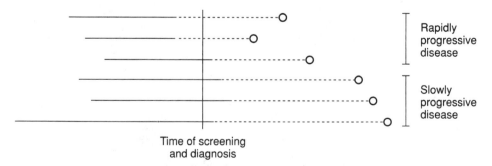

Time of screening
and diagnosis

Figure 19.2. Length bias demonstrating why more slowly progressive cases of disease may be detected by screening. Solid lines indicate preclinical phase; dotted lines, clinical phase; circles, death or other end-point.

[3]Length bias is less of an issue in randomized clinical trials if we can assume that the study and control groups have the same proportion of slow growers and rapid growers. Length bias assumes that disease that slowly progresses in the presymptomatic stage will remain slowly progressive once it enters the symptomatic phase. Length bias can be taken into account by studying groups that have previously undergone screening, thus removing from the group most of the long-standing cases of the disease.

ter 17, we illustrated the implications of using a test on a population with 1%, 10%, 50%, and 90% probability of the disease before conducting the test. The 1% example was used to illustrate a common pretest probability when risk factors for a common disease are present in a population to be screened. Even in this situation, it was evident that one test alone would not be adequate for diagnosis.

When the pretest probability is considerably lower, screening is even more difficult, as illustrated in the next example:

Suppose that the pretest probability of a disease is 1 per 1,000. Assume that we have available an excellent test with 99% sensitivity and 98% specificity. Using this test on a population with a pretest probability of disease of 1 per 1,000 produces the following predictive value of a positive test:

	Disease (+)	Disease (−)	Total
Test (+)	99	1,998	2,097
Test (−)	1	97,902	97,903
Total	100	99,900	

Predictive value of a positive test is:

$$99/2,097 = .047 = 4.7\%$$

Notice that even after we have obtained a positive test, the probability of disease is still less than 5%. Thus, even when screening with an excellent test, it is usually important that we apply our tests to groups of individuals who have pretest probabilities of disease greater than 1 per 1,000.

We can often identify risk factors for disease that allow us to characterize a group of individuals who have an adequately high pretest probability of disease. Age is the most common risk factor, because many diseases predominantly occur among particular age groups, such as premature infants or those older than 60 years. Other risk factors may be identified by such criteria as sexual history, past illness (*e.g.*, ulcerative colitis), occupational exposure (*e.g.*, lead), family history (*e.g.*, premenopausal breast cancer), and ethnicity or race (*e.g.*, sickle cell anemia).

How to Screen

Even if a high-risk group can be identified with perhaps a 1% pretest probability of disease, it is still usually necessary to use at least two different tests to diagnose the disease. If we apply our excellent test with 99% sensitivity and 98% specificity to a group with a 1% pretest probability of a disease, the predictive value of a positive test is obtained as follows:

	Disease (+)	Disease (−)	Total
Test (+)	99	198	297
Test (−)	1	9,702	9,703
Total	100	9,900	

Predictive value of a positive test is:

$$\frac{99}{297} = .33 = 33\%$$

The posttest probability or predictive value of a positive test is still less than 50%. This probability is certainly not adequate to make a diagnosis. Thus, in screening, the use of a second test is nearly inevitable, because even with an excellent test, most of the initial positives are actually false positives. Next, we need to consider the implications of using more than one test or combining tests.

There are two basic strategies for combining two tests. Using the first strategy label the results positive if the first test is positive and if a second test administered to all those who are positive on the first test is also positive. This strategy may be called POSITIVE-IF-BOTH-POSITIVE. With the second strategy for combining two tests, we label the results positive if either (or both) of the test results are positive. This strategy may be called POSITIVE-IF-ONE-POSITIVE.

With the positive-if-both-positive strategy, we usually administer the second test only to the individuals who are positive on the first test. The advantage of this strategy is that it requires second tests on only a small percentage of individuals. Thus, when feasible, the positive-if-both-positive strategy is often the most desirable.

With this strategy, a group that has been identified with two consecutive positives generally has a very high probability of disease. This is because the posttest probability of disease after performing the first test is used as the pretest probability of disease for the second test. This approach to calculating the posttest probability of disease after the second test is called the INDEPENDENCE ASSUMPTION.

The independence assumption assumes that the result of the second test, like the second flip of a coin, is not influenced by the result of the first test. The independence assumption is violated when two tests are actually measuring the same phenomenon and, therefore, the tests tend to have the same types of false-negative and false-positive results. If the independence assumption does not hold true, then the posttest probability of disease after obtaining two positives will often be less impressive than expected, as illustrated in the next example:

> A testing strategy for gastric cancer included an upper gastrointestinal (GI) X-ray film performed first. A technician then performed an endoscopy without biopsy if the upper GI test result was positive. The investigators expected that those with two positive results would have a very high probability of gastric cancer and the patient could then undergo biopsy by a gastroenterologist. The results of the study, however, demonstrated that this strategy was little better than using either test alone.

These results are not surprising, because the results of upper GI X-ray examination and endoscopy provide nearly the same type of information. They both rely on the gross anatomy. Thus, the results of the two tests are not independent, and individuals with two positive results will have a less than expected probability of having gastric cancer.[4]

The positive-if-one-positive strategy may be implemented by having all individuals initially undergo both tests. For instance, when screening for colon cancer, testing stool for blood as well as using a flexible sigmoidoscopy is an example of

---

[4]In general, tests that rely on different mechanisms of disease detection—such as exercise stress testing, thallium stress testing, and catheterization—will produce results that are more independent of each other than tests that rely on the same type of data such as gross anatomy.

a positive-if-one-positive strategy. This strategy is most useful when the two tests tend to detect different types of disease. For instance, flexible sigmoidoscopy is better for detecting left-sided colon cancers whereas stool blood testing is better for right-sided colon cancer. The need for the two tests to detect different types of disease when using the positive-if-one-positive strategy is illustrated in the next example:

> Mammography and sonography are being studied to determine whether a strategy that uses both of these test on all women older than 50 years will improve the outcomes of breast cancer. It was found that mammography detected 90% of the cancers, whereas sonography detected 60% of the cancers. The investigators expected to be able to detect nearly all breast cancers using both tests. They were disappointed when the results showed that performing the two tests did little better than using mammography alone.

If both mammography and sonography detect the same type of breast cancer, then administration of both tests will produce results that are no better than administration of mammography alone.[5]

One of the more confusing issues in screening using the positive-if-both-positive strategy is which test to use first. A common misconception is to use the test with the greater sensitivity first. Everything else being equal, the better test to use first is the one with the greatest likelihood ratio of a positive test. As we discussed and illustrated in Chapter 18, the test with the greatest sensitivity is not always the test with the greatest likelihood ratio of a positive test.

In practice, the issue of which test to use first is quite complicated because it also requires taking into account the relative importance of false-positive and false-negative results, safety of the tests, costs, and patient acceptance of the tests. A biopsy or angiography may be the best test to use first, for instance, but their side effects, costs, or lack of patient acceptance may limit their use to confirmation of other positive tests.

When to Screen

The frequency of screening is an important issue examined in the health literature. Screening frequency can greatly influence the cost and feasibility of screening large groups of patients. The longer the interval between screening, the more people who can be screened using the same resources.

Screening a group at one time and then rescreening them a second time, however, can be expected to produce very different results. The first time a group or population is screened, it is possible to detect disease that has been present for an extended period of time as well as disease that has developed recently. If there is a long presymptomatic stage, the initial screening may detect a large number of individuals with the disease. Once these individuals are treated, subsequent testing will only detect cases of the disease that have developed during the intervening period. Thus, we would generally expect subsequent testing to identify a much

---

[5]The positive-if-both-positive strategy has been called serial *or* consecutive positive testing. The positive-if-one-positive strategy has been called parallel *or* alternative positive testing. These terms may be confusing because most screening strategies ultimately require a subsequent confirmatory test. For instance, colon cancer screening that may be called parallel screening will ultimately require biopsy. Thus, we have adopted descriptive terms to label these two strategies.

smaller number of individuals with the disease. Failure to appreciate this principle may result in the following error:

> An initial screening program for gonorrhea in women conducted in the only women's health clinic in one community resulted in a 5% frequency of gonorrhea. The screening was continued each time patients returned to the clinic. Over the next several years, the percentage of cultures that were positive fell dramatically. The investigators concluded that the probability of developing gonorrhea had dropped dramatically in the community.

The reduction in the frequency of positive cultures may not reflect what is really happening in the community. Rather, it may predominantly reflect the fact that repeat testing only detects the newly developed cases of a disease rather than detecting new as well as long-standing disease.[6]

The recommended time interval between tests must also be considered in determining the frequency of screening. Ideally, the longer the presymptomatic stage, the less frequently screening needs to be performed. However, determining the frequency of screening based exclusively on knowledge of the natural history of a disease may not be a very reliable method, as illustrated in the next example:

> One reviewer who evaluated the results of the Papanicolaou (PAP) smear concluded that PAP smears should be done every 6 months to be sure that all new cases of disease are detected at an early stage. Another reviewer recommended screening patients every 5 years, arguing that cervical cancer is very slow growing and thus requires no more frequent screening.

Many screening tests depended on the adequacy of the sample obtained. In clinical practice, the PAP smear may not perform as well as expected in clinical studies because the sampling technique used in practice may inadequately sample the endocervical junction where cervical cancer is believed to originate. If this happens and the recommended interval is 5 years, then it can be 10 years or more before an adequate sample is obtained. Thus, in addition to the natural history of the disease, it is also important to consider the realities of testing in a clinical setting when evaluating the frequency of screening.

An additional factor affecting the frequency of screening relates to the types of individuals who seek screening tests in clinical practice. When screening depends on patients to initiate a visit, there are two types of patients: those who are screened repeatedly and those who rarely receive screening. This may result in SELF-SELECTION BIAS. Repeating screening tests at frequent intervals leads to rapidly diminished returns. Ensuring that those who rarely receive screening are included among those screened may produce far greater benefits. The trade-offs are illustrated in the next example:

> A pediatric lead screening program organizer needed to choose between testing patients every time they came in for follow-up and conducting home visits. Home visits would allow one test for all patients, even those who never made an appointment. The investigators found to their surprise that they could identify far more individuals with elevated lead levels by conducting home testing in which they tested every child once.

Often those who fail to seek care are the ones who need screening the most. Factors that increase the risk of disease may be closely linked to factors that keep

---

[6]This is different than length bias because it occurs even if all disease had the same natural history.

patients from seeking care. Social and economic factors often result in this self-selection bias.

Thus, to conduct an ideal screening program, three criteria must be established. First, we must establish that the disease detected early by screening would go on to cause substantial morbidity or mortality. Second, we need to establish that treatment is available that is most effective when used at the early stage before the development of symptoms. Third, we need to consider who, how, and when to screen to design a feasible screening program.

20 Testing a Test:

Questions to Ask and Flaw-Catching Exercises

The following checklist of questions to ask should help to reinforce the principles involved in testing a test:

1. Inherent properties of a test
   a. Precision: Do multiple repetitions of the test under the same conditions produce nearly identical results?
   b. Accuracy: Are the test results, on average, close to the true measure of the anatomic, physiologic, or biochemical phenomena?
   c. Clinical or field accuracy: Under usual conditions in which it is applied, has the test been shown to produce measurements that are close to the experimentally derived measurement?

2. Biologic variation: The concept of the reference interval to measure variability of disease-free individuals
   a. Has a reference interval been properly obtained to include a defined percentage, often 95% of those believed to be free of disease?
   b. Has outside the reference interval been distinguished from diseased?
   c. Has inside the reference interval been distinguished from disease-free?
   d. Is the reference sample group used generally applicable, or are there identifiable reference sample groups with different reference intervals?
   e. Have those who applied the test recognized that the reference interval is a description of a presumably disease-free group and that changes within the reference interval for any one individual may be pathologic?
   f. Has the reference interval been distinguished from desirable?
   g. Have the investigators justified moving the reference limits to accomplish specific diagnostic goals?

3. Variability of the individuals with the disease
   a. Have the investigators chosen the best available gold standard for defining which patients have the disease under study?
   b. Have the investigators included a broad enough cross-section of individuals with the disease to produce a realistic range of measurements for individuals with the disease?

4. Diagnostic performance: Distinguishing those with the disease from disease-free individuals
   a. How well does the test identify people with the disease? How high is its sensitivity? How often is it positive in disease?
   b. How well does the test identify people without the disease? How high is its specificity? How often is it negative in health?

    c. Has it been recognized that, despite the fact that sensitivity and specificity are theoretically not affected by the probability of disease in the group being tested, they may be different for early versus more advanced disease?

    d. Have the sensitivity and specificity of the test been distinguished from the predictive value of a positive test and the predictive value of a negative test?

5. Comparing tests

    a. Has the purpose for using the test been identified?

    b. If the test is designed to rule in a disease, has the test with the greater likelihood ratio of a positive been identified as the better test to use to rule in disease? If so, has the relative importance of a false-negative result and a false-positive result been taken into account?

    c. If the test is designed to rule out a disease, has the test with the smallest likelihood ratio of a negative been identified as the better test to use to rule out disease? If so, has the relative importance of a false-negative result and a false-positive result been taken into account?

    d. If the test is designed to monitor progression of disease, has the change from previous levels been used to establish criteria for a positive test?

    e. Have safety and cost been taken into account, as well as diagnostic performance when comparing tests?

6. Screening

    a. Is there evidence of substantial morbidity and mortality if the disease is not treated?

    b. Is there evidence that detection through screening and subsequent treatment produces better outcomes?

    c. Could lead-time bias explain an apparent improvement in outcome among individuals detected by screening?

    d. Could length bias explain an apparent improvement in outcome among individuals detected by screening?

    e. Can groups of individuals with risk factors for disease be identified, which enables screening of high-risk groups?

    f. Has a screening strategy been devised for initially screening individuals on the basis of the performance of two or more tests?

    g. Has the frequency of screening been identified on the basis of the natural history of the disease recognizing the potential for sampling error and self-selection?

Flaw-Catching Exercise No. 1: *Variability of the Test*
in Persons with the Disease and Persons without the Disease

Two investigations were conducted to evaluate the diagnostic usefulness of a new test for breast cancer. The test had previously been shown to have results that varied by less than 1% when repeated under the same conditions and read by the same individual.

In the first study, the investigators chose 100 women with metastatic breast cancer and 100 healthy women without any signs of breast disease. Results of the test for the healthy women were 30 to 100 mg/dL. Results for breast-cancer patients ranged from 150 to 200 mg/dL. Because this test perfectly separated the two groups, the investigators concluded that it could be considered an ideal test for diagnosing breast cancer and should immediately be applied to screening all women.

In a second study using the same test, another investigator compared 100 newly diagnosed breast-cancer patients with 100 patients with benign breast disease. The cancer patients' results ranged from 70 to 200 mg/dL, whereas results of patients with benign breast disease ranged from 40 to 180 mg/dL. The authors of this study noted the tremendous overlap between the two groups and concluded that the test was worthless.

A reader of these studies could not understand how two respected investigators could produce such inconsistent results. He concluded that there must have been errors in reporting the test results.

Critique: Exercise No. 1

To review these studies, it is helpful to organize the discussion by using the concepts of the variability of the test, the variability of the disease-free group, and the variability of those with the disease.

VARIABILITY OF THE TEST

Repeating the test under the same conditions provides information on the precision or reproducibility of the test. The study states that the test was previously shown to have only a 1% variation when repeated under the same conditions and read by the same individual. A measurement of precision requires repeat performance of the test in which the second results are not influenced by the results of the first test. In this case, the same observer performed the repetition of the test results; thus, it is possible that he or she was aware of and influenced by the initial results. If this was true, then the reproducibility or precision might be poorer than reported. In the rest of this discussion, however, assume that the authors are correct in believing the test is precise.

VARIABILITY OF THE DISEASE-FREE GROUP

The first study used healthy patients and found a range of numerical values from 30 to 100 mg/dL. In contrast, the second study used women with benign breast disease and found results of 70 to 200 mg/dL. These two studies may not be in contradiction; they may represent two different breast-cancer–free reference sample groups. It is possible that benign breast disease raises the levels of the test to intermediate numerical values.

The proper measure of the disease-free group is the reference interval, which usually includes 95% of the breast-cancer–free reference sample group. Results here, however, are presented as ranges that include 100% of the individuals; the total range tells nothing about how the results are concentrated. The results may be concentrated heavily between 70 and 100 mg/dL. Without all the data or at least a reference interval, it is difficult to use these studies to compare patients who do not have breast cancer with patients who do.

VARIABILITY OF PERSONS WITH THE DISEASE

The first study used patients with metastatic breast cancer and found a range of results from 150 to 200 mg/dL. The second study used newly diagnosed breast-cancer patients and found a range from 70 to 200 mg/dL. This discrepancy may not reflect error in reporting the data; it may reflect the different reference sample groups used. Newly diagnosed breast-cancer patients are likely to reflect a wider spectrum of persons with the disease. Individuals with early disease as well as metastatic disease are likely to be represented among newly diagnosed patients. Metastatic breast-cancer patients, however, may reflect only one end of the spectrum, that of severe disease. Thus, the wider range of numerical values found among the newly diagnosed patients may reflect the more representative breast-cancer group used in the second study.

DIAGNOSTIC PERFORMANCE

The data presented do not allow one to calculate the sensitivity or specificity of the test. The distribution of individual results is not mentioned, so it is not possible to obtain a reference interval and thus a cutoff line between positive and negative. Therefore, no conclusions are warranted about the diagnostic performance of the test.

In the first study, the investigators used individuals with a far-advanced disease and individuals who were free of any breast disease. It is not surprising that their test results appeared to separate the groups successfully. In the second study, the investigators included a wider spectrum of breast-cancer patients and compared them with women with benign breast disease. Therefore, it also is not surprising that there was more overlap of numerical values in this second study. The interpretations of the first study as a perfect test and the second study as a worthless test are both incorrect. The groups in the first study potentially provide information on the performance of the test among those with far-advanced disease, whereas groups in the second study could potentially provide information on the performance of the test among those with newly diagnosed breast cancer. The results, using these groups, are often quite different.

Flaw-Catching Exercise No. 2: *The Reference Interval*

An investigator attempts to derive the reference interval for a new test for diabetes in the following way:

1. He locates 1,000 hospital patients admitted for primary medical conditions other than diabetes.
2. He performs the new test on all 1,000 patients.
3. He plots the values for the new test, excludes the top 2.5% and the bottom 2.5%, and includes the other 95% as the reference interval.

The investigator now takes his new test to the community and performs screening tests on all volunteers. He tells all those who fall within the reference interval that they are free of diabetes and tells all those who fall outside the reference interval that they have diabetes. One year later, he retests several individuals whose values fell at the low end of the reference interval. He finds that they are now at the upper end of the reference interval, and he assures them that they are free of diabetes.

An obese male patient in his 20s with test results at the high end of the reference interval and a strong family history of diabetes asks for advice on how to avoid developing the disease. The investigator advises him that because he is within the reference interval, he has nothing to worry about.

Critique: Exercise No. 2

DEVELOPMENT OF THE REFERENCE INTERVAL

In developing the reference interval, an investigator should seek to include only individuals who are free of the disease under study. The investigator in the study here concluded that individuals admitted with primary medical conditions other than diabetes were free of diabetes. Diabetes, however, is a very common condition, and diabetic patients may develop a series of complications that increase their probability of being hospitalized. Therefore, it is likely that a proportion of individuals admitted with other primary diagnoses also had diabetes. The investigator may not have developed his reference interval from diabetes-free patients.

The investigator used the central 95% of the presumably disease-free group's results as the reference interval. This is the usual procedure, but it may not maximize the test's diagnostic performance. By altering the limits of the reference interval, it is sometimes possible to improve the test's ability to separate people with and without the disease. It must be remembered, however, that when we change the limits of the reference interval to produce fewer false-negative results, we then pay the penalty of producing more false-positive results, or vice versa. This penalty may be worthwhile, but further data are required before we can be certain. In any event, these data are inadequate for judging whether this new test helps to separate diabetic from nondiabetic persons. No external gold standard was used to define who actually had diabetes. All we know is the numerical values observed for the test.

APPLYING THE REFERENCE INTERVAL

The distinction between the concept of the reference interval and the concept of disease has not been maintained. The author has equated outside the reference interval with diabetes and within the reference interval as free of diabetes. No evidence is presented that supports the usefulness of the new test in separating diabetic from nondiabetic persons. It is possible that diabetic persons fall entirely within the reference interval for this test.

Even if this test had been shown to be useful in separating people with diabetes from those without diabetes, it is likely that there still would be a few individuals with diabetes whose measurements on the test were within the reference interval as well as diabetes-free individuals whose test results were outside the reference interval. Thus, the investigator cannot simply apply the test and label individuals as diabetic or nondiabetic.

CHANGES WITHIN THE REFERENCE INTERVAL

When an individual's results change but remain within the reference interval, it could indicate a manifestation of disease. The concept of the reference interval is developed primarily for individuals for whom no previous baseline data are available. When this is the case, it is necessary to compare an individual's current results with those individuals who are assumed to be free of the disease being assessed. If the individual has previously undergone the same test, this information can then be used as the basis of comparison.

A change within the reference interval may represent a large increase for a given individual; this is especially true if a patient previously was near the lower limits of the reference interval and then moved to the upper limits. For these individuals, changes within the reference interval may indicate early manifestations of disease.

REFERENCE SAMPLE GROUP

The reference sample group used in the study to develop the reference interval was composed of all hospitalized patients. Their reference interval may have been quite different from that of a younger, ambulatory, and otherwise healthy population. Thus, an error may have been introduced by developing the reference interval from one reference sample group and applying it to another group with different characteristics.

WITHIN THE REFERENCE INTERVAL VERSUS DESIRABLE

It is possible that all or some of those individuals whose results on the test were within the reference interval have numerical values that are higher than desirable. Remember that the reference interval reflects the way things are, not necessarily how they ideally should be. It is possible that losing weight and thus lowering the test results will prevent future problems. This assumes that the test in fact separates people with the disease from those without the disease, that losing weight will affect the test levels, and that lowered test levels indicate a better prognosis. The general point, however, is that results within the reference interval are not necessarily desirable results.

Flaw-Catching Exercise No. 3: *Diagnostic Performance of Tests*

The usefulness of a new test for thrombophlebitis is being evaluated. The traditional gold standard test for thrombophlebitis has been the venogram, with which the new test is being compared. To assess the precision or reproducibility of the new test, it is performed on 100 consecutive patients with positive venograms. The investigators found that 98% of the patients diagnosed as having thrombophlebitis had a positive test result. The investigators then repeated the test on the same group of patients. They again found that it was positive in 98% of the 100 patients. From this, they concluded that the new test was 100% precise or reproducible.

Having demonstrated the precision or reproducibility of the new test, the authors proceeded to study its diagnostic performance. The authors evaluated the success of the new test as measured against the venogram, the traditional gold standard.

They studied 1,000 consecutive patients with unilateral leg pain, of whom 500 had positive venograms and 500 had negative venograms. The investigators classified individuals as positive or negative and presented their data as follows:

New Test	Positive Venogram	Negative Venogram
Positive	450	100
Negative	50	400
	500	500

The investigators defined sensitivity as the proportion of individuals with the disease, as established by the gold standard test, who have a positive new test. Thus,

$$\text{Sensitivity} = \frac{450}{500} = 0.90 = 90\%$$

The investigators defined specificity as the proportion of individuals without the disease, as established by the gold standard test, who have a negative new test. Thus,

$$\text{Specificity} = \frac{400}{500} = 0.80 = 80\%$$

The investigators calculated the predictive value of a positive test for their study group. They defined this value as the proportion of persons with a positive new test who actually have the condition as measured by the gold standard test. Thus,

$$\text{Predictive value of a positive test} = \frac{450}{550} = 0.818 = 81.8\%$$

From these results, the investigators drew the following conclusions:

1. The new test is completely precise or reproducible.
2. The new test has a lower sensitivity and specificity than the venogram; thus, it is an inherently inferior test.
3. When applied to a new group of patients, such as a group with bilateral leg pain, a positive new test can be expected to have a predictive value of a positive test equal to 81.8%.

Critique Exercise No. 3

If a test is performed several times on the same individuals under the same conditions, the results for each individual should be nearly identical if the test is 100% precise or reproducible. The authors stated that the total number of positive new tests was identical when the test was repeated. They did not, however, indicate whether the same individuals were positive when the test was repeated as were positive the first time the test was performed. If the same individuals were not positive, the test could not be considered completely precise or reproducible. The authors also failed to indicate whether those who performed and interpreted the repeat test knew the results of the first test.

A gold standard is the measure of a disease against which new or unproved tests are compared, but the gold standard traditionally used may not be an ideal measure of the disease it is designed to diagnose. It is possible, however, for a new test to be a more useful measure of the disease than the accepted gold standard. When comparing the sensitivity and specificity of new tests with that of the gold standard, we must keep in mind that disagreement between the tests may result from a gold standard that is less than perfect rather than the inadequacy of the new test.

When the authors concluded that the new test had lower sensitivity and specificity than the venogram, they were making the usual assumption that the venogram had 100% sensitivity and 100% specificity. When we make this assumption, there is no way for the new test to have a higher sensitivity or specificity than the old test. Unless we can be sure that the venogram is always correct, it is premature to conclude that the new test is a less useful measure of thrombophlebitis. The authors, therefore, should have limited their conclusions about the sensitivity and specificity of the new test to a comparison with the venogram. If the new test is safer, cheaper, or more convenient than the venogram, it may come to replace the venogram in clinical practice. Clinical experience may eventually demonstrate that the new test is a better predictor of the consequences of thrombophlebitis than the venogram is, allowing the new test to be used as the gold standard. In the meantime, the best the test can do is to match the established gold standard test, assuming it has 100% sensitivity and 100% specificity.

The authors have used the correct definitions of the sensitivity, specificity, and predictive value of a positive test for their study group. As they stated, the predictive value of a positive test is the proportion of those with a positive new test who actually have the condition as measured by the gold standard. In this study group, the chance of thrombophlebitis or pretest probability is 50% (500 with thrombophlebitis, 500 without); thus, the predictive value of a positive test is 450 per 550, or 81.8%. The predictive value of a positive test, however, is different in different groups of patients, depending on the pretest probability of the disease in the group being tested. One cannot extrapolate a predictive value derived in one group of patients directly to another group with a different pretest probability of the condition. One would expect a group of patients with unilateral leg pain to have a different pretest probability of thrombophlebitis than a group of patients with bilateral leg pain.

The predictive values for bilateral leg pain cannot be estimated solely on the basis of the sensitivity and specificity of the test derived from patients with unilateral leg pain. However, if one can also estimate the percentage of those with bilateral leg pain who have thrombophlebitis, the pretest probability, then it is possible to estimate the predictive values of a test in patients with bilateral leg pain.

Because the probability of thrombophlebitis in a patient who presents with bilateral leg pain is much lower than 50%, the posttest probability of disease even after a positive test would be much lower than 81.8%.

Flaw-Catching Exercise No. 4: *Screening for Disease*

A newly discovered test, known as perfect screening antigen (PSA), was found to distinguish between individuals with prostate cancer and individuals without evidence of prostate disease. The test was so successful in separating these groups that investigators suggested it be used as a screening test for all men older than 50 years. Prostate cancer was known to be very unusual before age 50 years. Most cases occurred among men older than 60 years, with most being older than 70 years.

When PSA was used as a screening test, elevated levels were followed by biopsy. Biopsy had previously been shown to have both a specificity and a sensitivity of nearly 100% for prostate cancer when used to follow-up prostate nodules found on rectal examination. There were only a few mildly elevated PSA readings, which were deemed false positive on biopsy. The author thus regarded it as the ideal test to confirm or to rule out prostate disease among those with an elevated PSA.

When this test was first used in screening, the cases detected by screening were diagnosed with an earlier stage of disease compared with those diagnosed in the usual course of clinical care. The prostate cancer was almost always localized to the prostate, compared with the cases diagnosed in the usual course of clinical care in which a substantial number had spread beyond the prostate.

The investigators evaluated the combination of PSA testing followed by biopsy for persons with elevated PSA levels, using a group of 100 men 50 to 60 years old who had never been previously screened. They also assessed a group of 100 men, 70 to 80 years old, who had been examined every year by rectal examination for prostate nodules. The investigators found the following:

1. The 50- to 60-year-old men had as many definitively elevated PSA levels as the 70- to 80-year-olds. They found this surprising because of the known increase in the frequency of prostate cancer with age.
2. In subsequent screening efforts, it was evident that the PSA did not perform as well as it had when used to distinguish between men with prostate cancer and those without prostate disease. When used in screening, it produced a large number of minimal elevations, which usually turned out to be false positives.
3. The PSA also did not perform as well as expected in detecting early cancer in either age group. The sensitivity of the PSA was considerably lower than when it was used to separate patients with prostate cancer from those without prostate cancer.
4. Prostate biopsy also did not perform as well as expected when done following an elevated PSA rather than after a positive rectal examination. False negatives reduced the sensitivity of the test, which rarely happened when biopsy was used after rectal examination. The investigators could not believe these results because they knew that sensitivity and specificity should not change when a test is applied in a new situation.
5. Those individuals who were diagnosed through screening for prostate cancer on the basis of an elevated PSA and a positive biopsy were found to live longer from the time of diagnosis than those diagnosed in the usual course of health care. However, it was difficult to demonstrate an increased life span for the men diagnosed by screening, even with long-term follow-up.
6. Despite the difficulties in using PSA for screening, after diagnosis of prostate cancer, progressive increases in PSA over time were strongly associated with spread of prostate cancer. Thus, the investigators recommended using PSA as a test to follow the progression of prostate cancer.

The investigators were still optimistic about using PSA for screening and argued that the answer to these problems was to order the PSA twice and to proceed with biopsy if either test was positive.

Critique: Exercise No. 4

The findings observed by the investigator may be explained by the principles of screening we have examined. The investigators did not establish the criteria to demonstrate that PSA followed by biopsy was a useful screening strategy. Detection of disease at an earlier stage in the natural history may be useful if early detection is possible and, in addition, early treatment improved outcome. PSA testing may be able to detect disease at an earlier stage; however, these data do not, in and of themselves, establish that early detection improves outcome. It is possible that the cancers detected would remain clinically dormant and not progress to more advanced stages. It is also possible that cancers detected by PSA testing cannot be treated any more successfully than cancer detected at a later stage by rectal examination.

The results observed by the investigators may be explained as follows:

1. When a test is performed on a group of individuals such as the 50- to 60-year-olds who have not been screened before, cancers that have been present for an extended time may be detected. In a repeatedly screened group, such as the 70- to 80-year-olds, these cancers have generally been detected and hopefully removed. Thus, only a smaller number of newly developed cancers are detected when a previously screened group is rescreened.

2. When tests are first evaluated, they are often used on patients with clear-cut, often far-advanced disease. These individuals are compared with individuals who have no evidence of disease in the organ being assessed. In the case of prostate disease, common noncancerous conditions may affect test results. When tested in a population that contains some men with other forms of prostate disease, it is not surprising that the PSA test resulted in a greater number of slightly elevated measurements, most of which did not turn out to be prostate cancer.

3. The sensitivity and specificity of test results may not differ from population to population as long as the populations being compared have the same type and severity of disease. However, when comparing the use of tests among people with far-advanced disease and those with early disease, a difference in sensitivity and specificity should be expected. A test that can detect late disease may not be able to perform as well at detecting early disease. This may explain the results observed by the investigator.

4. The results of biopsy can be explained if we recognize the difference between a biopsy after a nodule is found on prostate examination and a biopsy after an elevated PSA. After a rectal examination detects a nodule, the biopsy is directed at the nodule itself. When there is no nodule, the biopsy may need to be done blindly (*i.e.*, without a clear-cut location to direct the biopsy). Thus, with a blind biopsy, it is not surprising that there would be some false negatives in which the wrong areas were sampled.

5. Successful screening programs require more than the ability to detect disease at an early stage. They require that early treatment improves outcome. Outcome may not be improved by early intervention for one of two reasons. First, the treatment may not be successful in preventing progression of the disease. Alternatively, early treatment may not be necessary because later treatment is also successful or because the disease does not frequently progress to more advanced stages. When earlier diagnosis leads to an increased time between

diagnosis and death (or other outcome) but does not alter the course of a disease, there is a lead-time bias. Lead-time bias results when screening merely detects the disease at an earlier point in the natural history but does not alter the course of the disease.

6. The problems that occur when the PSA is used as a screening test do not imply that it cannot be used as a test of prognosis. Once a disease is diagnosed, it may be possible to repeat the test and compare the new results to the individual's previous results. This offers the advantage of a comparison to the same individuals rather than to a reference interval made up of individuals who may or may not be similar to the person under study. In addition, tests that are useful for following the disease's progression aim to accomplish very different goals. They need to reflect the extent or severity of disease, not merely its presence. Thus, it should not be surprising that a test useful for following progression of disease may not be useful for diagnosis or screening.

Unfortunately, the solution is not merely to perform the same test twice. Performing the same test twice and then performing a second test if either test is positive is an example of a positive-if-one-positive screening strategy. This type of screening strategy is most useful if the two tests detect different types of disease. Using the same test twice is likely to detect, and also to fail to detect, the same type of disease each time.

Rating a Rate   III

21 Introduction to Rates

When you hear hoof beats, it is more likely to be a horse than a zebra. This maxim stresses the obvious but too often forgotten truth that common diseases occur commonly and rare diseases occur rarely. When we label one disease common and another rare, we are implying a difference in rates at which the diseases occur.[1]

All clinicians instinctively use a concept of RATES. We know that coronary artery disease is much more likely in a middle-age man than in a teenage girl. We know that pancreatic cancer is much more common in an elderly person than in a young person. We know that sickle cell anemia is much more likely in a black person than in a white person.

In our previous discussion of diagnostic tests, we showed that the lower the probability of the disease in a population (*i.e.*, the rarer the disease), the lower the predictive value of a positive test. For a rare disease, then, a positive test is much less likely to indicate disease. Clinicians automatically and perhaps subconsciously use this concept. We know that a young woman with T-wave changes on an ECG is unlikely to have coronary artery disease. We know that a young man with persistent abdominal pain is unlikely to have pancreatic cancer. We know that a white person with evidence of joint pain and anemia is unlikely to have sickle cell anemia. The clinician's appreciation of the rates of the disease may be based partially on clinical experience; however, it is helpful to be able to draw from research articles to gain a more objective and scientific assessment of the rates of disease. This section aims to assist you in acquiring the tools to understand how the rates of disease are scientifically measured and interpreted. Such an understanding helps in choosing the proper diagnostic methods and interpreting the results.

In addition to facilitating individual diagnosis, an appreciation of the rates of disease helps in the assessment of changes that occur over time or as a result of interventions. Rates of disease are an important tool for conducting the types of studies that were discussed in Part 1, *Studying a Study*. The ability to identify actual changes and true cause-and-effect relationships is dependent on an understanding of the principles of comparing rates. Finally rates of disease are becoming an important part of OUTCOMES RESEARCH. In outcome research rates are the measurements used to monitor and evaluate the results of clinical care.

It may not be obvious why it is necessary to study the rates of disease. Why not just compare how many times events occur? Let us look at the following example,

---

[1]Rate is used here to imply either a proportion or a rate as defined by epidemiologists and biostatisticians. A proportion implies that the numerator is a subset of the denominator. A rate technically implies that the denominator includes a measurement of time. Ratios are distinguished from rates and proportions because in a ratio the numerator is not necessarily a subset of the denominator. Probability is used to imply the special type of proposition in which the numerator contains the number of times an event occurs and the denominator contains the number of times the event could have occurred.

which illustrates the problems with comparing only the number of events that occur:

> A hospital review panel was evaluating the performance of clinicians at your hospital. For a procedure you frequently perform, they found five deaths among the 1,000 patients you treated at the hospital last year. The chief of staff had only one death among the 200 patients he treated. The panel decided that because you had five times more deaths than the chief of staff, you must have been using poor technique.

Instead of looking at the total number of deaths, it is fairer to look at the number of deaths that occurred in relation to the number of deaths that could have occurred. Your patients' chances of death and the chief of staff's patients' chances of death were identical: 5 per 1,000 equals 1 per 200. Rates of events have come to your defense. They are worth knowing about!

We have been using the term rate as a nontechnical, generic term to imply a measurement of an event's relative frequency of occurrence. However, it is important to recognize that, technically, a rate is distinguished from a PROPORTION or PROBABILITY. In both rates and proportion or probability, the numerator contains the number of times an event occurs. The denominators, however, are different. In proportions or probabilities, the denominator contains the total number of observations or opportunities for the event to occur. In a rate, the denominator also includes a unit of time during which the events could occur, such as per year. We use both rates and probabilities in deriving the three basic measurements of disease:

1. Incidence rate: The number of new cases that occur per unit of time
2. Prevalence: The probability of having a disease at some point in time
3. Case fatality: The probability of dying from a disease once it is diagnosed

INCIDENCE RATES are defined as follows:

$$\text{Incidence rate of a disease} = \frac{\text{Number of individuals who develop the disease over a period of time}}{\text{Total number of person-years at risk}}$$

Incidence rates measure the number of times the disease develops over a period of time, often 1 year, relative to the number of observations or opportunities for it to develop. The number of observations in the denominator is often measured in PERSON-YEARS. A person-year is one individual observed over a period of 1 year.

It is often difficult to know how many individuals are at risk of a disease at any point in time and how long they are at risk. Thus, incidence rates are commonly estimated by using the following formula:

$$\text{Incidence rate of disease} = \frac{\text{Number of individuals who develop the disease over a period of time}}{\begin{array}{c}\text{Number of individuals in the population}\\\text{at the midpoint of the time period of}\\\text{interest} \times \text{Length of the time period}\end{array}}$$

Imagine we wanted to study the incidence rate at which new cases of AIDS develop in New York City in 2000. Because individuals are constantly moving in or out of New York City, it is difficult to know the true number of persons who live in the city and how long they live there during 2000. However we can substitute data from the middle of 2000 to calculate an approximate incidence rate. In this situation it would be possible to use the census data to estimate the number of New York City residents. The approximate incidence rate of AIDS in New York City in 2000 then would be calculated as follows:

$$\text{Incidence rate of AIDS in New York City in 2000} = \frac{\text{Number of New York City residents who developed AIDS in 2000}}{\text{Number of New York City residents on June 30, 2000 as estimated by the 2000 census} \times 1 \text{ year}}$$

The incidence rate measures the new cases of a particular disease that develop per unit of time. This measurement may help in assessing the cause of a disease.[2] Once a disease occurs, it may be present for a long period. Thus, a second type of measurement frequently is used to estimate the probability of having a disease at a point in time. Known as PREVALENCE, it measures the relative frequency or probability of the disease at one point in time. The prevalence of disease is important in diagnosis because it is a starting point for estimating the pretest probability that a disease is present. The prevalence measurement provides an estimate of the probability of disease presence before evaluating an individual's history, physical examination, or laboratory tests. Thus,

$$\text{Prevalence} = \frac{\text{Number of individuals who have the disease at one point in time}}{\text{Number of individuals who are in the population at the same point in time}}$$

In the previous example, the prevalence of AIDS on June 30, 2000 in New York City would be calculated as follows:

$$\text{Prevalence} = \frac{\text{Number of New York City residents with AIDS on June 30, 2000}}{\text{Number of New York City residents on June 30, 2000 as estimated by the 2000 census}}$$

For most diseases, incidence rate and prevalence are related approximately as follows:

$$\text{Prevalence} = \text{Incidence rate} \times \text{Average duration of the disease}$$

In other words, the longer the average duration of the disease, the more individuals will have the disease at any particular time; therefore, the higher the prevalence. Chronic diseases with long duration, such as diabetes, may have a relatively low incidence rate of development of new cases but a high prevalence of the disease at any point in time. Acute, short-duration diseases like viral pharyngitis may have a high incidence rate of occurrence of new cases but a low prevalence of the disease at any point in time. Thus, it is important to appreciate that incidence rates and prevalence measure different phenomena. Incidence rates measure the rate at

[2]Biostatisticians and epidemiologists distinguish between cumulative incidence and incidence rates. Cumulative incidence contains in the denominator the number of individuals in the population at the beginning of the time period. The cumulative incidence is synonymous with risk. We can think of incidence rate as being analogous to the speed we are going over a short period of time and risk as the distance we have traveled over a large period of time, assuming the speed is maintained.

which a new case of the disease develops per unit of time. Prevalence measures the probability of having the disease at a particular time. Failure to appreciate this difference may lead to the type of error illustrated in the following example:

> A study of asymptomatic chlamydia in men was conducted by taking cultures from 1,000 randomly selected asymptomatic men. Ten of these men were found to have chlamydia. A second study observed a group of men from the same population over a 1-year period. This study found that over 1 year's time, only two of these men developed asymptomatic chlamydia. In comparing the studies, a reviewer concluded that one of them must be wrong because their conclusions were so widely divergent.

This seeming inconsistency is not inconsistent at all if one distinguishes incidence rates from prevalence. The first study of existing cases determined a prevalence; the second assessed the incidence rate. The fact that the prevalence of asymptomatic chlamydia was much higher than the incidence rate suggests that asymptomatic cases have a long duration. This may be explained by the fact that, although symptomatic cases usually receive treatment, asymptomatic cases may remain untreated in the community for a long period of time.

In addition to incidence rate and prevalence, it is necessary to define a third measurement to characterize the natural history of a disease. This measure is known as CASE FATALITY.[3]

$$\text{Case fatality} = \frac{\text{Number of deaths from a disease}}{\substack{\text{Number of individuals diagnosed with the} \\ \text{disease at the beginning of the time period}}}$$

Case fatality, unlike incidence rates, is affected by the success of clinical interventions designed to cure disease. Because case fatality measures the probability of failing to survive once the disease has developed, case fatality may be helpful in assessing prognosis. Case fatality over a period of time has an important relationship to mortality rates caused by a specific disease. Mortality rates measure the number of deaths from a disease in a particular year divided by the number of individuals in the population.[4] Mortality rate is related to incidence rate and case fatality as follows:

$$\text{Mortality rate} = \text{Incidence rate} \times \text{Case fatality}$$

This is a helpful relationship because mortality rates are often available. The data needed for the numerator of a mortality rate are available from death certificates, and population numbers for the denominator can often be estimated from census data.

Failure to appreciate this relationship may lead to the type of confusion illustrated in the following situation:

> In a study of the rates of duodenal ulcer disease, the authors properly obtained the mortality rates from duodenal ulcers in the United States in 1959 and 1999. In 1959, the yearly mortality rate was 5 per 1,000,000 person-years; in 1999, it was 1 per

---

[3]Case fatality is a proportion when referring to the probability of eventually dying from a disease. Case fatality is used as a proportion when it is multiplied by incidence rate to produce the mortality rate. Case fatality is a special form of risk that measures the cumulative probability of death from a disease.

[4]Technically mortality rates like incidence rates include person-years at risk in the denominator. However, like incidence rates the denominator is estimated by using the number of individuals in the population at one point in time, ideally the midpoint of the time interval under investigation.

1,000,000 person-years. Further study revealed that neither the incidence rate nor the prevalence of duodenal ulcers had changed. The authors could not make sense of these data.

Based on the relationship between incidence rates and mortality rates, the decline in mortality rate must have been due to a reduced case fatality. This decrease may reflect progress over 40 years in keeping alive those with duodenal ulcers even if there has been no progress in reducing the incidence rate of new duodenal ulcers.

Incidence rates, prevalence, and case fatality measure the chances of developing new cases of a disease per unit of time, the probability of having the disease at a point in time, and the probability of dying from the disease once it is diagnosed. In addition to these basic measures, the health literature often uses a measurement known as the PROPORTIONATE MORTALITY RATIO, which is defined as follows:[5]

$$\frac{\text{Proportionate}}{\text{mortality ratio}} = \frac{\text{Number of individuals dying from the disease}}{\text{Number of individuals dying from all diseases}}$$

The proportionate mortality ratio measures the probability that a death is due to a particular cause. Proportionate mortality ratios are a useful means of determining which are the most common causes of death in a particular group. They do not, however, tell us about the probability of death, as illustrated in the next scenario:

A well-designed study revealed that trauma was the cause of death in 4% of people older than 65 years and in 25% of children younger than 3 years. The authors concluded that those older than 65 years have a much lower probability of dying from trauma than those younger than 3 years.

The fact that people older than 65 years have a lower proportionate mortality ratio from trauma does not necessarily mean that the elderly have a lower probability of dying from trauma. Because many more deaths occur among people older than 65 years, even the 4% dying from trauma may represent a mortality rate from trauma that approximates the mortality rate among children younger than 3 years.

Having examined the types of measurements that are most commonly found in the health literature, let us turn our attention to the methods for obtaining measurements of disease.

[5]RATIO is a generic term used to indicate a measurement with a numerator and denominator. A proportion is a special type of ratio in which the numerator is a subset of the denominator. The proportionate mortality ratio is actually a proportion.

22 Sampling of Rates

Under some circumstances, it is possible to determine every case of a disease in a population. Mortality rates usually can be obtained on entire populations because death certificates are mandatory legal documents. It is often possible, therefore, to obtain the complete death rates or mortality rates from a disease for an entire population. For most diseases, however, it is not feasible to count every case of the disease in an entire population of interest; thus, the techniques of sampling are very helpful. SAMPLING ideally means that an investigator randomly selects a representative portion of the population, studies this sample, and then tries to extrapolate the results to the entire population intended for study.

Sampling Error

Even when properly performed, the process of sampling is not perfect. To appreciate the process and the inherent error introduced by sampling, one must understand the basic principle that underlies sampling techniques. This principle states that if many random samples are obtained, measures calculated from data in those samples on the average will be the same as the measurement in the original population. In other words, each sample may differ from the original population either by having a higher or a lower measurement. For example, the following shows an original population proportion of 10 per 1,000:

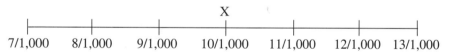

If samples of 1,000 persons were taken from this original population, the proportions might look like this:

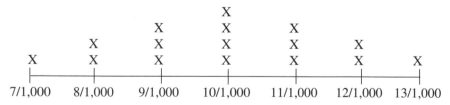

Notice that whereas some of the proportions obtained in particular samples are equal to the proportion in the original population, many of them are either higher or lower. Because samples are accurate only on the average, a single sample is said to possess an inherent sampling error. The spread or dispersion of the numerical values obtained from many samples can be summarized in a measurement known as a STANDARD ERROR. Thus, the standard error measures the size of the sample error. Failure to appreciate the existence of sampling error can lead to the following type of misinterpretation:

> A national organization attempted to estimate the prevalence of *Streptococcus* carriers by culturing a random sample of 0.1% of all school children in the nation. To verify their results, the same organization used a second random sample of 0.1% of the nation's schools and conducted a second survey using an identical protocol. The first survey revealed a prevalence of 15 per 1,000 positive strep cultures; the second survey revealed a prevalence of 10 per 1,000. The authors concluded that the inconsistent results were impossible because they had used the same methodology.

The authors failed to take into account the fact that sampling has an inherent error. This sampling error may explain the differences observed in the two samples. This example merely points out that two identically obtained samples may produce different results on the basis of chance alone. Remember that large numbers of samples, on the average, produce measurements that are identical with the true numerical value for the population, but any two samples may vary widely from one another and from the true numerical value in the larger population.

Sample Size

A second important principle in understanding sampling is that the more individuals who are included in a sample, the more likely a particular sample's measurement will closely approximate the numerical value in the larger population. Thus, it is the size of the sample that largely determines how close the sample's measurement is likely to be to the value in the larger population. This is not surprising because when everyone in the population is included in the sample, the sample's measurement is guaranteed to equal the population's value.

Let us look more closely at this principle. An important factor affecting the size of the sampling error is the size of the sample. Increasing the size of the sample decreases the effects of chance on the results. That is, it will reduce the random error and thus increase precision. Therefore, with a larger sample, the estimate obtained from the sample can be expected to be closer to the population's value. The relationship between the sample size and precision is not one to one; it is a square root function. As the sample gets larger, diminishing returns set in, and small or moderate increases in sample size may add little to the precision of the estimate. Investigators, therefore, attempt to balance the need for precision against the financial costs of increasing the sample size. The consequence of using small sample sizes is that the sample estimates may vary widely from one sample to another and from the true numerical value in the larger population. The following example illustrates the need to take into account the effects of the sample's size on the results of sampling:

> An investigator who sampled 0.01% of the nation's death certificates found that the mortality rate from pancreatic cancer was 50 per 100,000 person-years. A second investigator who sampled 1% of the nation's death certificates concluded that the true mortality rate for the nation was 80 per 100,000 person-years. To settle this dispute, the second investigator identified all deaths from pancreatic cancer in the country. He obtained a rate of 79 per 100,000 person-years. The second investigator concluded that the first investigator had performed his study fraudulently.

The first study used a sample size only one hundredth as large as the second study; therefore, it is likely that the sampling error of the first study was much larger. The fact that the second large sample turned out to be closer to the population's value is most likely due to its larger size rather than to fraud.

Random Sampling

In addition to the two important principles of sampling, one further point is left to consider. These two principles rest on the assumption that the sampling has been randomly obtained, meaning that all individuals in the population have an equal probability (or at least a known probability) of being chosen for inclusion in the sample. Unless random sampling is performed, one cannot accurately estimate how close the sample's results are to those of the larger population. The need for random sampling is illustrated in the following example:

> An investigator from one county hospital estimated that the community's rate of myocardial infarction was 150 per 100,000 person-years. An investigator at a private hospital in the same community estimated that the rate was 155 per 100,000 person-years. Because their results were similar, the investigators concluded that the rate of myocardial infarctions in their community must be between 150 and 155 per 100,000 person-years.

Neither of these studies attempted to obtain a random sample of the larger community or population. It is possible that myocardial infarction patients either selectively chose these two hospitals or selectively avoided them. If all the area hospitals were included in the sample, the rate of myocardial infarction might have been quite different. The rates in this example were calculated from conveniently available data known as CONVENIENCE SAMPLING. It is the simplest sampling to perform because the investigators merely calculate the rates for an easily available sample. The nonrepresentativeness of a convenience sample, however, means that it cannot be easily or reliably extrapolated to a larger population.[1]

When obtaining a random sample, investigators often permit all individuals in the population to have an equal probability of being selected for inclusion in the sample. This is known as a SIMPLE RANDOM SAMPLE. Many investigators have found that if they rely exclusively on simple random sampling, they fail to include enough individuals who possess the characteristics of interest for their study. For instance, if investigators are studying the rates of hypertension in the United States, they may be especially interested in the rates of hypertension for African-Americans or Asians. If they merely obtained a simple random sample of the population, it may not include many African-Americans or Asians.

Therefore, investigators could separately sample from American-Africans, from Asians, and from the rest of the population. This separate procedure of obtaining random samples from the different subsets or strata of the population is known as STRATIFIED RANDOM SAMPLING. It is permissible and often desirable as long as the sampling within each group is random. There are separate statistical methods for use with stratified samples.

---

[1]Occasionally, we are forced to make extrapolations from convenience samples. The most common example occurs when we want to extrapolate research observations to patients seen in the future. Time is one aspect of a population that cannot be randomly sampled.

Let us review the principles and requirements for sampling:

1. On the average, samples drawn from a population will have the same rate as in the original population. There is, however, an inherent sampling error introduced by using chance to select a portion of the population to be included in the sample.
2. The size of the sampling error is affected by the size of the sample obtained. Increasing the sample size decreases the size of the sampling error, but diminishing returns set in as we continue to increase the size of the sample.
3. The principles of sampling rest on the assumption that samples are randomly obtained. It is permissible to ensure adequate numbers in each category of interest by stratified sampling. However, sampling must be random within each category or stratum. If random sampling is not performed, no method exists for reliably relating the rate obtained in the sample to the true rate of the larger population from which the sample was drawn.[2]

[2]Inferences from samples are still obtained, even when random samples are not used in an investigation. When a nonrandom sample is used and inference is attempted, we are really drawing inferences about a population of individuals like those in the nonrandom sample.

23 Standardization of Rates

In the previous chapter, we outlined the requirements for obtaining rates using random sampling. In this chapter, we attempt to compare rates. We assume that the rates have been properly obtained and illustrate the precautions that must be observed in comparing rates, even those that are measured using proper random sampling techniques.

We compare rates from samples of two different groups. These groups may be two health plans, two cities, two countries, two industries, or the same health plan, city, country, or industry compared at different points in time. We compare rates to determine how much they differ between populations or how much they change over time. These comparisons are important for rates derived from sampling as well as for rates determined by using an entire population.

When using rates to compare probabilities or the chance of developing disease, it is important to consider whether the populations differ by a factor that is already known to affect the chance of developing the disease. This consideration is the same as adjusting for confounding variables, as discussed previously.

In performing a study, the investigator may already know that factors such as age, sex, or race affect the rate of developing a particular disease. The investigator should then adjust for, or standardize, the rates for these factors. The importance of what is called STANDARDIZATION can be seen in the incidence rate of lung cancer. Because age is a known risk factor for lung cancer, little is gained by discovering that a retirement community has a higher incidence rate of lung cancer than the rest of the community. Likewise, if one industry has a younger workforce than a second industry, it is misleading to compare the lung cancer incidence rate in the two industries directly, especially if one wishes to draw conclusions about the safety of working conditions.

To circumvent this problem, rates of disease can be adjusted to take into account the factors that are already known to greatly affect the rates through standardization of rates. Age is the most common factor used for standardization, but we can adjust for any factor that differs between groups and is known to affect the probability of developing the disease. For instance, to compare the rates of hypertension in two groups in order to study the importance of the mineral content of drinking water, one might adjust for race because blacks are known to have a higher rate of hypertension.

The principle used in standardizing rates is the same as that used to adjust for the differences in study groups discussed in Part 1, *Studying a Study*. Investigators compare rates among individuals who are similar in age or any other factor that is being adjusted. Before illustrating the method used for adjustment, let us see how misleading results can occur if standardization is not performed.

The incidence rate of pancreatic cancer in the United States was compared with the incidence rate in Mexico. The rate in the United States was found to be three times higher than the rate in Mexico per 100,000 person-years. The authors concluded that US residents have a rate of pancreatic cancer three times higher than the rate among Mexicans, assuming that the accuracy of diagnosis was equal in the two countries.

This interpretation of this study is superficially correct; if the data are accurate, the risk of pancreatic cancer is higher in the United States. However, pancreatic cancer is known to occur more often in older persons. It may be that the younger average age of the Mexican population accounts for the difference in rates of pancreatic cancer. This may be an important issue if we are examining the cause of pancreatic cancer. If the age distribution does not explain these differences, the investigators may have detected an important unexpected difference that requires further explanation. Thus, the authors should standardize their data for age and see whether the differences persist.

Standardization of rates is often performed comparing a special sample that is being studied to the general population. In performing this type of standardization, we often use the INDIRECT METHOD. This method compares the observed number of events, such as deaths in the sample of interest, to the number that would have been expected if the study sample had the same age distribution as the general population. When death is the outcome of interest, the indirect method produces a ratio known as the STANDARDIZED MORTALITY RATIO.

$$\text{Standardized mortality ratio} \ = \ \frac{\text{Observed number of deaths}}{\text{Expected number of deaths}}$$

The standardized mortality ratio is a useful means of comparing a sample from a population of interest to the general population. When interpreting this ratio, however, it is important to remember that a special population under study is often one that is not expected to have the same mortality rate as the general population.

For instance, when comparing a group of employed individuals to the general population, it is important to remember that employment often requires that individuals be healthy or at least not disabled. The need to take into account this employment effect is illustrated in the next example:

A study of new workers at a chemical plant found a standardized mortality ratio of 1 for all causes of death. The investigator concluded that because the standardized mortality ratio was 1, the chemical plant was free of health risks to the workers.

When interpreting this study, it is important to remember that new workers are often healthier than persons in the general population. This phenomenon is so common that it has been called the HEALTHY WORKER EFFECT. Thus, we would expect them to have a somewhat lower mortality rate than the general population or a standardized mortality ratio of less than 1. This standardized mortality ratio of 1 may fail to reflect hazards to these generally healthy workers.

When two groups from a population are under study or when changes over time in a population are being assessed, it is possible and desirable to use the direct method of standardization. The direct method works as follows: Suppose investigators wish to compare the incidence of bladder cancer in two large industries. The bladder cancer data for the two industries are shown in Table 23.1. Notice that the overall rates for both samples are 200 per 100,000 workers per year. Also, notice that the rates for each age group are as high or higher in industry A than in industry B. Despite the lower rates for each age group in industry B, it may at first seem surprising that the overall incidences are the same. However, looking at the number of individuals in each age group, it becomes apparent that industry A has a much younger workforce than industry B. Industry B has 60,000 workers from ages 50 to 70 years; industry A has only 30,000 workers in these age groups. Because bladder cancer is known to increase with age, the younger age of industry A's workforce reduces the overall rates in industry A. Thus, it is misleading to look only at the overall rates because industry B's overall rate is increased by its older age structure. This is especially true if we are asking about the safety of the industry environment itself.

To avoid this problem, the authors must standardize the rates to adjust for the differences in age and thereby compare the rates more fairly. To accomplish standardization, each sample is subdivided to indicate the number of individuals, the number of cases of the disease, and the incidence rate in each age group. When data are divided into groups using a characteristic such as age, each age group is known as a STRATUM. This is also shown in Table 23.1.

The authors then must attempt to determine how many cases of bladder cancer would have occurred in industry A if the age distribution was the same as in industry B. The steps in this process are as follows:[1]

1. Starting with the 20- to 30-year-old age group, the authors take the rate of cancer for that group in industry A and multiply it by the number of individuals in the corresponding age group in industry B. This produces the number of cases that would have occurred in industry A if it had the same number of individuals in that age group as industry B.
2. The authors then perform this calculation for each age group and calculate the total number of cases from the different age groups. This produces a total num-

Table 23.1. *Comparison of incidence rates of bladder cancer*

Age	Number of Individuals	Number of Cases of Bladder Cancer per Year	Incidence Rate of Bladder Cancer in Each Age Group[a]
Industry A			
20–30	20,000	0	0 per 100,000
30–40	20,000	10	50 per 100,000
40–50	30,000	20	67 per 100,000
50–60	20,000	80	400 per 100,000
60–70	10,000	90	900 per 100,000
Total	100,000	200	200 per 100,000
Industry B			
20–30	10,000	0	0 per 100,000
30–40	10,000	4	40 per 100,000
40–50	20,000	6	30 per 100,000
50–60	50,000	140	280 per 100,000
60–70	10,000	50	500 per 100,000
Total	100,000	200	200 per 100,000

[a]The incidence rate is obtained from the number of cases and the number of individuals in the age group. The incidence rates cannot be added down the column.

[1]The method illustrated is not necessarily the only or best method to use for standardization. For statistical purposes, it is common to weight the strata by the inverse of the variance of the estimate in each strata as is done in the Mantel-Haenzel method.

ber of cases that would have occurred if industry A had the same overall age distribution as industry B.

3. The authors now have standardized the rates for age and can directly compare the number of cases that occurred in industry B with the number of cases that would have occurred in industry A if industry A had the same age distribution as industry B. The authors have now age-adjusted industry A to industry B's age distribution.[2]

Let us apply these procedures to the bladder cancer data shown in Table 23.2.

If the age distribution was the same as industry B, 308 cases of bladder cancer would have occurred in industry A, but only 200 actually occurred in industry B. These figures are better measures for comparing the workers' risk of developing bladder cancer in each industry than are the unadjusted incident rates. The adjusted numbers accentuate the fact that, despite the equality of the overall rates, industry A has a rate as high or higher in each age group. Therefore, to make fair comparisons between populations that differ by age and where age is known to affect the incidence rate of developing disease, it is necessary to age-standardize the samples. If additional factors are also known to affect the rates, the same process can be applied to standardize or adjust for these factors.

Notice, however, that in performing standardization, the calculations give special emphasis to the largest strata. Thus, if there has been a substantial change in only one stratum, especially a small stratum, this effort can easily be lost in the process of standardization. In addition, progress may be made by delaying death. When death from a particular cause is moved from a younger to an older age group, this effect is not recognized by the process of standardization, as illustrated in the following study:

> A study of the mortality rates from cystic fibrosis was conducted to determine whether progress in therapy for children was reflected in these mortality rates in a large state with a stable population distribution. A comparison of data from 1969 and 1999 is shown in Table 23.3.

Notice in this example that the mortality rate from cystic fibrosis for those 0 to 10 and 10 to 20 years of age has fallen between 1969 and 1999. However, the

Table 23.2. *Method of age standardization*

Age Group	Incidence Rate of Bladder Cancer in Industry A	Number of Individuals in Industry B	Number of Cases That Would Occur in Industry A if It Had the Same Age Distribution as Industry B[a]	Number of Cases of Bladder Cancer That Actually Occurred in Industry B
20–30	0/100,000	10,000	0	0
30–40	50/100,000	10,000	5	4
40–50	67/100,000	20,000	13	6
50–60	400/100,000	50,000	200	140
60–70	900/100,000	10,000	90	50
Total		100,000	308	200

[a]This column is calculated by multiplying the previous two columns.

[2]It is also possible to age-adjust the opposite way, thus age-adjusting industry B to industry A's age distribution. The general conclusion would be the same; however, the estimates would be different.

Table 23.3. *Comparison of mortality rates from cystic fibrosis: 1969 and 1999*

Age (yr)	Mortality Rate per 100,000 Person-Years	Number in Age Group	Total No. of Deaths in One Year
		1969	
0–10	5/100,000	1,000,000	50
10–20	10/100,000	1,000,000	100
20–40	1/100,000	2,000,000	20
Total		4,000,000	170
		1999	
0–10	3/100,000	1,000,000	30
10–20	6/100,000	1,000,000	60
20–40	4/100,000	2,000,000	80
Total		4,000,000	170

mortality rate from cystic fibrosis among 20- to 40-year-olds has increased from 1969 to 1999. This increase is balanced by the decrease among younger individuals so that the overall crude mortality rates in both years were 170 per 4,000,000 or 4.25 per 100,000 person-years. It is attempting to try to standardize these mortality rates and obtain an adjusted measure of mortality rate. However, if we were to standardize by applying the 1999 age distribution to the 1969 mortality rates (or vice versa), the results after adjustment would be no different from the overall crude rates before adjustment. This occurs because the 1969 and 1999 populations have the same age distribution.

Unfortunately, standardization does not help us to see what is happening here. The unadjusted and the standardized rates both obscure the fact that a substantial decrease in mortality rates has occurred among 0- to 10-year-olds and 10- to 20-year-olds, whereas an increase has occurred among 20- to 40-year-olds. To recognize that this change has occurred, it is necessary to look directly at the actual data for each age group.[3]

It is important to appreciate that both crude and age-adjusted rates may fail to reveal differences or changes that occur in only one or a few age groups. Changes in one age group are especially likely to be missed when other age groups are changing in opposite directions.

These opposing changes frequently occur when death is being delayed until an older age but cure does not occur. This principle is important to understand to appreciate the error in the following study:

> An investigator studied a new treatment for breast cancer that prolonged the survival of women with stage II breast cancer by an average of 5 years. He confidently predicted that if his new treatment was widely applied, the overall age-adjusted mortality rate from breast cancer would dramatically fall over the next 20 years.

This investigator failed to recognize that when life is prolonged but death is moved to later years, this does not necessarily result in progressively improving overall age-adjusted mortality rates. Despite the success of this new breast-cancer therapy,

---

[3]The changes with age are an example of INTERACTIONS or EFFECT MODIFICATION between age and mortality rates. In general, standardization or adjustment for confounding does not necessarily take into account the effects of interaction or effect modification.

the authors are not claiming cure. When life is prolonged, individuals may die of the disease at an older age. When this occurs, the breast-cancer mortality rates in the younger age groups may fall, whereas the breast-cancer mortality rates in the older age groups may rise. Thus, the overall age-adjusted mortality rates may not reveal the progress that has been made. Therefore, adjusted mortality rates do not give us the entire picture. They are not an ideal way to compare populations or to compare the same populations at two or more points in time. In Chapter 25, we turn our attention to a better measure for making these comparisons, known as life expectancy. First, however, we examine how to compare rates to draw conclusions about differences or changes in rates of disease.

24 Sources of Differences in Rates

In this chapter, we will take a look at reasons for differences or changes in rates. We will assume that it has been established that two groups in a population have different rates of a particular disease or alternatively there has been a change in the rates over time in the same group.

Artifactual Differences or Changes

The differences in rates may be the result of real changes in the natural history of the disease itself, or they may reflect changes or differences in the method by which the particular disease is assessed. ARTIFACTUAL DIFFERENCES imply that, despite the fact that a difference exists, it does not reflect changes in the disease but merely in the way the disease is measured, sought, or defined.

Artifactual changes result from three sources:

1. Changes in the ability to recognize the disease. These represent changes in the measurement of the disease.
2. Changes in the efforts to recognize disease. These may represent efforts to recognize the disease at an earlier stage, changes in reporting requirements, or new incentives to search for the disease.
3. Changes in the definition of the disease. These represent changes in the terminology used to define the disease.

The following example illustrates the first type of artifactual change, the effect of a change in the ability to recognize a disease:

> Because of a recent increase in interest, a study of the prevalence of mitral valve prolapse was performed. A complete survey of the charts at a major university cardiac clinic found that in 1968 only 1 per 1,000 patients had a diagnosis of mitral valve prolapse, whereas in 1998, 80 per 1,000 had mitral valve prolapse included in their diagnoses. The authors concluded that the condition was increasing to an astounding prevalence.

Between 1968 and 1998, the use of echocardiography greatly increased the ability to document mitral valve prolapse. In addition, the growing recognition of the frequency of this condition led to a much better understanding of how to recognize it by physical examination. It is not surprising then that a much larger proportion of cardiac clinic patients was known to have mitral valve prolapse in 1998 compared with 1968. It is possible that if an equal understanding and equal technology were available in 1968, the prevalence would have been nearly identical. This example demonstrates that artifactual changes may explain large differences in the prevalence of disease even when a complete review of all cases is used to calculate the prevalence of disease.

Changes in the efforts to recognize disease may occur when the available treatment improves, as illustrated in the next example:

> A new treatment for migraine headache is approved for use and widely advertised in the medical journals and advertisements in major newspapers. The number of patients presenting for care with migraine headaches doubles in the year after approval of the new drug. These patients meet all the criteria for a diagnosis of migraine.

This apparent doubling of the prevalence of migraine is most likely due to the increased proportion of individuals with migraine headache who present for care after becoming aware of the new treatment. A high proportion of individuals with many self-limited or nonprogressive diseases do not seek health care. Changes in the types of patients who seek care can produce dramatic but artifactual changes in the rates.

The following example illustrates how the meaning of terminology may change over time and thus produce an artifactual change in the apparent rate of events:

> The incidence rate of AIDS increased every year between 1981 and 1990. In one year during the early 1990s, there was a sudden dramatic increase in the reported rate. One investigator interpreted this sudden increase as a sign that the epidemic had suddenly entered a new phase.

The dramatic increase may have been due to a change in the Centers for Disease Control and Prevention's definition of AIDS, which meant that more individuals with human immunodeficiency virus infection fell within the definition of AIDS. When sudden changes in the incidence rate of a disease occur, one must suspect artifactual changes, such as changes in the definition of a disease. In this case, one suspects that an artifactual change was superimposed on an actual change, complicating the interpretation of the data.

Actual Changes

Artifactual changes in rates imply that the true incidence prevalence or case fatality has not been altered even though superficially a change appears to have occurred. Actual changes, however, imply that the incidence, prevalence, or case fatality have changed. We first must ask whether any of the sources of artifactual differences are operating. If they are not operating or are not large enough to explain the differences, one can assume that actual differences or changes exist. Having concluded that actual differences or changes have occurred, we need to ask why these changes occur. Do they reflect a change in incidence, prevalence, case fatality, or a combination of these measurements?

The first step in understanding the meaning of an actual change in rates is to understand where in the natural history of the disease a change occurred. Then we can better appreciate the effects of the primary changes on the other rates of disease, as in the following cases:

1. The case fatality for Hodgkin's disease has dramatically decreased in recent years. Individuals are considered to have the disease until they demonstrate evidence of cure in long-term follow-up. Thus, the prevalence of Hodgkin's disease has increased. The incidence has remained stable; therefore, the mortality rates, which reflect the incidence rates multiplied by the case fatality, have fallen.

2. Lung-cancer incidence rates among women have increased dramatically over recent decades. The case fatality, however, has remained very high, with most patients dying within months of diagnosis. Thus, the mortality rates have also

increased dramatically. Because of the short duration of the disease, the prevalence has always been low; however, with the increased incidence rate of disease, it has risen slightly.

We might diagram these results as follows:

	Mortality Rates	Case Fatality	Incidence Rates	Prevalence
Hodgkin's disease	↓	↓↓↓	→	↑↑
Lung cancer	↑ ↑	→	↑ ↑	↑

These confusing patterns make sense when one recognizes that the primary change in Hodgkin's disease has been the decreased case fatality, whereas the primary change in lung cancer has been the increased incidence rate.

In addition to understanding the source of the differences or changes in rates, it is often tempting to use past changes in rates to predict future rates of disease.

Predicting future rates from current rates or recent changes in rates, or both, is extremely difficult. A recent change in rates may have any of the following meanings: (1) the changes may herald future changes in the same direction; (2) they may reflect predictable cycles or epidemics; or (3) they may be the result of unpredictable fluctuations representing an unusual frequency of events. Before concluding that observed changes in rates are likely to continue, one must consider the possibility of cyclic fluctuations. If a natural cycle occurs in the frequency of the disease, the incidence from year to year may look like that presented in Figure 24.1.

If investigators note the increase that occurred between 1990 and 1993, they may attempt to measure the changes between 1993 and 1996 and would again find an increase. It is important, however, that investigators realize that this actual change between 1990 and 1996 may be part of the natural cycle of disease. It does not necessarily imply that a further increase can be expected in future years.

As opposed to this predictable cycle of disease, there may be an unpredictable, random variation in the rate of disease from year to year (Figure 24.2). In this situation, if investigators select a year when the rate was higher and compare it with the next year, when by chance alone the rate was lower, they may believe they are documenting important changes when, in fact, they are merely discovering the statistical principle of REGRESSION TO THE MEAN. Regression to the mean or return to the average states that unusual values are by definition rare events, and the chances are against a repetition of a rare event twice in a row. In fact, by chance alone or random fluctuations, the next measurement is likely to be nearer the average value.

Subsequent values may be less extreme because of random fluctuation of events or because of biological, social, psychological, or economic adaptive forces that react to the unusual rate. Thus, both chance and reactive forces move the subsequent rate toward the average or mean. For instance, if one were studying how much an individual eats per meal, it is likely that the meal following a particularly indulgent one would be smaller than usual. Let us see how this principle may operate in a study of rates that produced actual differences, but differences that need to be carefully interpreted.

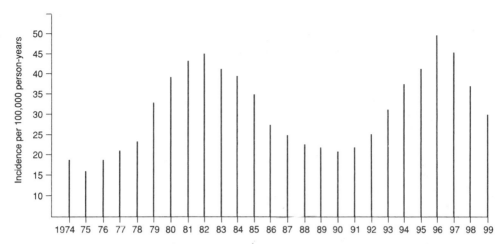

Figure 24.1. Predictable cycles or epidemics in the yearly incidence of a disease.

After a tragic accident that killed several men in a factory, an accident prevention program was initiated. Investigators found that the incidence rate of accidents at the time of the tragedy was unusually high: 10 per 1,000 worker-days. The rate fell to 2 per 1,000 worker-days when the program was established. The investigators concluded that the accident prevention program was an enormous success.

The investigators have shown that an actual change took place. They have not, however, shown that it was the accident prevention program that caused the change. It is possible that the 10 per 1, 000 worker-day rate was unusually high and by chance alone returned to a more usual rate of 2 per 1,000 worker-days. Even more likely, the fatal accident may have frightened the workers into taking more safety precautions. The authors started with an unusually high accident rate, and then a tragedy occurred that may have produced adaptive changes in behavior, which resulted in the rate dropping back toward the mean or average. It is premature to conclude that the accident prevention program would help other groups or even this group if it was instituted at another time. Thus, the principle of regression to the mean and adaptive changes may be the source of actual changes in rates

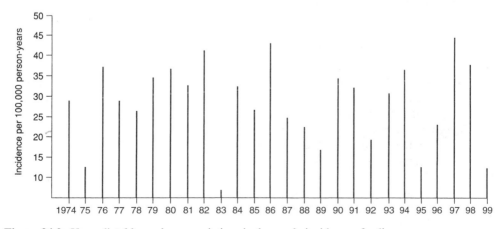

Figure 24.2. Unpredictable or chance variations in the yearly incidence of a disease.

in this example, but this source may imply that observed changes are not guaranteed to continue.

It is common for an investigation or an intervention to be initiated because of a suspicion that the rates of disease are increasing. Thus, it is important to recognize the phenomenon of regression to the mean and adaptive changes because they may start operating whenever short-term changes in rates are observed.

Another source of actual differences that affects prediction of future events is known as the COHORT EFFECT. A cohort is a group of individuals who share a common experience or exposure. If one or several cohorts in a population have had an exposure or experience that makes them particularly susceptible to disease at a future point in time, then the possibility of a cohort effect exists. The rates for a particular age group, which include the susceptible cohort, may be temporarily increased. This temporary increase is known as the cohort effect. When a cohort effect is present, one can expect the rates for this particular age group to fall again as time passes and the susceptible cohort moves beyond this particular age group. The importance of appreciating the cohort effect is illustrated in the following example:

> An investigator was studying the incidence rate of thyroid cancer. Concern existed that past pediatric head and neck radiation, frequently used until the 1950s, was a contributor to thyroid cancers. Using proper methods, the authors found that the incidence rate of thyroid cancer among 30- to 40-year-olds in 1960 was 50 per 100,000 person-years; in 1968 it was 100 per 100,000 person-years; and in 1980 it was 150 per 100,000 person-years. The authors concluded that by 1990, the rates would pass the 200 per 100,000 person-years mark. The authors were surprised to find that the incidence rate in 1990 was less than 150 per 100,000 person-years and continued to decline during the 1990s.

The authors have established that actual changes were occurring in the incidence rates of thyroid cancer in the 30- to 40-year-old age group. The source of these changes may be a cohort effect. The cohort of individuals who were radiated before 1950 carried an increased probability of thyroid cancer that did not necessarily affect those individuals who were born after 1950. By 1990, all individuals in the 30- to 40-year age group would have been born after 1950. Thus, it is not surprising to observe a decline in the incidence rate of thyroid cancer in 30- to 40-year-olds rather than a continued rise. The concept of a cohort effect not only helps predict the expected future rates, but it also helps to support the theory that past radiation increased the incidence rate of thyroid cancer.

Regression to the mean and the cohort effect are two reasons why it is dangerous to predict future rates of disease by direct extrapolation from recent changes in rates. In addition to the comparison of rates in samples from the same group over time, it is also possible to use rates to examine differences between samples from different groups. Comparison of rates in groups is often done to generate hypotheses that can then be evaluated by the types of investigations discussed in Part 1, *Studying a Study*. Investigators, for instance, might note differences in rates of coronary artery disease mortality among Alaskan Native Americans and Alaskan whites. From what they know about the diet of Alaskan Native Americans, they might hypothesize a group association between fish consumption and reduced coronary artery mortality even though they do not have data on the diet of individuals.

By comparing the rates of disease and adjusting for known risk factors, it is possible to establish that a factor is increased in one group and the probability of a disease is also increased in the same group. This allows us to establish GROUP ASSOCIATIONS. A group association means that in a particular group, the factor and the disease are both present at an increased rate. Note that a group association does not necessarily mean that those individuals with the factor are the same individuals as those with the disease.

Establishing the existence of a group association may lay the groundwork for subsequent studies that establish an association at the individual level and eventually a cause-and-effect relationship, such as in the case of cholesterol and coronary artery disease.

When using group data, the investigators frequently have little information about the individuals who comprise the group. Thus, when comparing rates to develop a hypothesis for further study at the individual level, investigators must be careful not to imply an association among individuals when only a group association has been established. This type of error, known as an ECOLOGICAL FALLACY, is illustrated in the following example:

> A study demonstrated that the rate of drowning in Florida is four times higher than in Illinois. The study data also demonstrated that in Florida, ice cream is consumed at a rate four times that of Illinois. The authors concluded that eating ice cream is associated with drowning.

To establish an individual association, the authors must first demonstrate that those who eat more ice cream are the ones who are more likely to drown. Relying on group figures alone does not provide any information about the existence of an association at the individual level. It may not be people who eat more ice cream who drown. The greater consumption of ice cream may merely reflect the confounding variable known as warm weather, which increases ice cream consumption and drowning. These authors committed an ecological fallacy. The establishment of an individual association between eating ice cream and drowning requires a demonstration that the relationship holds on an individual level.

When faced with differences in rates between groups or changes over time in the same group, the first step is to establish whether the difference or changes are artifactual or actual. If it is not likely that the differences or changes are due to the way the disease is measured, sought, or defined, the changes or differences should be considered to be actual or real. The source of the differences or changes is then sought in one or more of the three basic measurements: incidence, prevalence, or case fatality. Changes or differences in rates are often used to predict future changes and also to form hypotheses about the cause of disease to be used as the basis for studies of individuals. When predicting future rates, regression to the mean, adaptive changes, and the cohort effect must be taken into account. When using rates in groups to develop hypotheses, it must be recognized that the use of group rates establishes group and not individual association. Failure to appreciate the distinction between group and individual association may lead to an ecological fallacy.

25 Putting It Together:

Measuring Life Expectancy

Rates and proportions are the fundamental tools for comparing the health of populations. They can be used to compare the health of a population in one year with that of another. In addition, they can be used to compare the health of one population, such as a nation, with the health of another population, or nation.

Traditionally, the health of nations has been measured by taking into account only mortality. Data have not generally been available to incorporate morbidity and its impact on the quality of life. The fundamental measurement tool for comparing mortality is called LIFE EXPECTANCY. Unlike the other measurements discussed, life expectancy has the ability to take into account prolongations in life that still result in death.[1]

Life expectancy is a summary that combines the probabilities of death or mortality rates for each year of age in a population. Approximations of these mortality rates are available if a nation has two forms of data: (1) adequate data from death records in a particular year indicating the age of the individuals who died (*e.g.*, in each year, there must be death records available for everyone who died, indicating their age at the time of death); (2) data must be available from a census or other source estimating the number of individuals at each year of age at a point in time during the year.[2]

The number of deaths at a particular age divided by the total number of individuals of the same age in the population tells us the probability of death at each year of age. This probability is the key to the calculation of life expectancy. Life expectancy calculations usually also include data on gender and racial groups. Separate life expectancies are then calculated for each gender and racial group.

Life expectancy is calculated using what are called CROSS-SECTIONAL or CURRENT LIFE TABLES. These tables represent a snapshot view at one point in time. They are different than the life tables discussed in Chapter 9, which follow study and control groups over a period of time. Life tables that monitor patients over time are called LONGITUDINAL or COHORT LIFE TABLES to distinguish them from cross-

---

[1]If a measuring system and adequate data are available to assess morbidity, or the reduction in quality of life as a result of disease, then it is possible to construct what has been called a DISEASE-ADJUSTED LIFE EXPECTANCY.

[2]Ideally, the number of individuals is available from the beginning of the time interval because this number would indicate the total number of individuals who are at risk for death during the subsequent year. Approximations based on census data from other years are often substituted. Notice that the cause of death is not important for calculating life expectancy.

sectional life tables, for which data all come from the same year. Unfortunately, both types are often called life tables.[3]

We previously summarized cohort or longitudinal life tables using a survival plot. Survival plots can be used to display the data from a cross-sectional life table. Figure 25.1 displays a survival plot from a hypothetical cross-sectional life table. Notice that the vertical axis starts with a population of 100,000 individuals who are alive at time zero. That is, it starts with 100,000 births.[4]

Thus, in calculating 1999 life expectancies, we are assuming that these 100,000 live births will live out their lives experiencing the probabilities of death of each of the life-table's component age groups in 1999. Thus, in 1999 the 0- to 1-year age group will experience the 1999 probability of death of the 0- to 1-year-olds in 1999. In 2000, the 1- to 2-year-olds will experience the probability of death of the 1- to 2-year-olds in 1999. Similarly, in 2001, the 2- to 3-year-olds will experience the probability of death of the 2- to 3-year-olds in 1999, and so on. Despite the fact

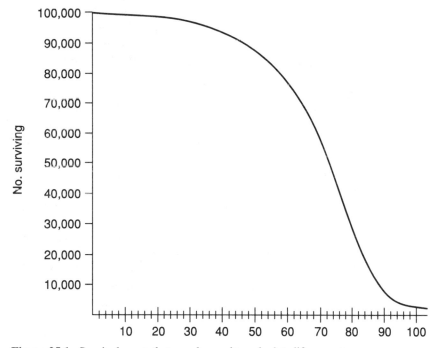

Figure 25.1. Survival curve that may be used to calculate life expectancy.

[3]Together, these two life tables can provide complementary information on life expectancy. Cross-sectional life tables provide information on life expectancy that is related to age, gender, and race, or the basic demographic data. Longitudinal life tables often provide information on life expectancy associated with a specific disease. These data together may be used to estimate the life expectancy for individuals of a particular age, gender, and race with a particular disease.

[4]The calculation of life expectancy requires us to visualize the existence of an imaginary population. This population is called a STATIONARY POPULATION. It consists of 100,000 individuals born alive in the year under consideration. These individuals are assumed to live out their lives in this population, leaving only because of death. No one is allowed to move in or out of this imaginary population. These 100,000 individuals are assumed to experience the probabilities of death observed for each age group during the year in which data are obtained.

Table 25.1. *Life expectancy for males in a developed country*

Age (yr)	Life Expectancy (yr)
0	75
20	57
40	38
65	15
75	10
80	6

that the individuals are aging, they are assumed to experience the probability of death of the year in which the data are collected.

The survival curve can be plotted by multiplying the probability of death at each age by the number of individuals who are still alive at the beginning of the time period. Thus, if .01, or 1%, of individuals have died during the first year, then 99,000 enter the second year of life. If the probability of death during the second year of life is .001, or .1%, then 99 individuals die during the second year, leaving 98,901 individuals entering the third year of life. Thus, it is possible to plot a survival curve indicating the number of individuals who are alive at the beginning of each year of age starting with a population of 100,000 live births.

The life expectancy can be calculated using the area under the survival curve. To calculate the life expectancy at birth, we can add together the total number of years of life lived by the original 100,000 live births and divide this number by the 100,000 live births to produce an average life span or what is called LIFE EXPECTANCY. Life expectancy at other ages such as 20 or 65 years or any other age can also be estimated in a similar way using the area under the curve starting at the age of interest. Thus, if we were trying to estimate the life expectancy at age 65, we would use the area under the survival curve for ages 65 years and older to calculate the number of years of life lived by those who have reached age 65 years. Then we would divide this number by the number of individuals who have reached age 65 years.[5]

The term *life expectancy* sounds like it should allow us to predict the future. However, the calculation of life expectancy assumes that everything in the future will remain the same; all individuals will remain in the same population; and the mortality rates will not change. This is unrealistic because the one predictable thing in life is the permanence of change. Thus, we must be careful in using life expectancy to predict the future just as we need to recognize that all probabilities calculated on the basis of current data may not hold true in the future. The implications for prediction are illustrated in the next example:

> The life expectancy in an underdeveloped nation was carefully obtained and calculated to be 45 years in 1975. Over the course of the next 25 years, using life expectancy to predict survival, the probabilities of death first indicated a survival

[5]Calculations are performed by starting with the stationary population of 100,000 and multiplying by the probability of death for the first time interval (usually the first year of life). Subtracting this number from 100,000 produces the number living at the beginning of the next age interval; that is, at age 1 year. This process is continued through each of the age intervals, producing a number living at the beginning of each age interval. Knowing the length of the age interval and the number of individuals alive at the beginning of the age interval, we can estimate the number of years of life spent in each age interval. We then add together the number of years spent in an age interval and all subsequent age intervals and divide this total by the number of individuals who enter that age interval. This allows us to calculate the life expectancy at any age we choose.

much better than expected and then indicated a subsequent decline over expected survival. The authors concluded that life expectancy measures have no value even if the data on which they are based are accurate.

Even if the data were accurately obtained, we would not expect it to predict the future perfectly. Perhaps the decline in infant mortality from diarrheal disease reduced the probabilities of death during the 1970s and 1980s. Then perhaps the AIDS epidemic took a high toll of deaths during the 1990s. Life expectancy measures are not designed to predict the future. They are useful for comparing one population with another in one particular year, such as 1999. They are also useful for comparing the same population in different years (*e.g.*, 1990 vs. 1999).

When life expectancy is calculated for different gender and racial groups, life expectancy measures may also be useful for comparing different groups within the same population. The presence of differences in life expectancy may be due to a variety of causes. Poorer quality or intensity of health services is one possible reason for these differences. They may also be due to genetic or socioeconomic effects which are not altered by health services.

When we speak of life expectancy, we usually mean the life expectancy at birth. Life expectancy at birth is the average number of years of remaining life for an individual born into our imaginary stationary population. Life expectancy at birth is not the only life expectancy that is usually available. Life expectancy at the beginning of any age can be calculated. For instance, examine Table 25.1, which might provide the life expectancies for males in a developed country.

Notice that the life expectancy at birth is 75 years. At age 65 years, the life expectancy is 15 years. If we add 65 years to the life expectancy at age 65, it is greater than the life expectancy at birth; the 15 years plus 65 years equals 80 years, which is greater than the 75-year life expectancy at birth. This phenomenon occurs because those who reach a particular age, such as 65 years, have already survived the potential for death at an earlier age. Whether they are biologically better survivors or just lucky, they will have a longer life expectancy than at the time of their birth when they face potential mortality during each year of life. Failure to appreciate this phenomenon can lead to the following misinterpretation:

> A conference on preventive health care for 80-year-olds proposed a series of health care procedures for all 80-year-olds in a nation with a life expectancy of 78 years. The national health system refused to consider paying for these preventive procedures, arguing that the individuals had already exceeded their life expectancy.

Remember, life expectancy for groups of individuals who survive to a particular age is greater than the life expectancy at birth. The life expectancy at an advanced age may be surprisingly long. For instance, note that in Table 25.1 the life expectancy at age 80 is 6 years.[6]

Using life expectancy to make recommendations for a particular individual is even more difficult than using life expectancy to make recommendations for the average member of a group, as illustrated in the next situation:

> A healthy 80-year-old man is considering elective surgery. Recognizing that the average life expectancy for 80-year-old men is 6 years, the physicians recommend against the surgery.

---

[6]Life expectancy at age 80 years may be a better predictor of the future for the average 80-year-old than life expectancy at a far younger age. This is the case because changes in the probability of death over a small number of years are usually modest compared with changes over a longer period of time.

The ability to predict the length of survival for a healthy 80-year-old man has very little to do with the average life expectancy of 80-year-old men. The life expectancy at 80 years for men takes into account all 80-year-old men, whether they are healthy or have life-threatening disease. Because of the high proportion of illness among 80-year-old men, those who are healthy constitute a very different group. Averaging the healthy and the sick together produces a life expectancy that may greatly underestimate the survival for the healthy individual.

In general, life expectancy is an average that combines data from the healthy and those with disease. The greater the proportion of those with disease, the less useful the life expectancy will be for making recommendations for the healthy individual.

The high probability of life-threatening diseases among the elderly can lead to another misinterpretation of life expectancy data. Reduction in one important cause of death among the elderly will not necessarily have a dramatic effect on life expectancy, as illustrated in the next example:

> A new cure for prostate cancer has nearly eliminated this frequent cause of death among elderly men. The investigators had expected a dramatic increase in the life expectancy among elderly men. To their surprise they found only a modest increase.

Unfortunately, among the elderly there are a number of competing causes of death. When one cause is reduced or eliminated, the other causes have the potential to increase in frequency. Other cancers or heart disease may increase and reduce the expected impact of eliminating one important cause of death. Thus, we must recognize the inherent limitation of life expectancy when dealing with the elderly and the healthy.[7]

Life expectancy is an average. Using averages to summarize the health status of a population has one additional feature that needs to be recognized. Let us review how averages are calculated. For instance, imagine that we want to calculate an average for the following numbers: 2, 21, 24, 26, 27. We would first add together all the numbers and obtain 100. Then we would divide by the number of data elements, that is, by 5. Thus, the average here is 100/5, or 20.

Notice that the average is below all the numbers except 2. The inclusion of 2 has pulled the average down. This is generally the case with averages. They are heavily affected by the extreme values, especially when the extremes are far removed from the other values.

When calculating life expectancies, a parallel phenomenon occurs. That is, the life expectancy at birth is most heavily influenced by what happens early in life. Thus, the influence on life expectancy of saving a healthy child is far greater than the influence of saving a healthy adult or a healthy 80-year-old. The implications of this phenomenon are illustrated in the next example:

> Reviewing the experience of a rapidly developing country, investigators noted that the nation rapidly gained years of life expectancy at birth when it controlled infectious diseases of the young. When it turned its attention to the diseases of the elderly

[7]On the other hand, life expectancy overestimates survival for those with disease. To accurately incorporate the impact of disease on life expectancy, we need to combine life expectancy measures using data based on age, gender, and race with life expectancy data based on disease-specific survival. One such approximation is known as the DECLINING EXPONENTIAL APPROXIMATION OF LIFE EXPECTANCY (DEALE). DEALE assumes that the life expectancy at a particular age is equal to 1 divided by the sum of the probability of survival on the basis of age, race, and gender (obtained from a cross-sectional life table) plus the probability of survival as a result of disease (obtained from a longitudinal life table).

and made rapid strides in controlling these diseases, there was much less impact on the life expectancy at birth. This contradiction could not be explained by the investigators, who concluded that life expectancy was a meaningless measure.

Life expectancy at birth is strongly influenced by mortality rates among the young. This is the case because saving a healthy child adds a large number of years to life, whereas saving a healthy adult or elderly person adds a much smaller number of years of life. Because life expectancy at birth reflects the average number of remaining years of life, it will be greatly influenced by the progress made among the young. To observe the impact on the elderly, it is necessary to calculate the life expectancy at older ages and see how they change from year to year.

Increases in life expectancy resulting from treatment of chronic disease or prevention of disease in adults may not appear to make a major impact. Increases of a few months in life expectancy from major advances in treatment may not seem very impressive. This is especially true if these months are viewed as occurring only at the end of life. In fact, a common misinterpretation of life expectancy data is to conclude that the extension of life expectancy implies that a brief period will be added on at the end of life. The impact of this misinterpretation may be seen in the following example:

> Coronary artery bypass surgery was shown to increase life expectancy by 6 months. A reviewer of this literature concluded that adding 6 months on at the end of life is not worth the hazards of surgery.

First, the benefits described here take into account the fact that surgery does have immediate hazards, which may produce immediate death. In addition, the benefits of extended life do not merely get tacked on at the end of life, distributed equally to everyone who undergoes bypass surgery. The benefits actually affect a small percentage of those undergoing surgery. These patients are the ones who do not die in the months and years immediately after the surgery but who would otherwise die.

Thus, it is important when interpreting an extension in life expectancy of 6 months to recognize that in this situation it is actually an impressive gain in life expectancy. In addition, its impact on some individuals may be dramatic and immediate, even though it may have little or no impact for many others.

Thus, life expectancy is a useful measure that summarizes the probabilities of death at different ages in a population. It is useful for comparing one population with another for the same year or for comparing how the same population changes from one year to another year. When data on gender and racial groups are available, life expectancy can be useful for comparing the mortality of these groups within a population.

It is important to remember, however, that life expectancy is not a good predictor of future survival; it combines survival for healthy and sick individuals; and it is strongly influenced by the mortality of the young. Thus, we need to be very careful when using life expectancy calculations to predict the future, to make recommendations for the healthy, and to apply these calculations to individuals.

26 Rating a Rate:

Questions to Ask and Flaw-Catching Exercises

The following set of questions for rating a rate is designed to review the areas covered and to provide an outline for critiquing a flaw-catching exercise or a real investigation of rates. It is divided into selecting a rate, sampling of rates, standardization of rates, sources of changes or differences in rates, and life expectancy.

1. Selection of rates
   a. Did the authors distinguish between and properly measure the basic measurements (*i.e.*, an incidence rate, prevalence, and case fatality)?
   b. Was the proportionate mortality ratio distinguished from the basic measurements?

2. Sampling of rates
   a. Was the entire population of interest included in the study, or were samples used?
   b. If samples were used, did the authors appreciate the inherent sampling error?
   c. If samples were used, was the sampling technique random or representative, or was bias introduced by the method of sampling?
   d. If samples were used, were the sizes of the samples adequate, or was it likely that a large variation was introduced by the small sample size?

3. Standardization of rates
   a. Was standardization necessary when comparing the rates of occurrence of an event in two different samples?
   b. If standardization was necessary, were the rates standardized for factors that are known to affect outcome so that the rates could be compared?

4. Sources of changes or differences in rates
   a. Were the observed changes or differences in rates artifactual as a result of changes in the ability to recognize the disease, efforts to recognize the disease, or changes in the definition of the disease?
   b. Were actual differences or changes the result of changes or differences in the incidence rate, prevalence, or case fatality?
   c. Do the changes or differences in rates predict future changes in the same direction, or will future rates be affected by the phenomenon of regression to the mean due to adaptive changes or a cohort effect?
   d. When using differences in rates to develop hypotheses for further study, was the distinction between group association and association at the individual level appreciated?

5. Life expectancy
   a. Was the life expectancy properly calculated?
   b. Was the life expectancy measurement used to compare the same population over time or to compare populations as opposed to efforts to predict the future?
   c. If the life expectancy was used for individual decision-making or group recommendations, was it recognized that life expectancy is based on data from healthy individuals plus those with disease?
   d. Were the factors that alter life expectancy appreciated, including the different impacts on life expectancy of intervention at different ages?
   e. Was it appreciated that small extensions in life expectancy may have a substantial immediate impact on some individuals and should not be viewed as occurring at the end of life?

The following flaw-catching exercises are designed to give you practice in applying the principles of rating a rate to simulated hypothetical research articles. The flaw-catching exercises include a variety of errors that have been illustrated in the hypothetical examples. Read each exercise. Then write a critique pointing out the types of errors committed by the investigators. A sample critique is provided for each exercise.

Flaw-Catching Exercise No. 1:

Changes in Cancer: What Is Progress?

A study of progress in survival after diagnosis of cancer in the United States compared the rates in 1969 with the rates in 1999 to assess changes. Data on incidence rates and mortality rates of cancer were collected. Incidence data were obtained from an intensive search of hospital records on a random sample of 1% of the nation's hospitals. Data on mortality rates were obtained from a complete review of all the death certificates in the nation. Case fatality was derived from the following formula for long-term changes:

$$\text{Mortality rates} = \text{Incidence rates of disease} \times \text{Case fatality}$$

The data from these studies are summarized in Table 26.1.

The researchers reviewed randomized clinical trials on cancers that caused nearly all of the cancer deaths among people 20 years and older. They found that among people with incurable cancers, the trials showed a 3-year increase in life expectancy when applying new therapies developed since 1969.

Finally, the researchers calculated the PROPORTIONATE MORTALITY RATIO based on a review of the cause of death from all death certificates. They found that the proportionate mortality ratio for cancer overall had increased from 22% to 24%.

Table 26.1. *Changes in cancer rates from 1969 to 1999*

Age (yr)	Incidence Rate	Case Fatality	Mortality Rate
0–19	No change	20% decrease	20% decrease
20–65	1% increase	1% decrease	No change
65+	15% increase	10% decrease	5% increase

The researchers confessed complete confusion, saying that it was possible to argue the following points:

1. There has been substantial progress on the basis of the decreased mortality rates for people younger than 20 years, the decreased case fatality for all age groups, and the increased survival rates in randomized clinical trials among those 20 years and older.
2. The situation is getting worse on the basis of the increased incidence rates among people older than 20 years. The increased cancer mortality rates among those older than 65 years and the increased proportionate mortality rates also support a worsening of the situation.
3. No change has occurred on the basis of the age-adjusted overall mortality rates.

The investigators throw up their hands and ask you, the readers, to explain how the data could support such inconsistent results.

Critique: Exercise No. 1

These rates are all compatible. They reflect different ways to look at and to argue about rates. Incidence rates reflect the rate at which new cases of the disease develop over a period of time. Case fatality reflects the probability of dying over a period of time if the disease develops. Thus, incidence rates and case fatality measure two very different phenomena. Incidence rates primarily reflect the underlying causes of disease. They may be artifactually changed by interventions that alter the effort to detect disease, the ability to detect disease, or the definition of disease. Primary prevention efforts, such as smoking cessation, may alter the underlying incidence. In general, however, incidence rates do not reflect the usual therapeutic efforts that are part of clinical care. Case fatality, on the other hand, is a measure of how successful therapy is at curing disease.

Mortality rates over a long period of time are related to incidence rates and case fatality as follows:

$$\text{Mortality rates} = \text{Incidence rates of disease} \times \text{Case fatality}$$

Thus, if the mortality rate and the incidence rate are known and stable, the case fatality can be approximated as follows:

$$\text{Case fatality} = \frac{\text{Mortality rate}}{\text{Incidence rate of disease}}$$

Therefore, the first table correctly used the relationship among incidence rate, mortality rate, and case fatality.

When an intervention successfully prolongs life but does not cure a disease, this intervention has no effect on the overall or long-term case fatality. Thus, the 3-year increase in life expectancy among people with incurable cancers is compatible with the more modest decrease in case fatality observed in the age-adjusted data. Life expectancy measures obtained from longitudinal life tables in randomized clinical trials can be used to take into account the prolongation of life in the absence of cure.

The increased proportionate mortality ratio tells us very little about the progress in survivals after diagnosis of cancer over those years. It does suggest, however, that mortality from other diseases is becoming less frequent compared with cancers. Proportionate mortality ratios are useful measures of the relative frequency of various causes of death. The increase in the proportionate mortality ratio suggests that deaths from cancer are becoming more common relative to deaths from other causes.

This exercise demonstrates how it is possible to argue for quite different conclusions from the same data. The argument presented by the researchers reflects different concepts about what is meant by progress. Is progress a reduced incidence of new disease? Is progress an increased cure rate for diagnosed disease? Alternatively, is progress a prolongation of life for people with disease?

Flaw-Catching Exercise No. 2:

Tuberculosis

An international group of tuberculosis (TB) experts decided to compare the mortality rate from TB in the United States with that of Mexico to determine whether anything could be learned. They knew that new cases of active TB were quite common in the United States before 1950, but that they had declined substantially until 1985. Since 1985, the overall incidence rate of active TB in the United States has gradually increased.

Using a carefully designed large random sampling technique, the investigators found that the mortality rate due to TB in 1999 was 200 per 100,000 person-years in Mexico versus 20 per 100,000 person-years in the United States. They also found that the mortality rate for individuals in the 65- to 80-year age group was 200 per 100,000 person-years in Mexico and 200 per 100,000 person-years in the United States in 1999.

Because the investigators knew that Mexico had a much younger population than did the United States and that age affects the incidence of active TB, they tried to age-standardize the rates. They applied the rates for each age group from the US population to the number of person-years in that age group in Mexico. After direct age adjustment, they found that 200 deaths occurred per 100,000 person-years from TB in Mexico in 1999. They found that there would have been 10 deaths per 100,000 person-years in the United States if the United States had the same age distribution as Mexico. Finally, they calculated the proportional mortality ratio for TB in the two countries. In Mexico, they found that TB has a proportionate mortality ratio of 1.5% versus 1% in the United States.

The authors drew the following conclusions:

1. The large difference in mortality rates between Mexico and the United States may have been due to chance.
2. The mortality rate in the United States for the 65- to 80-year-olds is much higher than the average US rate. Thus, as the average age of the US population gets older, TB will become more of a problem. This most likely explains the increase in the incidence of TB in the United States after 1985.
3. In comparing the unstandardized rates, it appeared that Mexico had 10 times the US incidence rate of TB. Once standardization was completed, it showed that Mexico had 20 times the incidence of active TB. Some mistake must have been made because rate standardization should not make the differences in rates look larger than prestandardized rates. Thus, contrasting the overall unstandardized rates is the fairest means of comparison.

4. The proportionate mortality ratios are the fairest way to compare the probability of death from TB. Thus, the probability of death from TB was 1.5 times higher in Mexico than in the United States.

Critique: Exercise No. 2

SELECTION OF RATES

Let us evaluate one by one the conclusions reached by the experts.

1. It is very unlikely that the differences between the United States and Mexico are due only to chance because of their great magnitude and the large sample size used in the investigation. However, before concluding that these differences are actual, we must consider whether artifactual differences either in effort or in ability to recognize TB occur between the two countries and whether these factors could explain the differences found. If we assume that Mexico is less able than the United States to recognize TB as the cause of death, this fact would actually increase the already large differences found. Thus, artifactual differences in the effort or ability to recognize deaths from TB are not likely to explain or to eliminate the differences found.

2. The authors have noted that the rates among 65- to 80-year-olds are identical in the United States and in Mexico. This suggests that the United States experiences a mortality rate among the elderly that is much higher than among the rest of the US population, which may be due to some permanent susceptibility among the US elderly. On the other hand, it may reflect a cohort effect. Remember, a cohort effect is a unique, temporary susceptibility among one group or cohort resulting from a special past experience. Historically, we know that TB was a much more common disease in the United States before 1950. In addition, we know that individuals who have been previously infected frequently control the infection but often do not eliminate it totally. These individuals have the possibility of subsequently developing active disease, especially when they become elderly. Thus, it is possible that the high incidence rate among the US elderly is related to their experience in an era when active TB was quite frequent. If the cohort effect explains the high TB incidence rate among the US elderly, then it is not likely that the high US rate among 65- to 80-years-olds will continue to increase as the proportion of elderly in the US population increases. The rates for this age group may actually fall as fewer susceptible cohorts, those who were not previously exposed to TB, advance into this age group. The overall increase in the incidence rate of active TB after 1985 was most likely not due to the aging of the population. Rather, it may have been associated with the increase in human immunodeficiency virus infection, which is known to predispose to the activation of TB.

3. The investigators correctly concluded that rate standardization for age was an important procedure if the rates were to be compared. Standardization is important because the populations have a markedly different age distribution, and age is related to the probability of dying from TB. The Mexican population is generally younger than the US population. Deaths from TB are concentrated among the old and the very young; thus, age standardization is necessary if a comparison is performed. The procedure for age standardization was correctly performed. By applying the rates for each age group in the US population to the

number of individuals in that age group in the Mexican population, the investigators were asking how many deaths would have occurred in the US population if there were the same number of individuals in each age group as in Mexico. This number can then be compared directly with the number of deaths that actually occurred in Mexico. Standardization may make the differences appear smaller or larger. There is no reason to believe that standardization will make big differences look smaller. As illustrated in the bladder cancer exercise in the discussion of standardization (Chapter 23), age adjustment may even reveal an important difference where none was apparent in the overall rates.

4. The proportionate mortality ratio reflects the number of individuals who die from a disease divided by the number who die from all diseases. Assuming the overall mortality rates are modestly higher in Mexico than in the United States, the denominator of the proportionate mortality ratio for Mexico will be higher. Thus, when calculating the proportionate mortality ratio for Mexico, we divide a much larger numerator by a modestly larger denominator. Therefore, it is not surprising that we come up with a proportionate mortality ratio for Mexico that is 1.5 times higher than the proportionate mortality ratio for the United States. The proportionate mortality ratio, however, should not be viewed as a measure of probability of death but rather as a measure of the relative importance of a disease in a particular population or group.

Flaw-Catching Exercise No. 3:

Life Expectancy in Econotiger and Developed Country

A developing country known as Econotiger compared its life expectancy with its own previous life expectancies and those of Developed Country. It found the following years of life expectancy:

	At Birth	At 65 Years	At 80 Years
Econotiger			
1979	50	15	5
1999	72	15	5
Developed Country			
1979	72	15	5
1999	75	18	5

The investigator drew the following conclusions:

1. A child born in Econotiger in 1979 will, on average, live until 2029 because the life expectancy in Econotiger in 1979 was 50 years.
2. The dramatic improvement in life expectancy at birth experienced in Econotiger will result in a far longer life expectancy at birth in Econotiger than in Developed Country during the 21st century.
3. The 1979 Econotiger life expectancy of 15 years at age 65 cannot be accurate because the life expectancy at birth is only 50 in 1979.
4. The life expectancy at age 65 years in Developed Country in 1999 represents a very modest improvement compared with 1979.

5. The identical life expectancies at age 80 in both countries in both years suggest that once an individual has lived to 80 years, life expectancy is 5 years regardless of whether health is good or poor.
6. Life expectancy is the only way to measure and compare the improvement in health because it is a measure that incorporates prolongations of life, even in the absence of cure.

Critique: Exercise No. 3

Life expectancy calculations require only accurate measurement of the number of individuals in each age group in a population and the number of individuals who die in that age group in the year being considered. Thus, they are a useful measure for comparing the same country over time and making comparisons between countries. However, life expectancy has a number of limitations and potential misinterpretations, some of which are illustrated in the six conclusions that were drawn from the previous data.

1. Life expectancy is not usually a useful measure for predicting the future. Life expectancy provides a snapshot view of the experience of each age group in a particular year. To use life expectancy to predict the future, we need to assume that nothing would change in the future. It is clear that many things are changing in Econotiger. Individuals born there in 1979 will not actually experience the probabilities of death at each age that were present in Econotiger in 1979. Rather, they will experience the reduced probabilities of death that are present in the subsequent years. Thus, the life expectancy at birth in 1979 of 50 years is a particularly poor predictor of how long the average person born in Econotiger in 1979 will actually live.
2. In general, extensions in life expectancy are most dramatically achieved by controlling infectious diseases of infants and children. By saving the life of an otherwise healthy infant or child, a large number of years of life expectancy is gained. Once these gains are obtained, further progress, as measured by life expectancy, is often more difficult to achieve. Improvement in longevity for the elderly may represent important progress, but it has only a modest effect on the life expectancy at birth. This progress is better reflected in the life expectancy at age 65 years. The data suggest that Developed Country has experienced this type of progress between 1979 and 1999. If Econotiger experiences this same progress in future years, the life expectancy at birth will still change very little by the early 21st century.
3. Life expectancy at age 65 years (or any other age) will not be the life expectancy at birth minus the age. Once individuals have survived to a particular age, such as 65 years, they have avoided a number of potential causes of death. Their total length of life will, on average, be greater than the life expectancy at birth. Even in a country where the life expectancy is only 50 years, some individuals will live to age 65 years and beyond. Their life expectancy is dependent on the probabilities of death at more advanced ages. These probabilities of death in a developed and a developing country may be quite similar.
4. In Developed Country, an improvement in life expectancy at age 65 of 3 years between 1979 and 1999 represents an impressive increase of 20%. The data suggest that the entire increase in life expectancy at birth that occurred in Devel-

oped Country is the result of the improved probabilities of death in people older than 65 years.

5. Life expectancy at advanced ages, such as 80 years, must be interpreted carefully. Life expectancy at all ages comprises the life expectancy of both the healthy and the diseased. At advanced ages, however, the proportion of people with disease is much greater than at younger ages. The smaller group of healthy individuals may have a much better prognosis than the larger number with disease. Thus, life expectancy should not be used to predict longevity for the healthy elderly.

6. Despite the usefulness of life expectancy in comparing a country's progress over time and making comparisons between countries, it also has important limitations. Life expectancy does not take into account improvements in the quality of life that are not also reflected in the length of life. Many of the benefits of health care are improvements only in the quality of life. Efforts to improve vision, mental health, and mobility, for instance, are not often reflected in increased life expectancy.

IV
Considering Costs and Evaluating Effectiveness

27 Introduction and Study Design of Decision-Making Investigations

For many years, the results of health research stopped at defining and measuring the probabilities of favorable and unfavorable outcomes. Traditionally, recommendations for decision-making were then made by experts who reviewed the outcome probabilities in the literature, added their own subjective judgments, and developed recommendations for clinical, institutional, and public health practice. Hidden in these recommendations were a series of subjective assumptions that rarely received scrutiny in the health research literature.

As decision-making in health care has become more complex, it has received greater attention. Explicit assumptions and quantitative measurements are increasingly replacing expert opinions. The health research literature increasingly includes decision-making research aimed at evaluating the effectiveness and considering the costs of preventive, therapeutic, and rehabilitative options. Quantitative decision-making research usually requires the investigator, at a minimum, to do the following:

1. **Model the decision:** This requires defining the alternatives that are being considered and the paths that eventually lead to potential outcomes. Decision-making investigations require the researcher to identify which options are being compared and what outcomes are being considered.
2. **Incorporate probabilities:** The investigator must determine which probabilities to use for measuring the favorable and unfavorable outcome. These probabilities may come from the research literature but they may need to be "guestimated" based on expert opinion.
3. **Incorporate utilities:** A measurement of the degree of preferences for each of the favorable and unfavorable outcomes is required. As we will see, these preferences are measured using what are called *utilities*.
4. **Incorporate costs:** As the cost of health care has increased along with the number of available options, researchers are also increasingly expected to measure and compare the financial consequences of each option being considered.

Thus, the health research literature now includes more than investigations that measure the probability of good outcomes and bad side effects. Increasingly, decision-making studies aim to measure or quantify the entire process of decision-making. They aim to structure or model the decision-making process, to measure each of the components, and to offer recommendations or guidelines based on the results. The results of these decision-making investigations now appear in most major medical, management, and public health journals and form the basis for what are called PRACTICE GUIDELINES. Thus this section, EVALUATING EFFECTIVENESS AND CONSIDERING COSTS, can be used as a guide to the guidelines.

In examining decision-making investigations we will focus on two hypothetical issues:

> There are three alternatives for treating single-vessel coronary artery disease. Conventional treatment is a combination of medications, angioplasty, and surgery. There are also two new treatments. One treatment is called transthoracic laser coronaryplasty (TLC). The third option is a new drug called Cardiomagic.

We will be looking at how we can compare these alternatives to decide which is the most effective for treatment and which is the most cost effective. We will also be examining options for approaching a disease that we will call PARALYSIS. We will examine the following situation:

> Paralysis is a common contagious disease of childhood that is usually self-limited. However a small percentage of children who experience the illness develop paralysis, and a few develop life-threatening complications. The disease produces serious short-term life-threatening consequences. Long-term paralysis and late complications can also occur. The conventional treatment for paralysis has been only supportive treatment which we will call a do-nothing approach. Recently an expensive vaccination has become available designed to prevent paralysis. We will discuss how we can compare the results of the vaccine to the do-nothing approach.

These types of decision-making investigations require a wide variety of information drawn from multiple sources. Thus, they can be very confusing to read and understand. However, decision-making investigations like the other types of studies that we examined in Part 1, *Studying a Study* can be understood by using the uniform framework. Therefore, we will return to the uniform framework and look at decision-making investigations step by step by examining the components of study design, assignment, assessment, analysis, interpretation, and extrapolation.

Study Question and Study Type

A variety of study questions can be addressed by decision-making investigations. The specific type of decision-making investigation used should depend on the question being addressed.

Let us begin by outlining the common types of decision-making investigations. Then it should be possible for you to determine whether the study type is appropriate to the study question.

Decision-making investigations can be divided into two general types. The first type includes efforts to consider favorable and unfavorable health effects. This type of investigation is often called a DECISION ANALYSIS.[1]

The second type of decision-making investigation is called COST-EFFECTIVENESS ANALYSIS. Cost-effectiveness analysis will be used as a general term here that

---

[1]The term DECISION ANALYSIS is often used even more generically to refer to all decision-making investigations that use a quantitative approach to decision-making under conditions of uncertainty. In this context, all investigation types discussed here, including those that incorporate costs, can be considered decision analyses. In addition, the term DECISION ANALYSIS has been used more narrowly than we use it here to imply the use of a decision tree as the method for modeling the options being considered.

includes all types of decision-making investigations that consider costs and relate them to a measure of favorable and adverse outcomes.[2]

Both decision analysis and cost-effectiveness analyses can be subdivided into several different types of investigations depending on the factors that are considered.

The first type of decision analysis that may appear in the literature is an OUT-COMES PROFILE.[3]

Table 27.1 shows the favorable and unfavorable outcomes shown to occur with TLC and Cardiomagic.

This profile provides considerable data that may be helpful in making decisions. However, it does not in-and-of-itself lead to recommendations. The outcome profile actually raises a series of questions that need to be considered in making decisions that can be incorporated into more complex investigations.

Let us examine Table 27.1 to see what information is provided and what is left out. First, note that the outcomes profile provides estimates of the probability of favorable and adverse outcomes. In an outcomes profile, however, the timing of the events are not necessarily made explicit. In addition, in an outcomes profile there is no attempt to combine or summarize the impact of favorable and adverse outcomes or long-term and short-term impacts. This process is left to the reader. An outcomes profile does not really provide a conclusion and cannot in-and-of-itself be used as the basis for recommendations. Therefore we may consider outcomes profiles to be a preliminary, partial, or incomplete decision-making investigation.

An outcomes profile may in-and-of-themselves provide enough information to make a decision if it is clear that both the harms and the benefits of a therapy such as TLC are more favorable than the harms and benefits of Cardiomagic. It is

Table 27.1. *Favorable and Unfavorable Outcomes with TLC and Cardiomagic*

TLC outcomes:

Successful 96%
Unsuccessful 3.9%
Death 0.1%

Cardiomagic outcomes:

Successful 80%
Unsuccessful 19.8%
Blindness 0.2%

[2]As we discuss later in this chapter, the term COST EFFECTIVENESS is also used to describe one particular type of decision-making investigation in which the investigator is interested in comparing different alternatives for obtaining the same outcome. In this special type of analysis, the results are stated as additional costs per additional outcome. The term EFFECTIVENESS as used in cost effectiveness has a somewhat different meaning than when used in the *Studying a Study* section of this book. Effectiveness in the context of cost effectiveness combines the favorable and adverse outcomes. When we viewed outcomes previously, we regarded effectiveness as including only favorable outcomes. Considerations of adverse outcomes or safety were discussed separately. Thus, in decision-making investigations, we should regard the term EFFECTIVENESS as implying net effectiveness.

[3]The term BALANCE SHEET has been used to describe this type of investigation, however, this term may be misleading. This is an accounting term that refers to assets and liabilities both measured in monetary terms such as dollars. The type of analysis being considered here does not imply the use of costs, and it is often not possible to directly compare the favorable outcomes with the adverse outcomes.

important to recognize, however, that the outcomes of TLC and Cardiomagic are not directly comparable. Looking at the adverse effects of these two treatments requires us to compare two outcomes: death and blindness. These have very different implications. We may need to quantitate the importance of outcomes such as death and blindness and incorporate these measurements into a decision-making investigation if we wish to compare TLC and Cardiomagic. In decision-making investigations, incorporating the relative importance of an event is accomplished by measuring utility.[4]

Utilities are designed to measure the preference of a rater for a particular health outcome or state of health. As we will see in Chapter 29 on assessment, there are a variety of methods for measuring utilities and considerable controversy about which is best. Regardless of the method chosen, the aim is to measure utilities on the same scale as probabilities. By doing so, it is possible to combine probabilities and utilities.

Thus, our goal is to measure the utilities of blindness and death on the same numerical scale. In addition, our goal is to combine the measurements of utilities that we obtain for blindness and death with the probabilities that they will occur. Thus, we use the same scale when measuring utilities and probabilities.

Remember that probabilities are measured using a scale of 0 to 1 which is often converted to percentages from 0% to 100%. On this scale, there are no measurements or values greater than 1 or less than zero. The utility scale generally defines 0 as death and 1 as full health or the state of health in the absence of manifestations of disease or other health-related conditions.

Once utility and probability are measured on the same scale the probability can be multiplied by the utility to produce what is called an EXPECTED UTILITY. We can consider expected utility to be the probability of an outcome adjusted for its value or utility. The calculation of expected utilities is an essential step in performing a decision-making investigation that attempts to compare options and draw conclusions. Thus, an investigation that measures utilities and combines them with probabilities is called an EXPECTED UTILITY DECISION ANALYSIS.

The possibility that death may occur raises an additional factor that also may be considered in a decision-making investigation. At times, we may want to consider the expected life span lost as the result of death. We have already encountered the measurement of life expectancy, which takes into account the life span. For cases in which we hope to return an individual to his or her state of full health, we can use life expectancy measures, as derived from the age or average age of the individuals being treated, to estimate average remaining life span.[5]

---

[4]At times, outcomes profiles may be adequate for decision-making when one option is clearly better than the other regardless of the utility that is placed on each outcome. For instance, in this case, regardless of how blindness and death are scored on a utility scale, TLC appears to have a more favorable outcome, everything else being equal, than Cardiomagic. In decision-making investigations, when one alternative is clearly more favorable than another, the alternative with the better outcomes is said to be DOMINANT.

[5]If the author is dealing with a women's disease, then life expectancy by age and gender should be used. Similarly, if the author is dealing with a disease generally limited to blacks, such as sickle cell disease, use of life expectancy by age and race would be appropriate. As discussed in the next chapter, the relevant life expectancy is not always the life expectancy derived from population data. For diseases that substantially reduce life expectancy, the appropriate life-expectancy measures take into account life expectancy for a particular disease as well as life expectancy defined by age and possibly gender and race.

Life expectancy can be incorporated into decision-making investigations along with utilities. When this is done, the investigation usually produces a measurement called QUALITY ADJUSTED LIFE YEARS (QALYs).[6]

Decision analyses that use QALYs to take into account life expectancy as well as utilities represent what many experts consider a fully developed decision analysis. We will call this form of decision analysis a QUALITY ADJUSTED LIFE-EXPECTANCY DECISION ANALYSIS (QALY decision analysis).

We have defined three types of decision analyses:

1. Outcomes profiles: This type of investigation merely states the probabilities of the known favorable and adverse outcomes from each of the alternatives being considered.
2. Expected utility decision analyses: This type of investigation combines the probabilities and utilities of each favorable and each adverse outcome and summarizes the results as overall expected utilities. Thus, expected utility decision analyses, as opposed to outcomes profiles, summarize the outcomes of each alternative and allow them to be directly compared.
3. Quality adjusted decision analyses: Like expected utility decision analyses, these allow direct comparison of alternatives taking into account the favorable and adverse outcomes. However, QALY decision analyses go beyond expected utility in that they incorporate life expectancy.

Cost-effectiveness analyses, in contrast to decision analyses, incorporate costs as well as consideration of favorable and adverse outcomes. Cost-effectiveness investigations, like decision analyses, can be divided into several different types.

As with outcome profiles, cost-effectiveness analysis may simply measure or describe the various costs as well as the probabilities of the potential outcomes. The reader's job is to combine these outcomes to reach conclusions. This type of investigation is called a COST-CONSEQUENCE ANALYSIS.

The data from a cost-consequence analysis might look like that in Table 27.2.

Cost-consequence analyses are really partial analyses since they do not generally allow us to directly compare two or more alternatives. To compare alternatives, the investigators need to bring in outside data or judgments.

A second type of cost-effectiveness analysis has unfortunately been called a COST-EFFECTIVENESS ANALYSIS. Using this term to describe a specific type of cost-effectiveness analysis can be very confusing. To minimize confusion, we will call this type of analysis a COST-AND-EFFECTIVENESS STUDY.

Table 27.2. Possible Data from a Cost-Consequence Analysis

Paralysis vaccine	
Outcomes:	Successful immunization 97% Unsuccessful immunization 2.9% Complications 0.1%
Costs:	$50 per use

[6]QALYs are the standard but not the only method for incorporating utilities and life expectancy. A method known as DISABILITY ADJUSTED LIFE EXPECTANCY or DALE is gaining recognition. Another measure gaining recognition is called YEARS OF HEALTHY LIFE.

A cost-and-effectiveness study looks at the costs required to produce an additional unit of desired outcome. For instance, imagine the following situation with paralysis:

> The cost of the new paralysis vaccine including the total costs of providing the vaccine and treating any complications is $15,000 per case of paralysis prevented.

This type of investigation compares the cost per additional desired outcome. It does not ask about the importance of the outcome or the life expectancy of the people saved. That is, cost-and-effectiveness studies do not consider utility or life expectancy. This type of cost-effectiveness analysis can be used to compare any outcomes, such as disease prevented, correct diagnosis, as well as lives saved. However, most comparisons of intervention options produce more than one outcome, most of which require consideration of utilities and life expectancy.[7]

Thus, a full cost-effectiveness analysis incorporates considerations of utility and life expectancy as well as cost. This type of cost-effectiveness analysis is called a COST-UTILITY ANALYSIS or a COST-EFFECTIVENESS ANALYSIS USING QALYs as the measure of effectiveness. Let us see what we mean by a cost-utility analysis:

> Paralysis vaccine was found to reduce the cost by $5,000 per quality adjusted life year saved when it was compared with the do-nothing option. The investigation took into account the utility of the outcomes as well as the life expectancy of people who received the favorable and adverse outcomes.

This form of cost-effectiveness analysis represents a fully developed analysis. It allows us to compare any alternative, taking into account all the relevant costs and health outcomes including the probability and utility of favorable and adverse outcomes as well as the life expectancy. Cost-utility analyses are increasingly considered the method of choice for most decision-making in health care. They allow us to directly compare alternatives and determine the costs relative to the health consequences.

At times, however, the question posed in an analysis does not relate to comparing the costs and health consequences of an intervention. Decision-making may at times require looking at trade-offs between money spent on health and money spent on other important outcomes such as environmental protection, economic growth, or education. To make these types of comparisons, it is necessary to translate effectiveness as well as costs into monetary terms.

The form of analysis that converts effectiveness as well as costs into monetary terms is known as a COST-BENEFIT ANALYSIS.[8] Let us examine how a cost-benefit analysis of coronary artery disease might look:

> An analysis was conducted to compare the economic costs and consequences of providing insurance coverage for paralysis vaccine compared with the alternative of providing college scholarships. The analysis assumes that a QALY could be converted to $30,000. The investigation found that coverage of the paralysis provided $2 in ben-

---

[7]At times, the key issue for an analysis is the relative costs. The effectiveness of two options may be comparable and the investigation is directed only at considering costs. This type of cost and effectiveness study is called a COST ANALYSIS.

[8]The term BENEFIT is also used to imply a favorable outcome. In the context of cost-benefit analysis, BENEFIT means net effectiveness measured in monetary units. Net effectiveness implies favorable outcomes minus unfavorable outcomes.

efits for every $1 in cost. The alternative of paying for college tuition provided $3 of benefit for every $1 of costs. Thus, paying for college tuition was considered the better alternative.

Note that cost-benefit analyses must make the conversion of quality adjusted life-year into dollars. This is a big step, and there is no agreement on the value of a year of life. Thus, this type of analysis remains very controversial. Fortunately, it is not often necessary to directly compare health expenditures with other uses of money. Therefore, cost-benefit analyses are not frequently seen in the health research literature.

We will not examine cost-benefit analyses. However, the conversion from a cost-utility study to a cost-benefit study is mechanically simple even though it represents a major intellectual leap. The key is determining the proper monetary value to place on a year of life. Once the monetary conversion of QALYs to dollars or other currency is agreed upon, that monetary figure merely replaces each QALY.

Thus, decision-making investigations can be classified as follows:

Decision Analyses

Outcomes profiles: Probabilities of favorable and unfavorable outcomes
Expected utility studies: Probabilities and utilities of favorable and unfavorable outcomes
Quality adjusted life expectancy (QALY) studies: Probabilities, life expectancy, and utilities of each outcome

Cost Effectiveness

Cost-consequence analysis: Costs and probability of favorable and unfavorable outcomes
Cost-and-effectiveness studies: Costs compared with a common unit of outcome such as lives saved
Cost-utility analysis: Costs compared to a unit of outcome that incorporate utilities and life expectancy such as QALYs

Cost-Benefit Analysis

Costs compared with outcomes converted to a monetary value of the outcomes

Study Population

As with all investigations, it is important to define the population being investigated. This is important because it tells us three things:

1. What type of individuals are being included and excluded;
2. What type of sources can be used to provide the necessary data; *and*
3. What types of extrapolations to similar populations will be possible if the results favor one of the alternatives.

The population that is the target of the decision-making study ideally should guide the investigator to the type of data to use. Unfortunately, data may not be available from the target population. To understand this, let us return to our examples and ask which population's data should be used to address the following study question:

> We are evaluating the costs and effectiveness of three types of treatments for single vessel coronary artery disease, conventional treatment, i.e., a combination of medications, angioplasty, and surgery.

When obtaining data to address the effectiveness or cost effectiveness of the three potential alternative treatments, it is important that the data come from individuals with single-vessel coronary artery disease. These treatments may also be used on patients with more extensive disease. Such individuals are likely to be older and have other related arterial disease. Thus, data derived from a population of patients with severe coronary artery disease would not be the type of data that should be used in addressing the study question:

> We are evaluating the costs and effectiveness of a new vaccine for paralysis, a common contagious disease of childhood that is usually self-limited but can produce short- and long-term complications.

When obtaining data to address the costs and effectiveness of this vaccine, the data should be obtained from a population in which the disease, paralysis, is common and usually self-limited. It would not be useful to obtain data from a population of severely ill children, especially if they had a high frequency of complications and required large expenditures if they did develop complications. Likewise, it would not be useful to obtain data from a population in which a high level of natural immunity already existed and therefore the disease was rarely experienced.

Thus when examining a decision-making investigation the reader must ask, "From what population (or populations) was the data obtained?" and "Is the population appropriate to the study question?"

Perspective

To evaluate whether appropriate data were included in an investigation, it is important to consider the study PERSPECTIVE. Perspective asks about how broadly we should look when measuring the effectiveness and the costs of an alternative. Let us examine some of the possible perspectives by returning to the use of paralysis vaccine. We could view the costs and effectiveness of the vaccine from at least the following perspectives:

- The patient who receives the vaccine and pays out of pocket
- The insurance company that pays for the vaccine as well as the short-term costs of treating paralysis
- The government insurance system that pays for the care for individuals who develop paralysis
- The society that, through one payment mechanism or another, receives the effectiveness and pays the costs of the administration of the vaccine and of the disease

The first three perspectives can be viewed as USER PERSPECTIVES. They reflect different ways for recipients or payors to view the costs and effectiveness of the vaccine. In theory, an investigation could be conducted from the perspective of the user of the investigation.

The final perspective is a SOCIAL PERSPECTIVE. A social perspective implies that we are interested in the impact of the effectiveness and the costs regardless of who obtains the effectiveness or who pays the costs. The choice of perspective guides the investigator in determining what should be included or excluded in the measurement of effectiveness and costs. Therefore, we can look at perspective as parallel to the inclusion and exclusion criteria used in other types of investigations.[9]

In general, decision-making investigations should use the social perspective. Other perspectives may also be used for additional analyses. There are two basic reasons for using the social perspective. First, it is the only perspective that never counts as a favorable outcome for one individual, an outcome that results from an adverse outcome for another individual. Similarly, the social perspective is the only perspective that never counts as a financial gain to one individual any event that poses a financial loss for another individual. Thus, social perspective is the only perspective that considers all the favorable and adverse outcomes and all the costs regardless of where they fall in society.

The perspective chosen should apply to both the effectiveness and the cost. If different perspectives are used for each, we cannot fairly compare or summarize the relationship between effectiveness and costs. Use of the social perspective thus considers all the favorable and adverse outcomes regardless of who they impact and all the costs regardless of who pays the bills. Using the social perspective allows us to compare effectiveness and costs in a consistent manner and to compare the results of one investigation with another.

As is often the case in study design, we do allow investigators to have it both ways. It is legitimate to conduct a decision-making investigation from the perspective of a potential user. If this is done, however, it is recommended that there also be a presentation from the social perspective. The social perspective is usually considered the ideal perspective for conducting a cost-effectiveness analysis. When a cost-effectiveness analysis is conducted from other perspectives, the results are often compared with or referenced to the results obtained using the social perspective. The use of the social perspective in cost-effectiveness analysis has been called the REFERENCE CASE.[10]

It is also important to recognize that many readers of a cost-effectiveness analysis do not look at the issue from a social perspective but rather from one or more user perspectives. Ideally, the data will be presented in such a way that it is possible for readers who want to take a user perspective to selectively use the data provided to reach their own conclusions from a user perspective.

Recognizing the perspective used in an investigation is especially important when we try to extrapolate the results or apply them to individuals or situations not included in the study. Thus, we return to the issue of perspective in Chapter 32 on extrapolating the results.

In summary, when reading a decision-making investigation, we first need to address the three basic questions of study design:

- What is the study question, and is an appropriate study type being used to address the study question?

[9]The perspective of the decision-making investigation should be distinguished from the identity of the decision-maker. For instance, a clinician may make a recommendation or a decision attempting to view the situation from the perspective of an individual patient, an institution, or even society as a whole.

[10]Throughout this section, we will rely on the reference case as the ideal method for conducting a cost-effectiveness analysis. The components of the reference case are derived from Gold, M. et al.: *Cost-Effectiveness in Health and Medicine,* Oxford University Press, New York, 1996.

- What is the study population?
- What is the study perspective?

Having addressed these questions, we can turn our attention to assignment and see what we mean by the decision-making model. In the next chapters in this section, we examine effectiveness using probabilities, utilities, and life expectancy, and we consider costs as well as effectiveness from the social perspective.

28 Assignment

Alternatives

The process of assignment in a decision-making investigation involves modeling, diagramming, or otherwise structuring the decision options. The selection of the alternatives to consider is under the investigator's control. As the reader, it is very important to review which options have been selected and, conversely, which potential alternatives have not been included.

First, let us examine what we mean by structuring or modeling the decision-making process. To conduct a decision-making investigation, the investigator needs to propose what is called a DECISION-MAKING MODEL. A decision-making model outlines the steps the investigator will consider in the decision-making process and the FINAL OUTCOMES that will be taken into account. By final outcomes we mean the outcomes that occur at the completion of the decision option. With TLC and Cardiomagic, the decision-making model may be described as follows:

> TLC and Cardiomagic will be compared. TLC or alternatively Cardiomagic may be chosen but not both. The outcomes of TLC are successful, unsuccessful, and death. No other therapy may be used if TLC is unsuccessful. Alternatively, Cardiomagic may be chosen. The outcomes of Cardiomagic are successful, unsuccessful, and blindness. If Cardiomagic is unsuccessful, surgery will be performed. The outcomes of surgery are successful, unsuccessful, and death. No other intervention will occur.

A common method for diagramming the decision-making process is a DECISION TREE. A decision tree graphically depicts the decision options and the choices that must be made to implement each option. The decision tree also depicts the events that occur through a chance process, outside the control of the decision-maker.[1]

Let us use our example of TLC and Cardiomagic to demonstrate the essential components of a decision tree.

Figure 28.1 represents a decision tree outlining the choice between TLC and Cardiomagic for patients with symptomatic single-vessel coronary artery disease. Note the following: First, there are two and only two alternatives to choose from, which are TLC and Cardiomagic. The choices of TLC and Cardiomagic are the decision options. Second, note that there is a square connecting the decision alternative called TLC and the decision option called Cardiomagic. This square is called a DECISION NODE. Decision nodes connect with the decision option by vertical lines. The decision-maker must choose between the available decision options connected to a choice node. That is, one and only one alternative can be chosen at any one time. TLC or Cardiomagic must be chosen, not both.

---

[1]The term DECISION-MAKER intentionally evades the question of who is making the decision. Thus, at times the decision-maker may be a clinician, a patient, an administrator, etc.

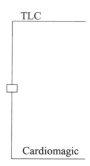

TLC

Cardiomagic

Figure 28.1. A decision tree outlining the choice between TLC and Cardiomagic for patients with symptomatic single-vessel coronary artery disease.

Once the choice of option is made, the decision tree depicts the subsequent course of events. There may or may not be subsequent choices to be made. In the decision tree for TLC depicted in Figure 28.2, we see only events that subsequently occur by chance.

For TLC, one of three outcomes occur: successful, unsuccessful, or death. Any individual can experience only one of these outcomes; that is, the outcomes are considered mutually exclusive.[2]

These three outcomes are connected by a CHANCE NODE. Chance nodes are represented by a circle. The outcomes called successful and death each brings us to the end of the TLC portion of the decision tree.

Figure 28.3 displays the option to use TLC and also the option to use Cardiomagic. Cardiomagic, unlike TLC, may be followed by surgery if it is unsuccessful. Thus, in the Cardiomagic alternative, there are two chance nodes that reflect the fact that the outcome is determined by the probability or chances that Cardiomagic will be successful followed by the probability that surgery will be successful, unsuccessful, or will result in death.

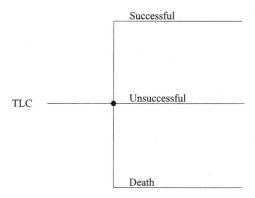

Successful

TLC

Unsuccessful

Death

Figure 28.2. Decision tree for TLC depicting only events that occur by chance.

[2]The mutually exclusive assumption may at times make the decision tree less than a true reflection of reality. In reality, any individual can experience both an unsuccessful procedure and an adverse effect. An outcome in which more than one outcome occurs can be included as an additional potential outcome. Often, combined outcomes are not included. Fortunately, at least from the social perspective, the unusual occurrence of more than one outcome often has little overall effect on the recommendations derived from the analysis. However, for the individual experiencing both an unsuccessful procedure and an adverse event, this is a particularly poor outcome.

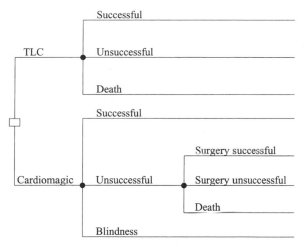

Figure 28.3. Decision tree displaying the options of using either TLC or Cardiomagic.

Relevant and Realistic Options

Now let us see what our decision tree has and has not achieved. When looking at a decision tree, we need to ask whether the options being considered are relevant to the study question and realistically modeled or displayed.

When looking at a decision tree, the first question to ask is: "Were the relevant alternatives considered?" Notice that there is no option to use conventional treatment such as surgery, angioplasty, or medications. Furthermore, observing the natural course of events without intervening is not an alternative. Whether or not these alternatives should be included in a decision tree depends on the question being asked and the current state of knowledge. The choice between TLC and Cardiomagic may be the appropriate issue if one of these must be selected for a particular group of individuals or both of these have been clearly shown to be superior to the other available options. When another alternative is considered conventional treatment, however, it should generally be included in a decision tree.

The other key question to ask in examining a decision tree is: "Does the decision process reflect realistic decision-making?" This question is more complicated than it first appears since all decision trees simplify the real decision-making process. Decision trees generally leave out unusual events, especially if they are not directly related to the therapy. For instance, a procedure that requires hospitalization may result in side effects unrelated to the therapy itself. For instance, hospitalization may increase the chances of developing hospital-acquired pneumonia or experiencing a medication error, yet a decision tree is not generally expected to incorporate these types of events. In addition, as we have already seen, a decision tree often skips potential choices. In the decision tree for our example, it was not permitted to stop after unsuccessful Cardiomagic treatment results. The greater the number of chance nodes, the more data that are needed to complete the decision tree. Thus, these types of simplification are usually necessary and acceptable to make the decision process model manageable.

The ideal way to construct a decision tree is to think of all possible final outcomes of the alternatives being considered and to display a decision tree that reflects all of these possible outcomes. This will usually include a large number of unusual outcomes and a number of similar outcomes. The researcher then combines outcomes that are similar and decides whether certain outcomes are so unusual or so inconsequential that they can be deleted from the decision tree. This very common practice is referred to as PRUNING THE DECISION TREE.

On the other hand, the reader must ask the bigger questions of whether the approach used in outlining the decision tree is a realistic reflection of clinical or public health decision-making. Remember that the decision tree in Figure 28.3 implied that the choice was between TLC and Cardiomagic. However, if there is an alternative to use Cardiomagic first, and if it is not successful to use TLC, then the decision tree in Figure 28.3 does not reflect realistic decision-making.[3]

Timing of Events

The timing of occurrence of potential outcomes is an important consideration in structuring the alternatives in a decision-making investigation. Some events occur immediately, and others may take years to occur. Some events may occur only once, while others may recur in the near or distant future. Whether or not to include events that occur in the future depends on the study's TIME HORIZON.[4]

The time horizon is the follow-up period that determines which outcomes are included in the model. The time horizon tells us how far into the future to look for favorable or unfavorable outcomes. The investigation may be interested only in short-term outcomes, such as hospital mortality, long-term outcomes such as late recurrences, or even consequences for the next generation. Notice that the TLC decision tree that we used only considers the immediate outcomes of the decision-making process. However, what if TLC could damage the coronary arteries and increase the probability of late complications? If this is the case, the decision tree for TLC with a longer time horizon would need additional chance nodes displaying additional potential outcomes.

Ideally, the time horizon should extend throughout the life of the individuals who potentially receive the intervention option. When shorter time horizons are used, the reader should ask: "Was the time horizon long enough to include all important favorable or adverse outcomes?"

The choice of appropriate time horizon may itself be quite complex. With genetic interventions, the appropriate analysis horizon may extend to future generations. Choice of time horizon may also be important in determining the proper structure of a decision tree, including which complications to consider. For instance, if the time horizon is extended long enough the disease may recur; that is, the treated coronary artery may experience restenosis or disease may develop in additional arteries. It is possible to construct more complicated decision trees incorporating recurrences and applying techniques known as MARKOV ANALYSES to incorporate recurrent events.

[3]When examining a decision tree, it is also important to identify the TIME FRAME of the analysis. The time frame is the period during the course of the disease when it is possible to use the intervention. Here, TLC and Cardiomagic are being used at the time when single-vessel coronary artery disease has become symptomatic. If the time frame of the analysis had extended to an earlier period in the course of the disease before symptoms had developed, it may have been possible to select preventive interventions. Thus, the choice of time frame can be very important in selecting decision options.

[4]The time horizon is also called the ANALYSIS HORIZON. Time horizon is used here because the issue is the time period that is considered in structuring the decision model. The time period for the analysis follows from the time period used to construct the model.

Other Factors in the Decision-Making Investigation

So far in this chapter, we have looked at the components of study design and assignment. In our example, we have described the choices to be considered (TLC and Cardiomagic) and the meaning of choice and chance nodes. Assume that TLC and Cardiomagic are the appropriate choices to consider and that TLC and Cardiomagic cannot be used together. Let us refer again to Figure 28.3 before we proceed to look at what is needed to complete the decision tree.

A decision tree is a particularly attractive model for decision making because it can be used as the basis for incorporating not only probabilities, but also utilities, life expectancies, and even costs. Now let us see how we can use a decision tree to incorporate the measurements needed for the various types of decision making.[5]

Utilities

Figure 28.4 includes the probabilities of each potential outcome in our example of TLC and Cardiomagic. Notice that the three potential outcomes of TLC are successful (0.96), unsuccessful (0.039), and death (0.001). The numbers included in parentheses are the probabilities that these events will occur, which together total 1. Figure 28.4 also outlines the potential outcomes and probabilities for Cardiomagic: successful (0.80), unsuccessful (0.198), and blindness (0.002).

It is possible to directly compare the successful and unsuccessful outcomes of TLC and Cardiomagic using probabilities alone. However, it is not possible to directly compare the consequences of death and blindness using only probabilities. Thus, to complete the decision tree it is also necessary to include a measure of the relative value of death and blindness. This is performed using utilities.

Figure 28.5 includes utilities for all the final outcomes. Success is given a probability of 1, which implies that the individual returns to full health. Death is given a probability of 0 which represents the lowest possible utility. Blindness is given a utility of .5, which implies that it is considered to be half way between full health

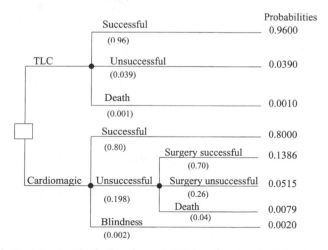

Figure 28.4. Decision tree including the probabilities of each potential outcome.

---

[5]Decision trees are not the only models that can be used as the basis for decision-making investigations. INFLUENCE DIAGRAMS can be used. These display the relationships between events and the factors believed to be relevant to decisions.

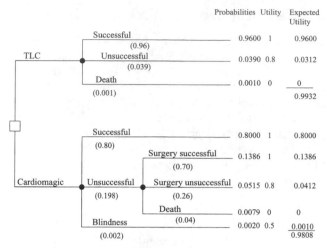

Figure 28.5. Decision tree displaying utilities for all outcomes.

and death. Later, we will examine methods for measuring these utilities and their implications in greater detail. For now, we examine how utilities are incorporated into the decision tree.

When utilities are used in a decision-making investigation, they must be measured on the same 0-to-1 scale as probabilities. Using the same scale allows us to combine probabilities with utilities. This is performed by multiplying probabilities and utilities to obtain EXPECTED UTILITIES. Expected utility can be viewed as a probability that is adjusted for or takes into account the utility or the relative value of the outcome. In expected-utility decision analysis, the expected utilities are compared. Let us see how the expected utilities would be calculated for TLC and Cardiomagic by looking at Figure 28.5.

The expected utilities of each outcome are obtained by a process known as FOLDING BACK THE DECISION TREE. With this process, we are calculating an overall probability that each of the final end-points or outcomes may occur in the decision process. Once this overall probability is calculated, we multiply the probability of the outcome by the utility of the outcome. For the Cardiomagic option in our example, the following outcomes may occur: (1) successful; (2) unsuccessful then successful surgery; (3) unsuccessful then unsuccessful surgery; (4) unsuccessful then death from surgery; (5) blindness.

Outcomes 2, 3, and 4 require combining two probabilities to reach an overall probability. For instance, the probability for unsuccessful Cardiomagic followed by successful surgery is obtained by multiplying the probability of being unsuccessful with Cardiomagic (0.198) by the probability of experiencing successful surgery (0.70). This equals .1386 which is the overall probability.[6]

Figure 28.5 summarizes the probabilities and utilities needed to complete the decision options. The decision tree now contains an expected utility for each potential outcome of TLC and Cardiomagic, the two decision options.

One more step must be completed before we can directly compare the final outcomes of the TLC and Cardiomagic options. This step summarizes each of the options

---

[6]Overall probabilities are calculated based on the INDEPENDENCE ASSUMPTION. This assumption implies that the probability of success at surgery is not influenced by whether or not Cardiomagic was successful. At times, the independence assumption may not hold in decision-making situations. It is possible that a factor that led to failure of Cardiomagic also influences the probability of unsuccessful surgery.

by adding together the expected utilities relevant to each option. This process is known as AVERAGING OUT THE EXPECTED UTILITIES. In averaging out the expected utilities for TLC and Cardiomagic, we would perform the following calculations:

$$\text{TLC expected utilities} = 0.9600 + 0.0312 + 0 = 0.9932$$

$$\text{Cardiomagic expected utilities} = 0.8000 + 0.1386 + 0.0412 + 0 + 0.0010 = 0.9808$$

Now we have folded back and averaged out to calculate overall expected utilities. For an expected utility decision analysis, these numbers represent the last step. They reflect a completed decision tree. This decision tree leads us to the conclusion that TLC is a better choice than Cardiomagic since it has a greater overall expected utility.

Life Expectancy

The questions addressed so far may be the only issues addressed in a decision-making study. If so, the study is an expected-utility decision analysis or a decision analysis adjusted for utility. That is, it considers only the probability of favorable and unfavorable outcomes and the utilities attached to these final outcomes.

As we indicated previously, decision-making studies can also include other factors. The two other key issues are whether the outcomes of the investigation use life expectancy and whether they include costs. When a decision analysis incorporates life expectancy measures, the results are usually presented using quality-adjusted life years (QALYs) as the measurement of effectiveness. To see how life-expectancy measures relate to the decision tree let us take a look at Table 28.1.

The QALYs are obtained by multiplying the probability of each final outcome, the utility of each final outcome, and the life expectancy of the average individual who experiences the final outcome. Table 28.1 shows the QALYs for each final outcome. Adding these together, we can average out and obtain the following results:

$$\text{TLC} = 17.44 \text{ QALYs}$$

$$\text{Cardiomagic} = 17.12 \text{ QALYs}$$

Once again, we can conclude that TLC is a better choice.[7]

Table 28.1. *Quality Adjusted Life Years (QALYs) for TLC and Cardiomagic*

	Probability	Utility	Life expectancy	QALYs
TLC				
Successful	0.9600	1	18	17.28
Unsuccessful	0.0390	0.8	5	0.16
Death	0.0010	0	0	0
Total QALYs				17.44
Cardiomagic				
Successful	0.8000	1	18	14.40
Successful after surgery	0.1386	1	18	2.49
Unsuccessful after surgery	0.0515	0.8	5	0.21
Death after surgery	0.0079	0	0	0
Blindness	0.0020	0.5	18	0.02
Total QALYs				17.12

[7]This approach to lining up life-expectancy measures along with utilities and probabilities as the outcomes of a decision tree is rarely used in the literature. It does, however, illustrate key issues. It also points out the need to define what is included in a utility. If life expectancy is included as a separate measure, utilities should not incorporate consideration of longevity. Unfortunately, this distinction is not always made in the literature.

Costs

Costs can also be added to the decision model. In the next chapter on assessment, we will discuss how costs are measured. Assuming they can be measured accurately, costs can be combined with measures of effectiveness based on the decision-tree model.

For instance, in our example, we have concluded that use of TLC results in 17.44 QALYs per use and Cardiomagic results in 17.12 QALYs per use. If the relevant cost of TLC is $116,600 per use and the cost of Cardiomagic is $50,000 per use, we can calculate COST-EFFECTIVENESS RATIOS. The cost-effectiveness ratio is defined as the cost per QALY.

Thus for TLC the cost-effectiveness ratio is:

$116,600/17.44 QALY *or* $6,686/QALY.

For Cardiomagic, the cost-effectiveness ratio is:

$50,000/17.12 QALYs *or* $2,921/QALY.

Thus, despite the fact that TLC produces more QALYs than Cardiomagic we can conclude that Cardiomagic produces more QALYs per dollar spent than TLC.[8]

For readers of the literature, the process of assignment requires us to look closely at how the decision is structured and what components are included in the investigation. This is usually reflected in a decision tree which defines the options, the chance events, and the relevant outcomes.[9]

The next step in the process is to look at how the data in the model were obtained. These issues are addressed in the assessment process, which is discussed in the next chapter.

---

[8]Occasionally, costs are directly incorporated into a decision tree as an outcome measure. When this is done, the outcome is called EXPECTED VALUE rather than expected utility.

[9]Often the decision tree itself may not be included in an article especially when the article is a form of cost-effectiveness analysis. Nonetheless, the choices and decisions that are the basis for the measurement of effectiveness can usually be outlined using a decision tree. It is possible to incorporate testing as well as therapeutic interventions into a decision tree. For instance, the decision to test can be included as a choice node with positive and negative results. The probability of a true positive and a false positive would then be incorporated as two chance consequences of a positive result. Similarly, for a negative result, the probability of a true negative and a false negative would be incorporated into the decision tree.

29 Assessment

Decision-making investigations require the investigator to obtain information from a variety of sources and to plug these pieces of information into a decision model that adequately describes the decision-making process.

As we found in the previous chapter on assignment, depending on the question being addressed and the type of investigation being conducted, we may need to obtain accurate and precise probabilities, utilities, life expectancies, and costs.

Probabilities

If possible, probabilities should be obtained from studies found in the research literature. Often, however, these estimates are not available and educated guesses must be used instead. These probabilities are referred to as SUBJECTIVE PROBABILITIES.

When using subjective probabilities, it is important to recognize that it is very difficult to accurately estimate probabilities, especially when the probability is very high (99% or more) or very low (1% or less). Thus, this problem often arises with estimates of the probability of adverse effects. In these situations, it is a common practice to either overestimate the probability, magnifying the chances of death for instance, or to underestimate the probability and therefore ignore the possibility of a rare side effect such as blindness.

Thus, the reader of decision-making literature needs to closely examine how the probabilities of rare but serious events were measured. When they are based on educated guesses or subjective judgments, these probabilities are especially prone to errors that need to be taken into account in the analysis.[1]

Utilities

As we have already discussed, utilities need to be measured on a scale of 0 to 1, the same scale used to assess probabilities. Utilities, unlike probabilities, are inherently subjective; they depend on how they are viewed by each individual. Each individual measures or scores utilities differently. Thus, there is no right utility.

What then are we measuring when we attempt to measure utilities? When decision-making investigations are conducted from the social perspective, the investigator is attempting to measure the average utility for individuals who are poten-

---

[1]Underestimating and overestimating the probability of events are even greater problems in the types of nonquantitative decision-making that is used for most decisions. One advantage of quantitative techniques, such as decision trees, is that they force the investigator to be explicit about which outcomes are being included and the probabilities that are attached to each outcome.

tially affected by the outcome. Let us see what we mean in the case of blindness.[2]

There are several techniques used to measure utilities. Currently, there is no consensus on which is best. The most straightforward method for measuring utilities is to ask individuals to indicate their own utility for blindness using a linear scale extending from 0 to 1 as seen in the following example:

> Imagine your quality of life if you became permanently and completely blind. Indicate on the following scale the relative worth of blindness. Notice that the scale extends from 0, which stands for immediate death, to 1, that stands for your state of full or complete health.

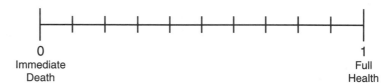

0
Immediate
Death

1
Full
Health

How did you score the utility for blindness?

When the scores of individuals are averaged, the utility of blindness is usually approximately 0.50. However, there is great variability from individual to individual. Perhaps you scored permanent and complete blindness as carrying a utility of 0.80 or as low as 0.20. This type of variability is not unusual. In addition, it is not always obvious why one individual perceives a condition as carrying a high utility and another perceives it as carrying a low utility. At times, an individual's profession or current state of activity may explain how they rate a condition's utility. More often, however, a large difference exists between similar individuals without obvious explanation. Thus, regardless of the utility that is used to represent the average utility for a decision-making investigation, it is important to recognize that wide variation may exist and this must be taken into account as part of the analysis.[3]

Regardless of the method used to estimate utilities, several issues are inherent in the scale used to measure utility. Remember, utilities are measured using a scale of 0 to 1. This creates issues at both ends of the scale. At the upper end, 1 is considered full health for the individual. For many medical conditions, it is impossible to bring an individual to full health. This is especially so for those with severe disabilities. Thus, when comparing an intervention designed for disabled people with one designed for people who can potentially be brought to full health, the disabled are at a disadvantage in terms of the extent of improvement that is possible as measured by utilities. An equally successful intervention may alter the utility score more among the potentially healthy compared with the disabled. To understand why this may be the case, consider the use of Cardiomagic in the following situation:

[2]The question often arises as to who should be asked to assess utility. Should the investigator ask people who are already blind and have thus gained experience with blindness or should we ask those who may become blind as a result of choosing the alternative to use Cardiomagic. The literature tells us that people who have already experienced a condition tend to score it with a slightly higher utility than those who have not experienced the condition. That is, people who have experienced blindness tend to adapt to its limitation and don't find it quite as bad as those confronted with potential blindness. The difference, however, is not great and studies of utilities may use either people who have experienced or those who have not experience the condition to obtain measures of utility.

[3]The technique demonstrated for directly scoring utilities on a scale of 0 to 1 is known as the RATING SCALE approach. There are a growing number of other methods for scoring utilities. The TIME-TRADE-OFF and REFERENCE GAMBLE METHODS are commonly used. There is considerable controversy over the best method to use. None of the currently available methods is ideal.

> Cardiomagic is being evaluated for use in otherwise healthy middle-aged men compared with its use in middle-aged men on dialysis. Despite its comparable probabilities of success, no success, and blindness, the procedure was found to produce greater expected utility when used on otherwise health individuals.

When dialysis patients return to their previous state of health, they do not return to a utility of 1. Rather, they return to the state of health for a dialysis patient who is doing well. This explains the greater expected utility when Cardiomagic is used on otherwise healthy individuals. When dialysis patients return to their previous state of health, their utility may only increase to approximately .6 compared to a previously healthy individual whose health may return to a utility of 1. As suggested in this example, decision-making investigations have been criticized as having a bias against the disabled.

There are also problems at the other end of the scale. In most decision-making investigations, 0 is defined as death. Considerable research and everyday experience tell us that, for many individuals, there are conditions worse than death. Prolonged vegetative states, severe mental incapacity, and intractable pain are typically viewed as having a utility worse than death. To use a scale that is the same as the one used for probabilities, it is not possible to incorporate negative utilities. However, it is possible to set death as greater than 0 and to set 0 as a state worse than death. Despite the possibility of performing this type of decision-making investigation, it is rarely seen in the decision-making literature.[4]

Life Expectancy

The measurements used to obtain life expectancy for a decision analysis can be very complex. The life-expectancy measurements we examined previously are designed as an average for all individuals of the same age and, sometimes, of the same gender or race. This type of life expectancy is not designed to take into account the consequences on life span of a specific disease that is being treated. Imagine the following:

> A decision-making investigation is being conducted to determine whether use of TLC or Cardiomagic is better for dialysis patients with coronary artery disease whose average age is 50. The average 50-year-old is assumed to have a life expectancy of 30 years.

The average 50-year-old may have a life expectancy of 30 years, but those on dialysis may have a much shorter life expectancy regardless of the success or failure of treatment of their coronary artery disease. Thus, the life expectancy that must be incorporated into each outcome of a decision tree is the life expectancy of the average individual to which the intervention is being applied. That is, if we are dealing with dialysis patients, the relevant life expectancy may be 10 years instead of 30.

The impact of life expectancy is even more dramatic when the goal is to compare two very different treatments—one aimed at young people and the other aimed at an older population. For instance, consider the following:

---

[4]There is an additional problem inherent in the utility scale. The utility scale is linear, that is the difference between 0.00 and 0.01 is the same as the difference between 0.50 and 0.51 or between 0.80 and 0.81. However, 0.00 is death and 0.01 implies continued life. Life and death are not measured on a continuous scale; they are discrete either/or conditions. Thus, it is important to recognize that the scale used to measure utilities cannot truly reflect the true situation, especially at the lower end of the scale.

QALY decision analysis examined the favorable and unfavorable outcomes of treating single-vessel coronary artery disease with TLC or Cardiomagic in individuals with an average age of 60. It compared these results with the prevention of paralysis by using a vaccine in children. The prevention of paralysis was shown to produce considerable more QALYs than the treatment of single-vessel coronary artery disease.

When comparing a treatment or a preventive intervention that is applied to very different age groups, it is important to recognize that a successful intervention among children results in a far greater improvement in life expectancy than an equally successful intervention among 60-year-olds. Thus, many more QALYs result from successful efforts to prevent paralysis in children compared with treatment of coronary artery disease among 60-year-olds. Decision-making investigations that incorporate life expectancy tend to favor the young. This tendency may or may not be justifiable, but the reader must recognize this tendency, especially when comparing different types of treatments aimed at different age groups.

Costs

To appreciate the costs that must be considered in a cost-effectiveness analysis, let us return to our example of paralysis:

Paralysis is a common contagious disease of childhood that is usually self-limited. However, a small percentage of children who experience the illness develop the complication of permanent paralysis, and a few develop life-threatening complications. The disease produces serious short-term life-threatening consequences. Long-term paralysis and late complications can also occur. The conventional treatment for paralysis has been only supportive treatment, which we will call a do-nothing approach. Recently, an expensive vaccination designed to prevent paralysis became available. A rare complication of the vaccine is development of a form of paralysis that is similar but usually less severe than the disease itself. We will see how we can compare the results of the vaccine with the do-nothing approach.

When assessing the costs of an intervention, it is necessary to consider the following types of cost.[5]

Health Care Costs

Health care costs include the cost of delivering the service and treating the short-term complications. For paralysis vaccine, this would include the costs of the vaccine and the associated costs of delivering the vaccine, as well as costs of treating the complications that develop as a result of administering the vaccine.

For the conventional treatment of symptoms and complications the costs include visits for health care and the cost of providing care for hospitalization and treatment of complications.

---

[5]These categories attempt to present the concepts incorporated into the recommendations of Gold et al. The separation of short-term and future health care costs is presented to clarify an important distinction for the reader. The omission of their use of the term DIRECT is an attempt to avoid confusion with other uses of this term, such as the use of *direct* and *indirect* to indicate program cost and institutional costs respectively. Both of these costs are included in the concept of direct as used in cost-effectiveness analysis. Note that this section does not attempt to define the methods used for actually measuring costs. The accuracy of the measurement of costs is an important issue, but one that is beyond the scope of this section.

Nonhealth Care Cost

Nonhealth care costs include that of time and the expense to access care by the patient as well as for anyone else who must provide paid or unpaid services. These especially include the costs of providing care outside the medical system even when this care is provided by family members without charge.

For paralysis vaccine, these costs include the time required from the parent or other caregiver to obtain the vaccine and time required to care for complications of the vaccine or the disease if the vaccine is not successful.

For the conventional approach, there are no costs of obtaining the vaccine but there will be considerable costs of taking care of the illness and the disease complications.

Future Health Care Costs

Future health care costs can theoretically be separated into costs that are and are not related to the treatment or the disease. The related costs of caring for long-term consequences of the disease or its treatment should be included in a cost-effectiveness analysis.[6]

For paralysis vaccine, future health care costs include the costs of ongoing care for all those who experience the complications of the vaccine and the costs of long-term treatment of those who experience the disease despite receiving the vaccine.

For conventional treatment, the future health care costs include the long-term cost of caring for those who experience the disease and survive the short-term life-threatening effects.

In this chapter, we have looked at what each of the variables needed to complete a decision-making investigation attempts to measure. Probabilities, utilities, life expectancy, and costs are included in the assessment. In the next chapter, we examine how the results are presented as part of the analysis.

---

[6]Unrelated costs include the cost of treating other diseases that occur unrelated to the disease being treated. For a condition like paralysis, these costs should be approximately the same for the vaccine and the conventional treatment. At the discretion of the investigator, these may be included for any added years of life. Gold recommends that the costs of treating unrelated disease be included during the years of life that would have been lived without the intervention and either included or excluded for the additional years of life. In addition, Gold's recommendations allow either inclusion or exclusion of nonmedical future costs, such as food and shelter (Gold RM, Siegel JE, Russell LB. *Cost-effectiveness in heath and medicine*. New York: Oxford University Press, 1996). We will assume that these are excluded as is increasingly the practice in most cost-effectiveness analyses.

30 Analysis

In Part 1, *Studying a Study,* we defined three analysis questions that apply to many forms of investigations. These are estimation, inference, and adjustment. The aim of estimation is to provide the best possible estimation of the strength of the relationship. Inference is an attempt to determine whether the results are likely to hold in a larger population. Adjustment aims to take into account differences between the alternatives being compared to see if they affect the results.

In decision-making investigations, certain approaches can be viewed as parallel to estimation, inference, and adjustment. Let us look at these one at a time.

Estimation

Estimation is a summary measure that results from an investigation. Each type of decision-making investigation produces one or more summary measurements. The measurement is different, however, if we are dealing with an expected-utility decision analysis, a QALY decision analysis, a cost-effectiveness study, or a cost-utility analysis.

The differences between the summary measurements used in different decision-making investigations depend largely on the factors that are used to measure the outcomes. Probabilities may be used, or life expectancy may be substituted. Cost may be used, or the investigation may focus exclusively on effectiveness.

To see what we mean by these different estimates, let us return to our TLC and Cardiomagic example.

Figure 30.1 reproduces the previous decision tree for TLC and Cardiomagic incorporating probabilities and utilities of each final outcome. The summary measurement or estimate for this decision-making study is the difference in expected utility:

$$0.9932 - 0.9808 = 0.0124$$

This measurement may have little meaning in-and-of-itself. However, an adjusted number-needed-to-treat can be calculated as 1 divided by this difference between the expected utilities. Here, the adjusted number-needed-to-treat equals the following:

$$1 \div 0.0124 \approx 80.0$$

This adjusted number-needed-to-treat tells us that on average 80 individuals need to be treated with TLC instead of Cardiomagic to produce one additional life at full health.[1]

---

[1]The adjusted number-needed-to-treat is being interpreted as the number of individuals who need to be treated with TLC as opposed to Cardiomagic to obtain one additional life at full health that would otherwise have resulted in an outcome with a utility of 0 (or death) if treated with Cardiomagic. That is how many individuals, who would have otherwise died, need to be treated to obtain the equivalent of one life saved at full health. As with all uses of expected utility, the meaning of the results assumes that we are willing to add together changes in utility from different individuals. Thus, we are assuming that preventing two cases of blindness, which provide two individuals an increase in utility from .5 to 1, is worth the same as providing full health at a utility of 1 compared with death at a utility of 0 for one individual.

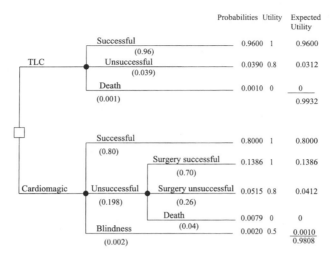

Figure 30.1. A utility decision tree incorporating probabilities and utilities for each outcome of TLC or Cardiomagic.

Now, let us look at the summary measurement that can be used when a decision-making investigation produces results measured in QALYs. The data from a QALY decision analysis are again presented Table 30.1.

This data allows us to easily present the difference in QALYs per use by subtracting the 17.12 QALYs for Cardiomagic from the 17.44 QALYs for TLC:

$$17.44 - 17.12 = 0.32$$

Again, this may not have very much meaning in-and-of-itself. In parallel to the measurement of expected utilities, we can calculate an adjusted number-needed-to-treat for QALYs as follows:

$$1 \div 0.32 \approx 3.0$$

Thus, on average, an additional QALY results from treating approximately three patients with TLC instead of Cardiomagic. The number-needed-to-treat to produce an additional QALY is thus a useful summary measure for cost-effectiveness as well as effectiveness. It tells us the number of individuals who need to receive the intervention of interest to produce one additional unit of desired outcome.

Table 30.1. *Quality Adjusted Life Years (QALYs) for TLC and Cardiomagic*

	Probability	Utility	Life expectancy	QALYs
TLC				
Successful	0.9600	1	18	17.28
Unsuccessful	0.0390	0.8	5	0.16
Death	0.0010	0	0	0
Total QALYs				17.44
Cardiomagic				
Successful	0.8000	1	18	14.40
Successful after surgery	0.1386	1	18	2.49
Unsuccessful after surgery	0.515	0.8	5	0.21
Death after surgery	0.0079	0	0	0
Blindness	0.0020	0.5	1.8	0.02
Total QALYs				17.12

Cost-Effectiveness Measures

In contrast to the measures of effectiveness, the estimates for cost-utility analyses are presented in two different ways that need to be understood and distinguished. Table 30.2 shows us the QALYs produced by TLC and Cardiomagic and also the costs of TLC and Cardiomagic. The table also shows this data for conventional treatment. These data allow us to calculate two types of summary measures. One is the cost-effectiveness ratio that has already presented. The other is known as INCREMENTAL COST-EFFECTIVENESS RATIOS.[2]

Let us examine the data for the decision using the three alternatives for single-vessel coronary artery disease (Table 30.2).

The cost-effectiveness ratio and the incremental cost-effectiveness ratios for the decision alternatives for single-vessel coronary artery disease would be calculated as follows:

$$\text{Cost-effectiveness of TLC} = \$116,600 \div 17.44 \text{ QALYs} = \$6,692/\text{QALY}$$

$$\text{Cost-effectiveness of Cardiomagic} = \$50,000 \div 17.12 \text{ QALYs} = \$2,920/\text{QALY}$$

Cost-effectiveness ratios measure the average cost of an alternative divided by the average health outcome if that alternative is used.

Incremental cost-effectiveness ratios as opposed to cost-effectiveness ratios make an explicit comparison between two alternatives. That is, they ask about the additional cost to obtain the additional effectiveness. Incremental cost-effectiveness ratios generally compare an alternative with conventional treatment. Using the data from Table 30.2, let us look at the incremental cost-effectiveness ratio of TLC compared with conventional treatment and Cardiomagic compared to conventional treatment.

$$\text{TLC vs. Conventional treatment} = (\$116,600 - \$20,000) / (17.4 \text{ QALYs} - 15 \text{ QALYs}) = \$96,600 / 2.4 \text{ QALYs} = \$40,000/\text{QALY}$$

$$\text{Cardiomagic vs. Conventional treatment} = (\$50,000 - \$20,000) / (17.12 \text{ QALYs} - 15 \text{ QALYs}) = \$30,000 / 2.12 \text{ QALYs} = \$14,151/\text{QALY}$$

Table 30.2. *Cost and QALYs of the TLC, Cardiomagic, and Conventional Treatment*

	Cost	QALYs
TLC	$116,600	17.44
Cardiomagic	$50,000	17.12
Conventional treatment	$20,000	15
Cost-effective Ratios		
TLC, $116,600 / 17.44 = $6,692/QALY		
Cardiomagic, $50,000 / 17.12 = $2,920/QALY		
Incremental Cost-effective Ratios		
TLC *vs.* Conventional = $40,000/QALY		
Cardiomagic *vs.* Conventional = $14,151/QALY		
TLC *vs.* Cardiomagic = $208,000/QALY		

[2]The special type of cost-effectiveness analysis called a cost-and-effectiveness study can also use cost-effectiveness and incremental cost-effectiveness ratios. However, for these studies, the cost-effectiveness ratio is cost per outcome, such as cost per life saved or cost per diagnosis made. The incremental cost-effectiveness ratio then measures the additional cost required to achieve an additional outcome such as a life saved or diagnosis made.

Notice that the incremental cost-effectiveness ratios are much greater than the cost-effectiveness ratios. This is the usual situation and reflects the different questions addressed by these two types of ratios. The cost-effectiveness ratio asks about the average cost of obtaining an outcome such as a QALY. This cost is really being compared with a DO-NOTHING OPTION. A do-nothing option is defined as not performing an active therapeutic intervention designed to change the outcome as opposed to the total absence of care. To the extent that do-nothing options are not very effective, an effective intervention can often produce additional QALYs at small to moderate costs.[3]

Incremental cost-effectiveness ratios on the other hand are usually comparing a new intervention with the existing conventional intervention. To the extent that the conventional intervention already has a reasonable degree of effectiveness, it should not be surprising that there are substantial costs per additional unit of effectiveness (i.e., per QALY). Thus, it is important to recognize that the incremental cost-effectiveness ratio is asking about the additional cost per additional unit of effectiveness measured as QALYs.

Incremental cost-effectiveness ratios can also be used to compare two new treatments, such as TLC versus Cardiomagic. When this form of comparison is made, however, we need to be aware of what is being compared; otherwise, considerable confusion can result. Let us calculate the incremental cost-effectiveness ratio comparing TLC with Cardiomagic:

$$\text{TLC vs. Cardiomagic} = (\$116,600 - \$50,000) / (17.44 - 17.12 \text{ QALYs})$$
$$= \$66,600 / 0.32 \text{ QALYs} = \$208,000/\text{QALY}$$

This very large cost-effectiveness analysis tells us that to produce an additional QALY using TLC instead of Cardiomagic will cost over $200,000 per QALY.

Which cost-effectiveness ratio to use depends on the question being asked. Usually the question has to do with a choice between alternative treatments. In these situations, the incremental cost-effectiveness ratios are the most informative. In fact, incremental cost-effectiveness ratios are now expected to be reported as part of a cost-effectiveness study. Which incremental-cost effectiveness ratio should be used? In general, comparing each new treatment to conventional treatment is the most helpful means of comparing different interventions for the same condition. In addition to providing a basis for comparison with other investigations, it also allows us to compare interventions for different conditions. At times, however, we may want to directly compare the impact of using two new treatments, such as TLC and Cardiomagic. In this situation, the incremental cost-effectiveness ratio comparing these two interventions may be useful.

Inference and Sensitivity Analysis

In Part 1, *Studying a Study,* we showed how confidence intervals can be used to perform inference. A similar approach, called SENSITIVITY ANALYSIS, is used in decision-making investigations. Sensitivity analysis is a general term used to

[3]The comparison group in a cost-effectiveness ratio is rarely specified. The costs are ideally being compared with the do-nothing approach but may in fact be compared with a zero cost alternative even if that does not in fact exist. When the do-nothing option carries costs such as custodial care, these costs may be reduced by the intervention being studied and thus may appear as costs reduced by the intervention.

describe a series of methods for isolating factors in a decision-making investigation and determining the influence each factor has on the results of the investigation. The analyses we have looked at so far use measures that are called BASE-CASE ESTIMATES. Base-case estimates represent the best available data or the investigators' best guess at the true value for the variable or factor. Sensitivity analyses are an effort to examine the consequences if the base-case estimate does not turn out to be accurate.

Sensitivity analyses are often classified as ONE-WAY or MULTIPLE-WAY SENSITIVITY ANALYSIS. In one-way sensitivity analyses, one factor at a time is examined to determine whether varying its level within a realistic range above and below the base-case estimate alters the conclusions of the investigation. Let us look at how a one-way sensitivity analysis might be performed:[4]

Table 30.3 summarizes the results of one-way sensitivity analyses that vary measures of the utility of blindness for the comparison of TLC and Cardiomagic. For this one-way sensitivity analysis, a high and a low estimate are used in addition to the base-case estimate that was used in the original analysis. The high estimate is designed to reflect the upper end of what is felt to be a realistic range of possible values while the low estimate is designed to reflect the lower end of this realistic range.

When looking at the results of one-way sensitivity analyses, we are interested in determining whether the relationships between the decision options change when the high or the low estimate is substituted for the base-case estimate. If using the low or the high estimate for a factor such as cost, probability, or utility alters the ranking of one option over another, then we say that the recommendation is sensitive to a particular factor. For instance, in constructing the decision tree for Cardiomagic, we used a base-case utility for blindness of .5. Now look at what happens in Table 30.3 if we alter the utility of blindness from a high of .9 to a low of .2. This change has very little impact on the expected utility, and the recommendation to use Cardiomagic is not affected.

Table 30.4 shows a one-way sensitivity analysis for Cardiomagic and cost. Notice that the impact of the high and low cost estimates on the incremental cost-effectiveness ratio is substantial. However, even the use of the high estimate produces an incremental cost-effectiveness ratio of $28,301/QALY, which is well below the $40,000/QALY incremental cost-effectiveness ratio for TLC. Thus, the conclusion that Cardiomagic is more cost effective than TLC is not sensitive to the estimates of cost.

Table 30.3. *Cardiomagic* vs. *Conventional Therapy:*
One-Way Sensitivity Analysis for Utility of Blindness

	Incremental cost (base-line)	Incremental QALYs	Incremental cost-effectiveness ratio
Blindness utility 0.9 (high)	$30,000	2.13	$14,133
Blindness utility 0.5 (base-case)	$30,000	2.12	$14,151
Blindness utility 0.2 (low)	$30,000	2.11	$14,179

[4]Other one-way sensitivity techniques are used for special purposes. One is THRESHOLD ANALYSIS, which varies key factors to determine the level of these factors that would alter the conclusions obtained from a particular decision-making investigation. Threshold analyses aim to determine the toss-up point or thresholds at which a different recommendation would be made.

Table 30.4. *Cardiomagic* vs. *Conventional Therapy:*
One-Way Sensitivity Analysis for Costs

	Incremental cost	Incremental QALYs (base-line)	Incremental cost-effectiveness ratio
Cardiomagic cost high	$60,000	2.12	$28,301/QALY
Cardiomagic cost base-case	$30,000	2.12	$14,151/QALY
Cardiomagic cost low	$20,000	2.12	$9,501/QALY

It is important to look one at a time at key factors and examine how their realistic high and low values may influence the recommendation. However, these one-way sensitivity analyses underestimate the uncertainty that exists because in practice, variation in more than one factor is at work at the same time. Thus, it is often important for the investigators to perform a multiple-way sensitivity analysis, altering two or more factors simultaneously.

An extreme but commonly used and easy to understand form of multiple-way sensitivity analysis is called the BEST CASE/WORST CASE ANALYSIS. Best case/worst case analysis reflects the investigators' attempt to create scenarios in which key factors are all favorable within a realistic range (best case) or unfavorable within a realistic range (worst case). These scenarios are not designed to reflect the very worst or very best possible outcomes but rather the extremes of realistic range.[5]

Table 30.5 shows how a best case/worst case analysis might look for comparing the cost-effectiveness ratio of TLC with conventional treatment. Two potentially important factors, the probability of success and the cost, are initially both set at the most favorable realistic estimate and then both are set at their least favorable realistic estimate.

When the probability of success and the cost for TLC are set at their most favorable realistic level (best case), the incremental cost-effectiveness ratio is $31,202/QALY. This best case situation for TLC is far greater than the $14,151/QALY base-case estimate for Cardiomagic, and it is greater than the high estimate of $28,301/QALY for Cardiomagic we obtained using our one-way sensitivity analysis. This provides convincing evidence that Cardiomagic is more cost effective than TLC.

Table 30.5. *Cost Effectiveness of TLC* vs. *Conventional Treatment:*
Best Case/Worse Case Analysis

	Incremental cost	Incremental cost-effectiveness ratio
TLC best case success = 0.98	$85,000	$31,202/QALY
TLC base case success = 0.96	$96,600	$40,000/QALY
TLC worse case success = 0.90	$120,000	− $500,000/QALY

[5]The best case/worst case sensitivity analysis is often considered too demanding an approach since it is unlikely that uncertainties in multiple key variables will act in the same direction. Other forms of multiple-way sensitivity analyses are increasingly being used to calculate confidence intervals or CREDIBILITY INTERVALS. A number of complicated mathematical approaches are used to obtain these estimates. The best known is the MONTE CARLO SIMULATION which aims to establish confidence intervals by randomly selecting levels of each of the key variables using computer simulations. By performing a large number of these simulations, a distribution of results can be obtained and used to calculate a confidence interval or credibility interval.

When the probability of success and the cost of TLC are set at their least favorable realistic level (worst case), the incremental cost-effectiveness ratio is −$500,000. The negative number implies that, given these unfavorable assumptions, TLC is now less cost effective than conventional treatment. If these unfavorable assumptions are true when compared with the base-case for conventional treatment, then by spending $500,000 on TLC, we are reducing the effectiveness by 1 QALY compared with using conventional treatment. Thus, our multiple-way sensitivity analysis has raised some degree of uncertainty as to whether TLC is actually a better treatment than conventional therapy.

Adjustment and Discounting

Adjustment is performed to take into account differences in alternatives that can affect the results. The timing of events is one very important factor that we have not identified until now but which usually needs to be taken into account or adjusted for as part of the analysis in a decision-making investigation. Timing of events is important for both decision analysis and cost-effectiveness analysis.

To understand the impact of the timing of events, let us take another look at TLC. Recall that using the base-case, TLC has been found to be effective in treating single-vessel coronary artery disease compared with conventional treatment. It produces a substantially greater probability of favorable short-term outcomes despite its slight increase in adverse outcomes.

Short-term net effectiveness in comparison with conventional treatment still leaves open questions regarding TLC's impact on favorable outcomes in the long term as well as possible long-term adverse outcomes. Assume that the following information is now available:

> More than a decade after the widespread use of TLC began, it was recognized that late effects on the coronary artery made it more likely to close, producing a higher incidence of late myocardial infarction.

In most decision-making situations, not all events occur at the same time. The impacts of treatment may be immediate or delayed for many years. Even in the absence of an intervention, a disease may not have an impact for many years in the future. Note that people who experience the late effect on the coronary artery have still received the advantage of the favorable short-term outcome. That is, on average, they have lived longer.

The most common and accepted method for taking into account the consequences of the timing of events is DISCOUNTING.[6] Discounting considers the fact that the benefits, harms, and costs that occur in the future are given less importance than those that occur immediately. The concept of discounting comes from economics and is most easily understood in terms of costs. However, it is important

---

[6]The two basic approaches to taking into account the effects of timing are discounting and incorporating the timing of events into utilities. Most experts consider discounting of costs, favorable outcomes, and adverse outcomes to be the proper approach for decision analysis and also for cost-effectiveness analysis. In decision analysis, however, timing of events is often incorporated into utilities. Note that decision trees are structured to reflect the sequence of events, but they do not tell much about the time intervals between events. Long-term consequences are not necessarily distinguished from short-term consequences in a decision tree. Unless explicit discounting occurs, outcomes are usually dealt with as if they occur simultaneously. That is, a discount rate of 0% is used or the impact of timing is incorporated into the measurement of utilities.

to recognize that discounting or taking into account the timing of events needs to be conducted for costs, favorable outcomes or benefits, and adverse outcomes or harms. An adverse outcome in the distant future is not as bad as an adverse outcome that occurs in the immediate future. Similarly, a favorable outcome in the distant future is not valued as highly as a favorable outcome that occurs in the immediate future. For instance, with paralysis vaccine, the favorable outcome of prevention of paralysis does not necessarily occur immediately. A case of paralysis prevented may occur a number of years in the future.

The concept of discounting can be understood by recognizing that most people prefer to receive $100 today rather than $100 a year from now. This is the situation even if the pay-off a year from now takes into account inflation. That is, most people prefer $100 now to receiving $100 plus a guaranteed adjustment for inflation a year from now. As economists see it, if you receive $100 today, you generally can invest the money and, on average, receive a REAL RATE OF RETURN. The real rate of return means that 1 year from now, you will have more than $100 even after adjusting for inflation.

Looked at the other way, most people would prefer to pay $100 a year from now rather than today. A dollar paid in the future is not as costly as a dollar spent today. In fact, when performing discounting, the investigator is really calculating the amount of money that needs to be invested today to pay bills that are not due until a future time. The amount of money that needs to be invested today is called the DISCOUNTED PRESENT VALUE or PRESENT VALUE. To calculate the discounted present value, the investigator needs to choose what is called a discount rate. Choosing a 3% annual discount rate implies that approximately $97 dollars need to be put aside today to ensure the availability of an inflation adjusted $100 a year from now. If the discount rate is 5%, only about $95 needs to be put aside today to ensure the availability of an inflation adjusted $100 a year from now.[7]

What is the proper discount rate? Economist generally agree that costs should be discounted to reflect the real rate of return, which is the rate that can be expected on average from investing money even after taking into account the impact of inflation. There the agreement ceases since the real rate of return is neither constant nor predictable. However, the accepted range of discount rates is between 3% and 5%. A 3% discount rate is recommended as the base-case when performing a sensitivity analysis. A second analysis to determine the consequences of using a 5% discount rate can also be performed.

The discount rate for favorable and adverse effects should generally be the same as the discount rate used for costs. If different rates are used, the following situation can occur:

> In discounting cost, favorable outcomes, and adverse outcomes for paralysis vaccine, costs were discounted at 5% but favorable outcomes were discounted at 3%. The authors concluded that since interventions that could be implemented in the future were much less expensive, it is desirable to wait to implement a paralysis vaccine campaign.

---

[7]Note that if the discount rate is 0%, then $100 needs to be put aside to ensure the availability of $100 a year from now. Thus, if discounting is not performed the investigator is really assuming a discount rate of 0%.

Discounting costs at a greater discount rate than favorable outcomes always encourages delay. In fact, every year it looks desirable to wait until the next year when costs look more affordable compared with favorable outcomes. Thus, regardless of the discount rate that is used, it is important to discount cost, favorable outcomes, and adverse outcomes at the same discount rate. It is not enough just to discount costs. It is generally accepted that favorable and adverse outcomes also need to be discounted and at the same discount rate.

31 Interpretation

Meaning of Cost-effectiveness Ratios

As with all types of investigations, interpretation is designed to evaluate the implications of the results for the types of individuals who are included in the investigation. With decision-making investigations, no individual or group is actually included in the investigations. Rather, the investigator usually creates a model designed to simulate the situation facing a particular type or group of individuals. Thus, the interpretation of a decision-making investigation should address the investigation's implications for the types of individuals for which the investigation was designed.

Often, the most important and confusing interpretation in a decision-making investigation is the meaning of the cost-effectiveness ratios. Let us take a close look at how we interpret these ratios for the types of studies on coronary artery disease and paralysis that we have already examined. To obtain comparable measures, we use incremental cost-effectiveness ratio comparing each option with the do-nothing treatment.

As we have seen, the base-case results of the three alternatives for treating single-vessel coronary artery disease and use of paralysis vaccine are as follows:

TLC: $116,600 ÷ 17.44 QALYs
Cardiomagic: $50,000 ÷ 17.12 QALYs
Conventional treatment: $20,000 ÷ 15 QALYs

For paralysis vaccine, there is only one option since the conventional treatment is the same as the do-nothing options:

Paralysis vaccine: −$5,000 ÷ 1 QALY

To compare this cost-effective ratio to TLC, we can calculate
the cost of 17.44 QALYs as follows:

Paralysis vaccine: −$87,200 ÷ 17.44 QALYs

To examine the implications of these cost-effectiveness ratios, they can be plotted together on a cost–QALYs graph. Figure 31.1 is a cost–QALYs graph. Notice that Figure 31.1 contains four potential areas, or quadrants, labeled A, B, C, and D. The zero point for the graph is the do-nothing option with which all other options are compared. Figure 31.2 includes the plotted costs and effectiveness on our cost–QALYs graph.

A location in each of the four quadrants has a different implication. Quadrant D, where paralysis vaccine is located, is the ideal quadrant. Here, there is increased effectiveness as measured by QALYs and reduced cost as measured in dollars. The incremental cost-effectiveness ratio in quadrant D is thus negative. When an option

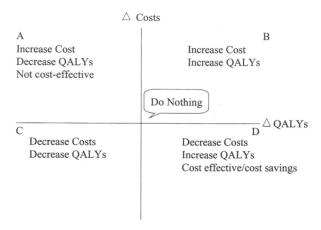

Figure 31.1. A cost–QALYs graph.

is located in quadrant D it is cost-saving/effectiveness-increasing. This is a special situation where we can unequivocally say that the results are cost effective.

At times, this situation is called COST SAVINGS. Use of this term results in considerable confusion since, as we shall see, cost savings can also result when the number of QALYs are reduced. This is the situation when the results are in quadrant C, in which there is also a cost reduction accompanied by an effectiveness reduction as measured by reduced QALYs. Quadrant C is more accurately labeled cost-reducing/effectiveness-reducing.

When interpreting decision options that fall into quadrant C, it is important to recognize that these may be labeled cost-effective if the decision-maker concludes that a relatively small reduction in QALYs is worth the substantial reduction in cost. At times, it may be reasonable to substantially reduce costs even though effectiveness is also reduced. However, calling this approach cost effective obscures what is happening. It is better to label this cost-reducing/effectiveness-reducing and then to separately determine whether the substantial reduction in cost justifies the reduction in effectiveness.

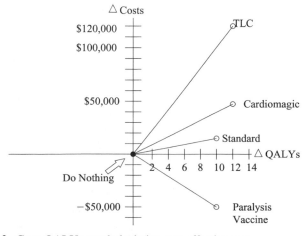

Figure 31.2. Cost–QALYs graph depicting cost effectiveness.

Quadrant A is also a clear-cut result. In this quadrant, the costs are increased and the effectiveness is decreased. Therefore, neither costs nor effectiveness support a decision option that falls in quadrant A and such options should be labeled as not cost effective.

Most alternatives being considered by cost-utility or QALY cost-effectiveness studies end up in quadrant B. These decision alternatives increase both cost and effectiveness. When an alternative is located in quadrant B, it is very important to determine the magnitude of the cost-effectiveness ratios and to be sure their meaning is clear.

Defining Cost-effective

When treatments are located in quadrant B, where both costs and effectiveness are increased, we are faced with the difficult questions of where to draw the line. Let us review the data we have obtained on incremental cost-effectiveness ratios for TLC and Cardiomagic:

> The incremental cost-effectiveness ratios for TLC compared with standard treatment is $40,000 per QALY and the incremental cost-effectiveness ratio for Cardiomagic compared with standard therapy is $14,151 per QALY. The incremental cost effectiveness of TLC compared to Cardiomagic is $208,000 per QALY. Which treatment(s) should be considered cost effective?

The answer depends on how cost effectiveness is defined. Considerable controversy exists regarding the methods for interpreting these results and deciding which treatment(s) should be labeled cost effective. A variety of methods have been used to try to categorize the results of incremental cost-effectiveness ratios to be able to declare a level which is considered cost effective. This has been very controversial since determining what dollar figure to use to draw a line requires placing a monetary value on a QALY.[1]

Despite the considerable controversy surrounding the best method to use, many cost-effectiveness studies act as if there were three categories of results:

1. Those that are clearly within the cost-effective range for a QALY from the social perspective
2. Those that are clearly outside the cost-effective range for a QALY from a social perspective
3. Those that are in a borderline cost-effectiveness range for a QALY from a social perspective

In the United States, the clearly cost-effective range in the literature has been approximately $30,000 per QALY or less. The clearly outside the cost-effective

---

[1]One method used to place a monetary value on a QALY is the HUMAN CAPITAL APPROACH, which attempts to convert a QALY into a dollar value based on recipient's ability to contribute economically. This approach has been criticized because it only includes activities that result in financial payments and thus undervalues those who work without monetary payments, the retired and low-wage groups. Efforts have been made to use what economists call a WILLINGNESS-TO-PAY APPROACH. These approaches are attractive to economists but have been very difficult to implement, and special situations such as legal cases may distort the data. Two other approaches with less theoretical foundations are also used. Past practice with drawing lines and refusing to pay may be used as evidence of where a society is willing to draw the line. A simple approach that takes into account the ability to pay is to use the per capita income, or the per-capita gross domestic product of the nation in which the investigation is conducted or to which the results will be applied.

range has been considered $100,000 per QALY or more. This approach makes it clear that the $14,151 per QALY for Cardiomagic is considered cost effective. However, this leaves a large borderline zone in which the $40,000 per QALY for TLC clearly lies.[2]

In general, results that fall within the borderline range should not be declared cost effective. In addition results in the borderline range should not be classified as not cost effective. Decisions on how to treat these borderline incremental cost-effectiveness ratios need to be left to the actual user and the specific situation.

TLC has been found to be slightly more effective but considerably more expensive. If we are faced with a choice between using Cardiomagic or TLC, the incremental cost-effectiveness ratio tells us the additional cost which must be incurred to provide the additional benefit. Using the methods increasingly applied in cost-effectiveness analysis, TLC would not be considered cost effective from the social perspective if Cardiomagic can be used instead.

What are the implications when an intervention falls clearly outside the range of cost effectiveness from the social perspective? First, it is important to note that when an intervention is clearly outside the cost-effective range, it may still be more effective than the alternatives. In fact, TLC has been found to be slightly more effective than Cardiomagic, producing 17.44 QALYs per use compared with 17.12 QALYs for Cardiomagic. These additional QALYs, however, are very expensive to achieve. The incremental cost-effectiveness ratio of $208,000 per QALY is telling us that from the social perspective, no society can afford to generally provide everyone in need with QALYs that cost this much.[3]

It is important to recognize that an intervention that has been declared not cost effective from a social perspective may look quite different from an individual perspective. An individual who has the personal resources or adequate insurance coverage may well favor the use of TLC rather than Cardiomagic despite the extremely high cost per extra QALY that results.

Distributional Effects

We have already seen that cost-effectiveness analysis may be viewed as being biased in favor of the young over the old. In addition, we have seen that a bias exists in cost-effectiveness analysis towards the healthy as opposed to the permanently and severely disabled. In particular situations, there may be additional tendencies to favor one group over another. To understand these impacts, it is important to examine the results of a decision-making investigation to determine what types of individuals receive the favorable outcomes and what types experience the adverse

[2]Acceptable and unacceptable ranges depend heavily on a society's ability to pay. The gross domestic product is one method for helping to define this range. The $30,000 figure is clearly within the per capita income for North America and most of Europe and Japan. This is not the case if the same application was used in a nation with a per capita income of $1,500. However, in nations with low per capita incomes, the costs may also be substantially lower. When a definitive value is set on a QALY, the investigation is really a cost-benefit analysis since equating a QALY with a set monetary figure allows all outcomes to be converted to dollars. Remember that the essential difference between cost-effectiveness analysis and cost-benefit analysis is that in cost-benefit analysis, outcomes and costs are measured in the same monetary units.

[3]The fact that a country cannot afford to generally provide everyone in need with QALYs that cost this much does not preclude a society from paying for specific services that would otherwise be considered not cost effective from the social viewpoint. A number of political, economic, and even research rationales may be made for heavily subsidizing a limited number of expensive services.

outcomes. In addition, it is important to focus on the types of individuals who bear the financial costs.

The process of interpreting the results of a decision-making investigation is not limited to interpreting the summary measures such as incremental cost-effectiveness ratios. Summary measures, by definition, are averages. They are designed to summarize the average results. Average results do not tell the whole story for two fundamental reasons. First, the average does not in-and-of-itself say much about what types of individuals experience the favorable outcomes and what types experience the adverse outcomes or must pay the additional costs. Examining the types of individuals who experience the favorable and adverse outcomes and pay the cost is known as examining the DISTRIBUTIONAL EFFECTS of the intervention.

To illustrate the distributional effects, let us return to the paralysis example and consider an aspect of the vaccine that we have not focused on previously. That is, which type of individual experienced the favorable and the adverse outcomes of the vaccine.

> The favorable outcomes of the paralysis vaccine are the prevention of paralysis. The adverse outcomes are the rare occurrence of a paralysis-like illness among children of parents who have voluntarily had their children vaccinated.

It is unfortunate whenever anyone experiences the adverse outcomes of an intervention. However, when children (or their parents) voluntarily agree to accept the treatment after they are made aware of known adverse effects, they are accepting the adverse outcomes as part of the treatment. However, that is not the situation if the treatment is not accepted voluntarily. Imagine that the following new information is available on the impact of the paralysis vaccine:

> It has been found that the virus contained in the vaccine can spread to other children. Children exposed to their vaccinated peers are often protected while a few children unknowingly exposed to vaccinated children may experience the paralysis-like illness.

Thus, here the impact of the adverse effects of the vaccine may fall on persons who never voluntarily agreed to receive the vaccine. Some may argue that submitting individuals to harm without their (or their parents') agreement is not an acceptable approach even if it results, on average, in improved outcomes at reduced costs. Regardless of how you view this controversy, it is important to recognize the distributional effects.[4]

Risk-taking Attitudes

In addition to the distributional effects of the potential outcomes and costs, it is helpful to look not only at the average outcome but at how much and how often the results are especially good or especially bad. Decision-makers may be less interested in the average result than in the less frequent but important outcomes that are especially good or especially bad. At times, these favorable outcomes may greatly improve the quality of life for an individual and, conversely, adverse outcomes may be devastating.

[4]Distributional effects often raise issues of social justice related to the impact on groups in society who have a lower socioeconomic status or are otherwise disadvantaged. Disproportionate negative impacts on groups who are already at a social disadvantage are often seen as violating principles of social justice.

When the outcomes that may occur are quite variable, decision-makers may well be attracted by the possibility of an especially favorable outcome or repelled by the possibility of an especially bad outcome. In these situations, the decision-maker may be willing to take risks to achieve the favorable outcomes or wish to avoid risks to avoid experiencing the unfavorable outcome.

When interpreting the results of a decision-making investigation, it is important to recognize that these studies usually assume what is called RISK NEUTRALITY. Risk neutrality implies that the choice of alternatives is not influenced by a tendency to gamble to achieve a desired outcome (*i.e.,* RISK SEEKING). Similarly, risk neutrality implies that the decision is not influenced by a tendency to avoid choosing an alternative that poses the potential of an unacceptable adverse outcome (*i.e.,* RISK AVOIDING).[5]

Individuals vary in their risk-taking attitudes and behavior, but for most people, there are conditions under which they are likely to gamble and under which they are very cautious and try to avoid taking chances. Before accepting the recommendation of a decision-making investigation based on risk neutrality, it is important to examine the situation and decide whether risk-taking or risk-avoiding behavior is likely to be a common tendency.

Let us see what we mean by risk taking and risk avoiding by looking at the following situation that requires a choice between two options:

Assume you have coronary artery disease that has resulted in a quality of health equivalent to 0.8 compared with your previous state of full health (*i.e.,* 1). Imagine that you are offered the following pair of options but you can select only one of the two. Which do you prefer?

Option 1.   Select a treatment with the following possible outcome:

- 50% chance of raising the quality of your health from 0.8 to 1 and
- 50% chance of an outcome that reduces the quality of your health from 0.8 to 0.6

Option 2.   Refuse the treatment and accept a quality of your health of 0.8.

This decision is a classic "toss-up." That is, according to the expected utility, both choices are the same. To see why this is the case, Figure 31.3 shows a decision tree

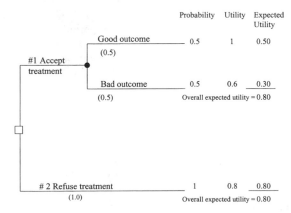

Figure 31.3. A decision tree depicting a risk neutral toss-up decision.

[5]Decision-making investigations do not usually indicate their risk-taking approach. When nothing is mentioned, the reader can reasonably conclude that the approach is risk neutral. Expected utility approaches, for instance, are inherently risk neutral. For that reason, the results of expected-utility decision analyses must be used with care when applied to a particular individual since that individual may be a risk seeker or a risk avoider in any one particular situation.

depicting this decision and calculates the expected utility for options 1 and 2. Notice that the expected utilities for the two decision options are the same. Although these options are considered a toss-up, most people do not view the outcomes as identical.

In this situation, some individuals will be risk takers who favor option 1 in order to have the possibility of improving their health. Faced with the same choice, other individuals will refuse the treatment. They are risk avoiding and unwilling to accept the possibility that their health would be worse as a result of the treatment. Risk neutrality is unusual in individual decision making where the individual only has one opportunity to choose between alternative treatments. This is one reason why decision-making investigations that examine average results are more useful for groups and populations than for individual decision making.[6]

In this chapter, we have examined how the results of a decision-making investigation can be applied to the type of individual included in the decision-making model. Finally, as with other types of investigations, we turn our attention to effort to extend or extrapolate the data. Thus we will next examine how decision-making investigations can be used as the basis for Practice Guidelines that apply what has been learned to new situations.

---

[6]Risk-taking and risk-avoiding situations are important in clinical as well as population or public health decision making. In clinical situations, risk-seeking attitudes generally occur when the clinical condition is severe and the outlook is poor. Patients are frequently willing to take a "long shot" when they are severely ill or faced with enduring a poor quality of life (*i.e.,* a low utility). On the other hand, when individuals have what they perceive to be a minor impairment (*i.e.,* a utility close to 1), they are likely to be risk avoiding or risk averse.

32 Extrapolation

In Part 1, *Studying a Study,* we examined several types of extrapolation, including extrapolation of results to individuals like those included in a study. For decision-making investigations, we first need to consider the impact of extrapolating the results to all individuals who are similar to those included in the investigation.

To Similar Populations

The process of extrapolation to similar populations is the basis of what are called PRACTICE GUIDELINES. Practice guidelines ideally extrapolate from what has been learned from decision-making investigations and use them to make recommendations for clinical, institutional, or public health practice.

Practice guidelines can make any of three different types of recommendations called *standards, guidelines, and options.* STANDARDS imply a recommendation that should be implemented for all individuals to whom the practice guidelines apply. A standard may state that an intervention should occur or alternatively that an intervention should not occur. GUIDELINES imply a recommendation for using one of the alternatives that applies to a substantial majority of the individuals whom the practice guidelines address. However, the recommendation may also include specific exceptions indicating when another alternative should be used.

Practice guidelines that include what are called OPTIONS suggest there is no single alternative that can be recommended. This often means that differences in patients' utilities can alter the most desirable alternative. The inclusion of options may also imply that the data are not adequate to recommend one intervention over an alternative.

Let us imagine that the following practice guidelines were proposed for single-vessel coronary artery disease. See if you can identify standards, guidelines, and options included in the following recommendation:

> Cardiomagic is indicated for initial treatment of single-vessel coronary artery disease. Surgery is contraindicated for initial therapy. If Cardiomagic fails, conventional treatment should be used unless it has already been unsuccessful. In these cases, TLC should be used. If Cardiomagic, TLC, and conventional therapy are all unsuccessful, either immediate surgery or observation followed by surgical intervention for increasing symptoms may be used.

When the practice guidelines state that Cardiomagic is indicated without presenting any contraindications, this implies that using Cardiomagic as initial treatment is a standard; that is, it is the expected treatment. The fact that surgery is contraindicated reinforces that standards can imply what should not be done as well as what should.

The recommendation for treatment if Cardiomagic fails is a guideline. It states what should generally be done for the majority of individuals to whom the practice guideline apply, but it makes an alternative recommendation for a specific situation (*i.e.,* if cardiomagic fails conventional treatment should be used unless it has already been unsuccessful. In these cases TLC should be used.).

If Cardiomagic, TLC, and conventional therapy have all been unsuccessful, the practice guidelines present options for immediate surgery or observation followed by surgical intervention for increasing symptoms. The use of options implies there is no clear-cut advantage of one approach over the other or that the data is not available to support one approach over the other.

Two additional issues should be considered when extrapolating to similar populations. When additional QALYs result from an intervention, we need to consider their meaning and their overall impact.

First, it is important to recognize that the QALYs being added are not added equally to all individuals who undergo the treatment. Some will experience a major positive outcome, some will experience no change, and some will experience only an adverse effect. In addition, depending on the timing of outcomes, some of the outcomes will be immediate, some will occur in the not too distant future, and others will be experienced many years in the future.

An appreciation of the impact of additional QALYs helps to avoid the following common but incorrect extrapolation of the results of a cost-effectiveness study:

> A reviewer of the cost-effectiveness literature noted that the effectiveness of Cardiomagic was 17.12 QALYs per use compared with 15 QALYs per use for conventional therapy. The reviewer concluded that this was a quite small difference, especially because the impact occurs by adding years at the end of life.

The additional 2.5 QALYs gained per use are actually quite impressive. Few interventions provide this large an increase in QALYs. In addition, Cardiomagic is being used to treat single-vessel coronary artery disease, a condition that can be immediately fatal in middle-age patients. For those who experience the benefit, the impact is immediate and substantial. That is, when it is effective, it can be expected to prolong the life of younger individuals although it may not influence the longevity of the elderly.

In addition, to understand the impact of a decision-making study on a target population similar to the one included in the investigation model, it is important to appreciate the overall or AGGREGATE EFFECTS. When extrapolating to a target population that has similar characteristics to the population modeled or displayed in the decision tree, the investigators are often interested in the overall impact or aggregate effect. The overall impact or aggregate impact will depend on the size of the target population.

In decision analysis using QALYs, for instance, aggregate effectiveness may be reported as the total number of QALYs that would result if the intervention was applied to all individuals in a particular population who are similar to those included in the model used in the investigation.

Let us see the potential impact of considering the aggregate effects by comparing the results of TLC and paralysis vaccine:

> A reviewer of the Cardiomagic and paralysis cost-effectiveness literature noted that Cardiomagic provides on average 2.5 additional QALYs per use while paralysis vaccine provides far less than 1 QALY per use. Nevertheless, he noted that in the United States, using Cardiomagic for all patients with single-vessel coronary artery disease will save 1.5 million QALYs compared with standard treatment while using the

paralysis vaccine for all children will provide 2 million QALYs. Therefore, he concluded that paralysis vaccine is more effective than Cardiomagic.

Care must be taken when using measures of aggregate effectiveness to compare two different types of interventions, such as paralysis vaccine and treatment of single-vessel coronary artery disease that are applied to two very different target populations. Aggregate effectiveness addresses a different question than do the cost-effectiveness studies. Aggregate effectiveness, like population attributable risk, asks questions that depend on the particular composition and size of a target population. Aggregate effectiveness does not compare one procedure or approach with another. Rather, it compares the impact of the procedure plus the characteristics and size of the target population. This approach may be useful at times for making population-based decisions but it requires additional data and additional assumptions that are not part of the results of cost-effectiveness analysis.

Beyond the Data

Extrapolation often requires that we extend the results to situations for which we do not have data. This is called EXTRAPOLATION BEYOND THE DATA. An investigator may conduct this form of extrapolation using LINEAR EXTRAPOLATION. That is, the investigator may assume that more effort will produce more results in direct proportion to the increased effort. This linear assumption may not hold true, especially when extending beyond the range of the data.

Cost, for instance, may not increase in a linear or straight-line fashion as volume increases. The costs of increasing the scale or volume of services provided are referred to as MARGINAL COSTS. Let us see what we mean by marginal costs in the following example:[1]

> As paralysis vaccine programs were implemented, it was found that the cost per vaccine delivered fell initially as the program grew and could more efficiently use personnel and publicize the program using mass media. However, as the program continued to expand, costs per vaccine delivered began to rise again as extra efforts were needed to identify and to obtain access to the most difficult to reach individuals.

Economists refer to ECONOMIES AND DISECONOMIES OF SCALE. The initial reduced cost per vaccine delivered is an example of an economy of scale whereas the eventual increase in cost per vaccine delivered is an example of a diseconomy of scale.

To Other Populations and Other Perspectives

As we noted in Part 1, *Studying a Study,* extrapolation to populations with different underlying assumptions or different characteristics can lead to very misleading results. Let us first look at the potential for problems when we extrapolate the results of a decision-making investigation to a new population, nation, or culture.

> Paralysis vaccine was introduced into the rural areas of a developing country where a dependable source of electricity for refrigerating the vaccine could not always be assured. In this setting, the results of the intervention were very different in that the

---

[1]The term MARGINAL COSTS is sometimes incorrectly equated with incremental costs. It is important to distinguish between these two very different concepts.

cost was considerably reduced but so was the effectiveness. Once the problems with handling the vaccine were addressed, the intervention was found to cost only $500 per QALY. Unfortunately, this was considered more than the developing nation was able or willing to pay.

This example illustrates many of the problems with extrapolating from one population to another. The costs of labor and of delivering services may be much less in a developing country. However, if special training or equipment is needed for effectiveness, then effectiveness may also be reduced. Even if the cost-effectiveness ratios are substantially lower in a developing nation, the developing country may not have the ability or willingness to pay. Thus, it is a very difficult task to extrapolate cost-effectiveness data and results from one society to another.

Extrapolation to groups with different characteristics can also produce wrong or misleading conclusions. For instance, imagine the following extrapolation of the TLC and Cardiomagic results:

> The successful use of Cardiomagic for single-vessel coronary artery disease was so convincing that the results were widely extrapolated to recommend use of Cardiomagic for patients with severe coronary artery disease in two or more vessels. The favorable outcomes were not as great and the adverse outcomes were greatly increased when Cardiomagic was applied to this new group of individuals.

It is not surprising that the outcomes will be different when an intervention is applied to groups with more severe or different types of disease. Therefore, just as in other types of investigations, it is very important in decision-making studies to carefully examine the types of individuals who are included in the alternatives being compared. Extrapolation to other groups carries assumptions that may not hold true among the new group of individuals to whom the results are extrapolated.

In addition to extrapolation to societies and new groups within the same society, we need to consider what happens when we extrapolate to a different perspective. This is a tempting but difficult form of extrapolation that is especially relevant to decision-making investigations. To understand the difficulty in extrapolating from the social perspective to a payer perspective, imagine the following situations.

> A health insurance administrator for an insurance system that provides coverage for individuals until they are 65 years old examined the cost-effectiveness study of TLC and Cardiomagic. He concluded that despite the fact that Cardiomagic was more cost effective from the social perspective than TLC, from the perspective of his insurance plan, TLC was more cost effective and should be the only alternative covered under that plan.

This situation demonstrates the potential consequence of trying to apply cost-effectiveness studies conducted with a social perspective to a payer perspective. If a health insurance system has only limited responsibility for paying for care or has responsibility for a limited number of years, the administrators may view costs quite differently than if they have life-long comprehensive responsibility as is assumed from the social perspective.

For instance, if responsibility for costs only lasts until age 65 years and the average age of those who undergo the procedure is 60 years, the insurance company may be especially concerned with short-term costs. Thus, it is important to recognize that the payer perspective on cost often looks very different from the social perspective.[2]

Another user perspective that may be taken when viewing the results of a cost-effectiveness analysis is the provider or institutional perspective. Let us see how TLC and Cardiomagic might look from this perspective:

> A reviewer of TLC and Cardiomagic as well as the paralysis vaccine literature looked at the relative costs and effectiveness of these two types of interventions from the social perspective. He concluded that for the same expenditure of funds, more QALYs could be obtained by providing all children with paralysis vaccine and reducing the use of TLC. A hospital administrator whose hospital performed large number of TLC procedures argued in response that from the hospital's perspective, if TLC procedures were reduced in half, it would only serve to substantially increase the cost of performing the remaining TLC procedures.

The provider or institutional perspective is reflected in the approach of the hospital administrator. From his perspective, costs are seen quite differently than from the social perspective. For instance, institutions have fixed costs, such as equipment, that remain regardless of how many TLC procedures they perform. The social and institutional perspectives may both be true as seen from different points of view.[3]

As we have indicated, cost-effectiveness investigations are ideally conducted from the broadest perspective, the social perspective. All other types of perspectives can be viewed as subtypes of the social perspective. The social perspective is not only broader than the perspective of any one individual, institution, or group, but it is even broader than the population perspective that takes into account all people in the current population. The social perspective ideally also considers future populations and the impacts of change over time.[4]

Finally, it is important to remember that cost-effectiveness investigations like all studies are conducted assuming a set of current alternatives and data. The alternatives may change rapidly, and unfortunately, cost-effectiveness analyses may sometimes be considered out of date by the time they are completed.

[2]Note that the government and the social perspective are not the same. Often, government has a payer perspective. If a government provides insurance coverage, it may have a payer perspective. When comprehensive lifetime benefits are provided, including Social Security, that provide living expenses for the elderly, the tendency is even to go beyond the social perspective to try to include the additional living expenses for the additional years of life. Inclusion of these costs has been controversial, but they are not generally included from the social perspective. Payer perspectives may also be influenced by the special characteristics of the subgroup of individuals for whom they are responsible. Insurance companies that cover generally healthy individuals may look at recommendations quite differently than an insurance plan that covers the general population or individuals who have advanced disease.

[3]In addition, institutions may have personnel costs that can't be reduced for lower volume since they need the equipment to be staffed regardless of volume of services. In addition, change itself involves economic (and psychological) costs. Institutions may have special concerns regarding the effect that the change will have on its reputation, cash flow, or other local effects. The social perspective views all costs and outcomes as averages for the future and does not take any of these factors into account. Thus, any one provider or institution looking at a cost-effectiveness study will not necessarily agree that the conclusions drawn from the social perspective apply to them.

[4]We can think of perspectives as being individual, institutional or target population, and social. The first three are static in that they look at the world as it currently exists and examine an intervention's impact at different levels of aggregation (*i.e.,* one individual, a group, the target population). In contrast, the social perspective ideally is dynamic. It looks not only at the current state of affairs but tries to incorporate changes over time. These changes are only partially predictable so it is often difficult to fully reflect the social perspective. Nonetheless, policies aimed at encouraging innovation, funding research, or making other investments that are not likely to pay off for many years reflect the dynamic component of the social perspective.

Despite the potential problems and difficulties in conducting decision-making investigations, it is important to recognize the contributions that these types of investigations make to clinical care and public health. The requirements to measure and express results quantitatively can improve communication. Decision-making studies require the investigator to apply numbers to vague terms such as rare and common and likely and unlikely. The need to explicitly define the decision-making process means that consequences must be defined and uncertainties recognized. Uncertainty always exists in decision making. Formal decision-making investigations help us to measure and to determine the impact of uncertainty.

The decision-making literature is an important part of the movement toward evidence-based decision making in health care and public health. Decision-making investigations require the investigator to spell out in great detail the available evidence and the assumptions that have been made in filling the holes where evidence is not available. In decision-making investigations, the investigator must be able to respond to the demands to show the evidence and justify the assumptions.

Finally, the forms of decision-making studies that incorporate costs have added an entire new dimension to the health research literature. Previously, clinical and public health decision-making relied almost exclusively on issues of favorable and adverse outcomes. Technological advances in recent years have opened up so many therapeutic and preventive alternatives, no society can afford to do everything that has even a small degree of effectiveness. Cost-effectiveness studies despite their many limitations often present the best available method for systematically choosing between the available alternatives. For this reason, cost-effectiveness studies are now widely published in the health research literature.

33 Questions to Ask and Flaw-Catching Exercises:

Decision-Making Investigations

Questions to Ask in Decision-making Investigations

Study Design
- What is the study question and the type of decision-making investigation?
- What is the study population?
- From what perspective is the investigation being conducted?

Assignment
- What alternatives are being evaluated and what chance events are included?
- Are the alternatives relevant and realistic for the study question?
- Was the time horizon appropriate for the timing of events?

Assessment
- How are the probabilities and the utilities obtained, and are they accurate and precise?
- How are the life-expectancies obtained, and are they accurate and precise?
- How are the costs obtained, and are they accurate and precise?

Analysis
- *Estimation:* Were the results appropriately expressed as cost effectiveness and/or incremental cost effectiveness to measure the size of the effect?
- *Inference:* Was an appropriate sensitivity analysis conducted?
- *Adjustment:* Was an appropriate method of discounting for present value used?

Interpretation
- Are the cost-effectiveness ratios correctly interpreted?
- How was cost effectiveness defined? Did the definition take into account distributional effects?
- Are issues of risk taking and risk aversion considered?

Extrapolation
- *To similar populations:* Are issues of aggregate effects considered?
- *Beyond the data:* If this occurred were marginal costs and effectiveness considered?
- *To other populations and perspectives:* If this occurred did the investigators recognize the differences that need to be taken into account?

Flaw-Catching Exercise No. 1: Pulverizer—Evaluating Costs and Effectiveness as a Treatment for Kidney Stones

An evaluation of the costs and effectiveness of pulverizer, a newly approved method for treatment of calcium-containing kidney stones for otherwise healthy individuals, was investigated. Pulverizer has been shown to have a high probability of breaking apart first kidney stones of 2 cm or less and allowing them to pass down the ureter. Immediate side effects are minimal, but there is a concern that use of pulverizer increases the probability of recurrence of kidney stones over the following decade.

An investigator decided to compare the use of pulverizer at the time of diagnosis with the conventional method using a decision-making investigation. The conventional method consists of treating symptoms and observing the natural course of kidney stones and intervening. Surgery, which includes an average of 4 days in the hospital, is performed only if the stones do not pass after a week.

In the decision alternative to use pulverizer, this treatment was assumed to have a 95% chance of success and a 5% chance of failure. Failure is immediately followed by surgery, which is assumed to have a 99.5% success rate and a 0.5% chance of death. Pulverizer is assumed to be used at the time of diagnosis, thus avoiding hospitalization and returning the patient to work an average of a week earlier.

The alternative to use conventional treatment is assumed to require an average of 4 days in the hospital during which 80% of the stones pass. Surgery is performed on individuals whose stones do not pass in a week or who develop complications. Surgery is assumed to have a 99.5% success rate but to result in death in 0.5% of the patients. Under the above assumptions and assuming that successful treatment returns the patients to full health, the two treatments were found to be equally effective.

The costs considered for pulverizer are the cost of treatment, surgery, and subsequent hospitalization. The costs considered for conventional treatment are the costs of hospitalization, medication, and medical care. Costs are included regardless of who pays the bills.

The conventional treatment was found to cost $15,000 per successful outcome, whereas pulverizer was found to cost $10,000 per successful outcome. A sensitivity analysis taking into account the length of hospitalization required for the conventional treatment found that if hospitalization could be shortened from an average of 4 days to an average of 2 days, the cost per successful outcome would be identical.

The investigators concluded that since both methods cost less than $30,000 per use, they were both cost effective but pulverizer was more cost effective. They concluded that pulverizer was the best treatment available and should be tried on all stones at the time of diagnosis.

Figure 33.1 displays the decision tree used in this investigation. Figure 33.2 includes the probabilities and utilities and calculates the expected utilities.

Critique: Exercise No. 1

Study Design

- What type of decision-making investigation was being conducted?

The results of this investigation are measured in costs per successful outcome. This approach makes the assumption that the two methods are equally effective. When

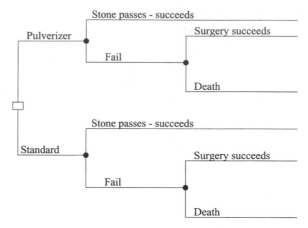

Figure 33.1. Decision tree used in pulverizer investigation.

the results are expressed as cost per successful use or other outcome measure, it is called a cost-and-effectiveness study as opposed to a cost-consequence study or a cost-utility study. In a cost-consequence study, the outcomes are merely described rather than combined. A cost-utility investigation expresses the results incorporating utilities and often incorporating life-expectancy measures, therefore expressing the results as QALYs.

• What was the study question and what population did it address?

The investigators were trying to evaluate the relative cost and effectiveness of pulverizer versus conventional therapy for initial calcium-containing kidney stones in otherwise healthy individuals when pulverizer is used at the time of diagnosis. Recognition of the study question directs the investigator to the type of population that should be used to collect the necessary data for the decision-making investigation. In this case, the data should reflect effectiveness and costs for healthy individuals with kidney stones of moderate size and should not consider stones not containing calcium.

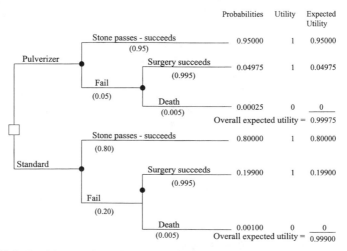

Figure 33.2. Decision tree including probabilities, utilities, and expected utilities.

• From what perspective is the investigation being conducted?

The investigators do not explicitly state the perspective being used in this investigation. However, the fact that costs are calculated regardless of who pays the bills implies that the investigation is conducted from the social perspective.

Assignment

• What alternatives are being considered? Are any alternatives for using pulverizer omitted?

The decision alternatives chosen include only use of pulverizer or the conventional combination of treatment of symptoms and surgery for stones that do not pass. Other alternatives are not considered. For instance, there is no mention of the alternative to use pulverizer as a substitute for surgery after stones fail to pass.

• Was the time horizon appropriate for the timing of events?

The investigation only considers effectiveness and costs during the duration of the initial stone episode. The investigators do not consider the possibility of recurrences. Recurrence could be handled in a number of ways including use of a Markov process that allows the investigators to vary the probability, timing, and cost of recurrences.

Assessment

• What utilities are being used in calculating effectiveness?

The investigators explicitly state the utilities they are using, with successful outcome equal to 1 and death equal to 0. As is often the situation, the investigators do not distinguish utilities for different routes to the favorable or the unfavorable outcomes.

• Was the assessment of costs complete?

The measurement of costs is incomplete. To include all the appropriate costs from the social perspective requires consideration of nonmedical expenses, such as the cost of accessing care, as well as the future costs, such as treatment of recurrences.

Analysis

• What is the adjusted number-needed-to-treat for this investigation?

The overall expected utility for pulverizer is 0.99975 compared with 0.99900 for the conventional treatment. The adjusted number-needed-to-treat is equal to:

$$1/(0.99975 - 0.99900) = 1/0.00075 = 1,333$$

This adjusted number-needed-to-treat tells us that, on average, over 1,000 individuals need to be treated using pulverizer rather than conventional therapy to produce one additional favorable outcome, that is full recovery rather than death. This represents a large number-needed-to-treat, but it indicates that the investigators should not have assumed the two treatments were equally effective.

- What type of sensitivity analysis is being conducted?

The investigators conducted a sensitivity analysis for cost by varying the number of days of hospitalization needed for the conventional treatment. This sensitivity analysis varied one factor at a time and thus is an example of a one-way sensitivity analyses. The investigator used this analysis to conclude that if the hospitalization could be shortened to 2 days, the cost per successful outcome would be identical. When an investigator uses a sensitivity analysis to determine the toss-up point, the sensitivity analysis is called a threshold analysis. The fact that decreasing hospital days to less than two could reduce the costs of conventional treatment below that of pulverizer implies that the recommendations are sensitive to the length of hospitalization.

- Is discounting performed to adjust for the timing of events?

The investigators act as if all the outcomes of interest occur in the immediate future. The investigators do not consider future events such as recurrence. Here as with many decision-making investigations, it is important to consider the occurrence and timing of future events. If recurrences were included in the decision-making investigation, it would be important to discount the costs as well as the harms and benefits of the treatment of the recurrence to take into account their occurrence years into the future.

Interpretation

- Does this investigation establish that pulverizer is cost effective for treatment of first kidney stones of 2 cm or less in otherwise healthy individuals?

Whenever the results of a one-way sensitivity analysis suggest that the recommended alternative is sensitive to a modest change in a variable, such as length of hospitalization, the investigators need to be especially careful in interpreting the results. In addition, the results of this investigation are expressed as cost per successful treatment. By indicating that the costs per case were less than $30,000 the investigators are interpreting the results the same way they would if the results were expressed as incremental cost per QALY. Incremental cost per QALY would have required the results to explicitly incorporate life expectancies as well as utilities.

Approaches for declaring an intervention to be cost effective remain controversial unless the treatment reduces cost and also increases QALYs compared with the conventional treatment. The investigator might have concluded that given the base-case estimate for pulverizer, it was found to be slightly more effective and reduced the cost compared with conventional treatment. Thus, if and only if the base-case assumptions are true, pulverizer can be considered more cost effective than conventional treatment when used as described in this investigation.

Extrapolation

- What assumptions need to be made to conclude that pulverizer should be tried on all stones at the time of diagnosis?

The investigators have extrapolated the results from otherwise healthy individuals with kidney stones of 2 cm or less to all patients with kidney stones. This extrapolation assumes that pulverizer has the same probability of favorable outcomes, probability of adverse, and costs when applied to patients with larger stones, non-calcium stones, and additional conditions that may complicate treatment. Since pulverizer is being investigated for patients with stones of 2 cm or less, it may already be known that pulverizer's impact on larger stones is different than its impact on these smaller stones. In addition, there are likely to be other less obvious assumptions that are violated in this extrapolation. Patients with other complications, for instance, may have very different probabilities of death at surgery than the probabilities used in this decision-making investigation.

Flaw-Catching Exercise No. 2: GREAT Dialysis versus Hemodialysis—A Cost-Effectiveness Study

A new dialysis method commonly known as GREAT dialysis (gradient re-entry abdominal thoracic dialysis) is being evaluated to compare its cost and effectiveness with hemodialysis, which is conventional treatment for adult patients. The cost and effectiveness are being evaluated based on use of the treatments for the lifetime of the dialysis patient who requires dialysis beginning at an average age of 60 years.

Both methods of dialysis are assumed to be paid for by a comprehensive health care system that pays for approved methods of dialysis as long as the patient lives. The system is part of a government health care insurance system that covers the cost of all necessary medical care but requires patients and families to cover the costs of access to care and other nonmedical costs of care. The investigation aims to include all alternatives that would provide favorable outcomes to patients while controlling the costs of the health insurance system.

Hemodialysis requires twice weekly outpatient dialysis treatment that lasts an average of 3 hours. Hemodialysis results in hospitalization, on average, for 1 week per year as a result of complications. Based on extensive experience with hemodialysis, the life expectancy of the average person undergoing hemodialysis is estimated to be 10 years with death occurring throughout the follow-up period.

GREAT dialysis is a new method in which a dialysis device is implanted in the abdomen and thorax and provides dialysis which is as good as the kidney's dialysis for an average of 10 years. On average, surgery is assumed to be required every 10 years for replacement with an average of 1 replacement per patient. There are no known side effects of GREAT dialysis except the 3% chance of death that results from the initial surgery and the 1% chance of death that results from the replacement surgery. Since GREAT dialysis is believed to function as well as the patient's own kidney, the life expectancy of the average person using GREAT dialysis is estimated at 20 years, except for those who die at surgery. However, since GREAT dialysis is a relatively new procedure, a low estimate of 10 years life expectancy was also made.

Utilities for hemodialysis have been established by asking hospitalized dialysis patients to rate the quality of their health. The average utility was 0.5, and this was used as the base-case utility for hemodialysis patients. Ninety-five percent of the patients had a utility between 0.9 and 0.3. The utility for GREAT dialysis was set at 1 since, if successful, GREAT dialysis returns patients to their former states of health.

The costs of hemodialysis include yearly medical care costs of the procedure and the 1 week of hospitalization. The costs of GREAT dialysis include the medical care costs of the device and the surgery plus follow-up care for the initial implant and for one replacement. Future costs of hemodialysis and GREAT dialysis were discounted at 3%.

The investigators found that the incremental cost-effectiveness ratio of GREAT dialysis was −$2,000 per QALY compared with hemodialysis reflecting increased QALYs and decreased costs. After performing one-way sensitivity analyses for utilities and life expectancy, a best case/worst case sensitivity analysis was conducted to see the impact of assuming that the utility of hemodialysis was 0.9 and the life expectancy of GREAT dialysis was 10 years. The best case/worst case sensitivity analysis found that the incremental cost-effectiveness ratio for GREAT dialysis compared with hemodialysis varied from −$5,000 per QALY (best-case) to +$1,000 per QALY (worst case).

The investigators concluded that GREAT dialysis could save the system several billion dollars per year. However, they concluded that despite any cost advantages, they could not recommend a procedure with a 3% death rate when an effective alternative exists.

Based upon the sensitivity analysis, they also concluded that GREAT dialysis may increase costs as reflected in the worst case situation and therefore recommended that it not be included as a covered service. A reviewer of this article agreed that GREAT dialysis may cost more based on its use in this investigation but argued that it should be covered since once implemented on a large scale, the costs would be lower. In addition, the review suggested that GREAT dialysis should be used on all dialysis patients including children.

Critique: Exercise No. 2

Study Design

• What type of decision-making investigation is being conducted?

The results of this investigation are expressed as incremental cost per QALY, Thus, the investigators were conducting a cost-utility study, or specifically, a cost-effectiveness analysis using QALYs.

• What is the study question and to what population is it being addressed?

The investigation is addressing the costs and effectiveness of GREAT dialysis compared with hemodialysis for a population of adult patients who already need dialysis.

• From what perspective is the investigation being conducted?

As indicated by the investigators, both methods of dialysis are assumed to be paid for by a comprehensive health care system that pays for approved methods of dialyses as long as the patient lives. The payor is a government health care insurance system that covers the cost of all medical care but requires patients and families to cover the costs of access to care and other nonmedical costs of care. Thus the perspective is that of a payor of comprehensive medical services and not a social perspective.

Assignment

- What alternatives are being evaluated?

The only alternatives considered are GREAT dialysis and hemodialysis. Neither transplantation nor a combination of treatments is considered.

- Are the alternatives relevant and realistic for the study question?

If hemodialysis is commonly combined with transplantation, this alternative might have been included as well to ensure that the decision-making investigation reflected realistic decision making. Similarly, if GREAT dialysis can be and is being combined with hemodialysis, that alternative would also be important.

- Was the time horizon appropriate for the timing of events?

The time horizon is the duration of follow-up that is included in the decision-making investigation. In this investigation, follow-up was assumed to occur until the death of the patient, which is usually an appropriate time horizon.

Assessment

Figure 33.3 displays the decision tree that appears to have been used in this investigation including the probabilities, utilities, and life expectancies.

- Are the probabilities, utilities, life expectancies, and costs precise and accurate?

The probabilities used for hemodialysis are based on extensive experience. However, since GREAT dialysis is a new procedure, much greater uncertainty exists regarding the probability of its outcomes. Thus it would have been desirable to make realistic low and high estimates for the probability of favorable and adverse outcomes of GREAT dialysis in addition to including a low estimate for life expectancy.

Asking patients undergoing the procedure to estimate their utilities is an acceptable method of obtaining utility scores. However, the utility of hemodialysis was estimated from inpatients undergoing dialysis. This is not the best group to use in

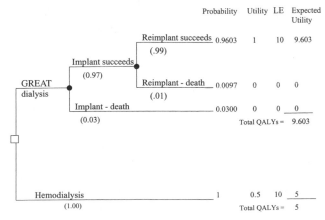

Figure 33.3. Decision tree used in GREAT dialysis versus hemodialysis cost-effectiveness investigation.

estimating utilities because they may be more seriously ill than the group of patients undergoing outpatient hemodialysis.

The investigators included medical care costs and future costs but did not include the nonmedical costs required from the patient or others, such as family members, to obtain the medical care.

Analysis

- Were the results appropriately expressed in terms of cost-effectiveness ratios?

The investigators appropriately presented the results of effectiveness as QALYs and calculated an incremental cost-effectiveness ratio. Since hemodialysis is considered conventional therapy, it is appropriate to compare GREAT dialysis with hemodialysis.

- Was an appropriate sensitivity analysis conducted?

The use of a best case/worst case analysis is an acceptable but demanding method for conducting multiple-way sensitivity analysis. Additional one-way sensitivity analyses would ideally have been presented indicating whether the results of GREAT dialysis are sensitive to such factors as the cost of GREAT dialysis and the time interval prior to replacement. Both of these factors may be subject to change as more experience is gained with GREAT dialysis.

- Was an appropriate method to discount present value used?

The use of a 3% discount rate is the accepted discount rate though the additional use of a 5% rate as a form of sensitivity analysis is also recommended. A more serious error is the discounting of costs without the discounting of effectiveness. Costs and effectiveness must be discounted at the same rate. Discounting of costs without discounting of effectiveness means that delaying use of a procedure is seen as desirable because each year the costs become less while the effectiveness remains the same. This is not realistic in the case of dialysis since the patients cannot wait.

Discounting for effectiveness is important in this investigation not only because costs are discounted. GREAT dialysis carries a probability of death only during surgical implants, whereas hemodialysis carries a probability of death throughout the period of follow-up. This difference in the timing of the events implies that discounting needs to be conducted to compare the effectiveness of these two treatment alternatives.

INTERPRETATION

- Are the cost-effectiveness ratios correctly interpreted?

The investigators correctly concluded that the results of their base-case estimate showed that GREAT dialysis is cost saving. If this base-case estimate was performed correctly, it can be used as the basis for interpreting the results of the investigation. Thus, it would have been acceptable for the investigators to declare GREAT dialysis not only cost saving but cost effective on the basis of the increased QALYs and decreased costs. They would need to limit this interpretation to the base-case conditions and the assumptions of this decision-making investigation.

• What definition is being used in this investigation to establish cost effectiveness?

The investigators seem to be equating cost saving and effectiveness increasing with cost effective and seem to require the sensitivity analysis as well as the base-case estimates to demonstrate reduced costs and increased effectiveness. This is too difficult a criterion to meet. The results of the best case/worst case sensitivity actually strengthen the argument that GREAT dialysis is cost effective compared with hemodialysis because even under the demanding condition of a best case/worst case analysis, the incremental cost per QALY is not more than +$1,000. Using cost reducing and effectiveness increasing as the criterion for coverage is very demanding since new procedures that increase effectiveness while reducing costs are rare. Much more common are new procedures that increase costs while increasing effectiveness or that reduce costs while maintaining current levels of effectiveness.

• Are issues of risk taking and risk aversion considered?

This decision-making investigation is conducted, as are most such studies, assuming risk neutrality. However, when interpreting the results, the investigators indicate that the immediate death associated with the use of GREAT dialysis should be given considerable weight. They actually indicate that they could not recommend GREAT dialysis on the basis of the 3% risk of death from initial insertion. This recommendation indicates that the investigators have incorporated a strong risk-aversive assumption when interpreting the results. Consideration of risk-taking or risk-avoiding attitudes are not part of most decision-making investigation, though they are often part of real clinical and public health decision making.

Extrapolation

• How did the investigator extrapolate to similar populations? Were aggregate effects considered?

The investigators drew conclusions about the aggregate effects or overall impact when they concluded that the use of GREAT dialysis would save the system several billion dollars per year.

• Did the reviewer extrapolate beyond the data?

The reviewer has extrapolated beyond the data. By concluding that changes in volume will alter the costs, they are making a statement about marginal costs as opposed to incremental costs. Marginal costs reflect the economies of scale or diseconomies of scale associated with the widespread use of a procedure. This extrapolation takes the reviewer beyond the data and thus carries assumptions that may or may not hold true. It is possible to argue for coverage of GREAT dialysis on the basis of the data contained within this investigation without having to extrapolate beyond the data.

• Did the reviewer extrapolate to other populations?

By drawing conclusions about children as well as adults, the reviewer extrapolated to another population. Children may or may not experience the same effectiveness and the same costs as adults undergoing GREAT dialysis. Extrapolation to children relies on a series of new assumptions that are not discussed as part of this investigation.

Selecting a Statistic

V

34 Basic Principles

Statistics have three purposes in the analyses of health research studies:

1. To make estimates of the strength of relationships or the magnitude of differences
2. To be used in statistical significance testing. These tests allow us to draw inferences about a population from samples obtained from the same population, taking into account the influence of chance.
3. To adjust for the influence of confounding variables on those estimates and inferences.

In this Part 5, *Selecting a Statistic,* our goal is to provide insights about how statistics can be used to serve these purposes.

We must first recognize that the measurements taken on individuals in an investigation are a subset or SAMPLE of a larger group of individuals who might have been included in the investigation. This larger group is called the POPULATION.[1]

If we can plot the frequency with which different measurement values occur in the population, this provides a graphic representation of the POPULATION'S DISTRIBUTION OF DATA. A population's distribution of data tells us how frequently various data values occur in the larger population from which samples are drawn for observation (Fig. 34.1). Data in this graphic form, however, are difficult to assimilate or communicate.

Rather than describe a population distribution graphically, statistical methods are concerned with a numerical summary of the distribution of data. Every type of population's distribution has a limited number of summary values, called PARAMETERS, that are used to completely describe the particular distribution of data. For example, to completely describe a GAUSSIAN DISTRIBUTION,[2] two parameters are needed—one measuring what is called LOCATION and the other measuring what is called DISPERSION. These two parameters are called the MEAN[3] (the distribution's location along a continuum, or more specifically, its center of gravity) and

---

[1]In health research, we usually think of measurements being taken on persons rather than on animals or objects. This might lead us to the mistaken impression that the statistical use of the term POPULATION is the same as its use to describe a politically or geographically distinct collection of persons. Although the term population in statistics might be that type of collection, it is not limited to such. Rather, a POPULATION is defined as the collection of all possible measurements (not necessarily of persons) from which a sample is selected.

[2]The gaussian distribution is also known as the NORMAL *distribution.* We avoid using that term because NORMAL has an alternative meaning clinically. The gaussian distribution is the most commonly assumed population distribution in statistics.

[3]The term AVERAGE is often used as a synonym for the mean. In statistical terminology, these are not the same thing. A mean is calculated by summing all the measurements and dividing by the number of measurements. An average, on the other hand, is calculated by multiplying each of the measurements by particular values, called weights, before summing them. That sum is then divided by the sum of the weights. A mean is a special type of average in which the weight for every measurement is equal to 1.

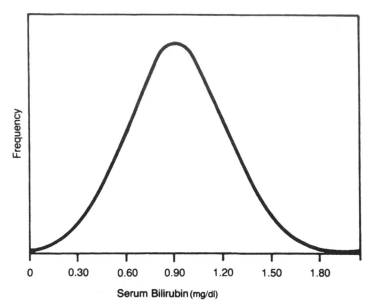

Figure 34.1. A hypothetical population distribution for serum bilirubin measurements.

the STANDARD DEVIATION[4] (the dispersion or spread of the distribution as indicated by how far from the mean individual measurements occur). Figure 34.2 shows a gaussian distribution with the mean indicated as the measure of the distribution's location and the standard deviation as the measure of dispersion.

To demonstrate what is meant by the location of a distribution, let us assume that the mean serum bilirubin in the population is 1.2 mg/dL instead of 0.9 mg/dL. Figure 34.3 shows what the gaussian distribution of serum bilirubin would be in this case.

Notice that the general shape of the distribution in Figure 34.3 is unaltered by changing the mean, but the position of the center of gravity of the distribution is moved 0.3 mg/dL to the right. If we changed the dispersion of the distribution in Figure 34.2, however, the shape of the distribution would be altered without changing its position. For example, compare the distribution in Figure 34.2 to Figure 34.4, in which the standard deviation has been changed from 0.3 mg/dL to 0.4 mg/dL.

We seldom are able to observe all the possible measurements in a population. Using measurements observed in a sample from the larger population, however, we can calculate numerical values to estimate the value of the larger population's parameters. These samples' estimates of a population's parameters are the focus of statistical methods. In fact, those estimates are called STATISTICS. A single statistic used to estimate the numerical value of a particular population's parameter is further known as a POINT ESTIMATE. These point estimates are the statistics we use to make estimates of the strength of relationships or magnitude of differences in the population.

---

[4]The standard deviation (σ) is the square root of the variance (σ^2) The variance is equal to the mean square deviation of data (χ_i) from the mean (μ). Therefore, the population standard deviation is equal to the square root of: $\Sigma(\chi_i-\mu)^2\sigma \div N$

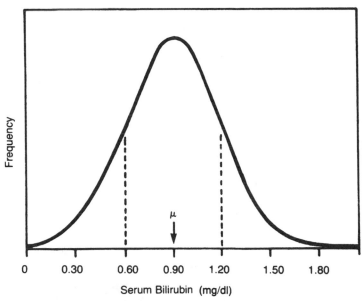

Figure 34.2. A hypothetical gaussian distribution of serum bilirubin with a mean of 0.9 mg/dL and a standard deviation of 0.3 mg/dL. The broken lines indicate values equal to the mean ± 1 standard deviation.

As stated previously, a sample is a subset of all possible measurements from a population. For all statistical methods, it is assumed that the sample is a random subset of the population from which it is derived. Although random subsets can be obtained in several ways, in this section we consider only the simplest (and most common), called a SIMPLE RANDOM SAMPLE. In a simple random sample, all

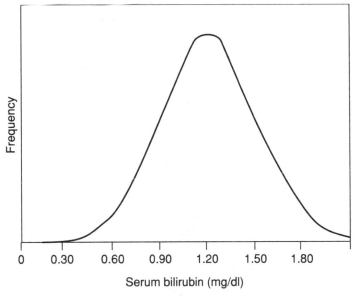

Figure 34.3. A hypothetical gaussian distribution of serum bilirubin with a mean of 1.2 mg/dL and a standard deviation of 0.3 mg/dL. Comparison of this distribution with Figure 34.2 shows what is meant by different locations of a population's distributions of data.

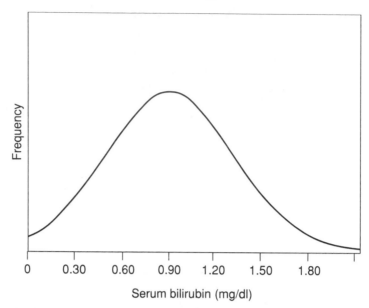

Figure 34.4. A hypothetical gaussian distribution of serum bilirubin with a mean of 0.9 mg/dL. Comparison of this distribution with Figure 34.2 shows what is meant by different dispersions of a population's distributions of data.

measurements in the population have an equal probability of being included.[5] Chance, then, dictates which measurements are actually included.

When a population's parameters are estimated using a sample's statistics, chance selection of the particular measurements to be actually included in the sample influences how close the sample's estimate is to the actual numerical value of the population's parameter. Unfortunately, we can never know how closely a particular statistic correctly reflects its corresponding population's parameter because we would have to measure the entire population to know the actual value of a parameter. What we can determine, however, is how much the statistics or estimates are expected to vary, on the basis of chance variations among random samples. That knowledge forms the basis of statistical inference or statistical significance testing.

The framework of statistical inference was described in Part 1, *Studying a Study*. We noted that statistical significance testing is performed under the assumption that the null hypothesis is true. The null hypothesis provides us with the hypothetical value with which our observed estimates can be compared.

We also noted in Part 1 that the bottom line in statistical significance testing is the *P* value.[6] *P* values are calculated from research observations by first converting the sample's estimate to an appropriate STANDARD DISTRIBUTION. We use standard distributions to simplify calculations because the *P* values corresponding to

---

[5]In a general sense, a RANDOM SAMPLE implies that any one individual in the population has a known probability of being included in the sample. Here, we are limiting those known probabilities to the condition that they are all equal to each other. Thus we are using a simple random sample.

[6]Recall that the *P* value is the probability of obtaining a sample at least as different from that indicated by the null hypothesis as the sample actually obtained if the null hypothesis truly describes the population. It is not, as often assumed, the probability that chance has influenced the sample observations. That probability is equal to 1 (*i.e.,* we are certain that chance has influenced our observations).

any location in these distributions can be obtained from statistical tables. Much of what we consider to be the methodology of statistics is related to converting estimates to a standard distribution.[7]

As we discussed in Part 1, an alternative to using statistical significance testing to investigate the influence of chance on sample estimates is to calculate an interval estimate or confidence interval.[8] Within a confidence interval, we have a specified degree of confidence (often 95%) that the larger population's parameter value is included.[9] Commonly, confidence intervals are found by algebraically rearranging calculations used to perform statistical significance tests.[10]

When performing statistical significance tests or calculating confidence intervals, a ONE-TAILED or a TWO-TAILED procedure can be used. A two-tailed statistical significance test or interval estimate is used whenever the researcher is not sure whether the population's parameter is greater than or smaller than the value implied by the null hypothesis. That is the usual circumstance, but occasionally one encounters ONE-TAILED statistical significance tests or interval estimates in the health research literature. A one-tailed test or confidence interval is applicable when the investigator is willing to assume that the direction of the relationship being studied is known and analysis is concerned only with examining the size or strength of the relationship.

To illustrate the distinction between one- and two-tailed statistical procedures, imagine a randomized clinical trial in which we measure diastolic blood pressure for a group of individuals before and after treatment with an antihypertensive drug that has previously been demonstrated to be effective. Before examining the data resulting from the study, we might assume in our hypothesis that diastolic pressure will decrease when patients are on the drug. In other words, we might assume that it is impossible for the drug to cause an increase in diastolic blood pressure. With that assumption, statistical significance testing or interval estimation can be one-tailed and the statistical power of our analysis increased. If, on the other hand, our study hypothesis is that a new antihypertensive drug will lower diastolic blood pressure, statistical significance testing or interval estimation should be two-tailed. This is because we consider it to be possible, even though it might be unlikely, that a new antihypertensive drug would cause an increase in diastolic blood pressure.

Selecting Statistical Methods

When selecting a specific statistical method, statisticians must think about VARIABLES. Variables express or represent data in the mathematical procedures that are part of statistics. For example, if we included measurements of age in our research, age would be expressed or represented by one of the variables in our statistical analysis. Once we understand what the variables are, we must make two decisions:

[7]Examples of standard distributions include the standard normal, Student's t, chi-square, and F distributions. These distributions are discussed in later chapters.

[8]This interval is sometimes referred to as CONFIDENCE LIMITS. In statistical terminology, confidence limits are the numerical values that bound a confidence interval.

[9]In classic statistics, an INTERVAL ESTIMATE means that if we examine an infinite number of samples of the same size, a specified percentage (e.g., 95%) of the interval estimates would include the population's parameter. A more modern view among statisticians is that this is tantamount to assuming there is a specified chance (e.g., 95%) that the value of the population parameter is included in the interval. The latter interpretation is usually the one of interest to the health researcher.

[10]When confidence intervals are calculated from the same data as statistical significance testing they are said to be test-based.

(1) what is the function of each variable and (2) what type of data is represented by each of those variables. First, let us see what we mean by the function of a variable.

Most statistical methods distinguish between DEPENDENT and INDEPENDENT variables. These are indications of the function or purpose of a variable in a particular analysis. Usually, a collection of variables that is designed to investigate a single study hypothesis contains only one dependent variable. That dependent variable can be identified as the variable of primary interest or the outcome or end-point of a study. We generally wish to test hypotheses or make estimates, or both, about that one dependent variable. There may be more than one outcome or end-point in an investigation; however, we usually analyze one outcome at a time.[11] On the other hand, that collection of variables might contain no, one, or several independent variables. The independent variables reflect the study hypotheses plus potential confounding variables, which need to be taken into account when hypotheses are to be tested and estimates are to be made. Remember that in a case-control study, however, the dependent variable is the previous characteristic that is being assessed.

To illustrate the distinction between independent and dependent variables, consider a cohort study in which the relationship between smoking and the probability of coronary heart disease is investigated. Suppose only two variables are measured on each individual: smoking (vs. not smoking) and coronary heart disease (vs. no coronary heart disease). To analyze those data, we first recognize that our primary interest is to estimate or to test a hypothesis about the probability of coronary heart disease. Thus, coronary heart disease is the dependent variable. Further, we wish to compare the probability of coronary heart disease among nonsmokers. Hence, smoking status is the independent variable.

After identifying the one dependent variable, number of independent variables determines the category of statistical methods that is appropriate to use. For instance, if we are interested in estimating the probability of coronary heart disease in a community without regard to smoking status, or any other characteristic of individuals, we would apply statistical procedures known as UNIVARIABLE ANALYSES. These procedures are applicable to a set of observations that contains one dependent variable and no independent variables. To examine the probability of coronary heart disease relative to smoking status, however, we would use methods called BIVARIABLE ANALYSES. These methods are applied to collections of observations with one dependent variable and one independent variable. Finally, if we were interested in the probability of coronary heart disease for individuals of various ages, genders, and smoking habits, we would apply MULTIVARIABLE ANALYSES.[12] These methods are used for sets of observations that consist of a dependent variable and more than one indepen-

---

[11]The focus on one hypothesis at a time with collection of other data to perform adjustment and subsequent statistical significance testing has traditionally been the end of the process. It is advisable however, to regard the process as a first step in which the most important variables affecting an outcome are recognized. It is then possible to examine the impact on the study sample, or similar target population, of introducing the intervention being studied given the distribution of those most important variables in the study sample. This process can be called INTERVENTION MODELING. Simulation techniques may be used in intervention modeling to make point estimates and confidence intervals for the expected impact on populations either similar to or different than those represented in the study sample.

[12]A common error in the use of statistical terminology is to refer to procedures designed for one dependent variable and more than one independent variable as MULTIVARIATE ANALYSES. This term, however, properly refers to procedures designed for more than one dependent variable. The use of multivariate procedures, such as discriminate analysis, is typically rare in health research. We have not attempted to include multivariate procedures in our flowchart.

dent variable such as age, gender, and smoking habit. Multivariable methods are frequently used to accomplish our third goal of statistical methods: to adjust for the influence of confounding variables.

Health research investigations often include several sets or collections of variables. For example, suppose we have conducted a randomized clinical trial in which subjects received either drug X or a placebo and are cured or not cured of a particular disease. Because we were concerned about the influence of age and gender on cure (*i.e.,* we were concerned that age and gender differences might be confounding variables), we included them in our research records. Therefore, our study contains four variables: treatment (drug X or placebo), cure (yes or no), age, and gender. The collection that includes all four variables would have cure as the variable of interest; thus, cure would be the dependent variable. Treatment, age, and gender would be independent variables, reflecting our interest in examining cure relative to the specific treatment received and the subject's age and gender. Even before testing hypotheses or making estimates about cure, however, we would likely be interested in whether randomization achieved similar age distributions in the two treatment groups. The collection of variables that would allow us to compare age distributions contains age as the dependent variable and treatment as the independent variable. Here age is the variable of interest and treatment group is the condition under which we are assessing age. Thus, the decision about which is the dependent variable and which is the independent variable depends on the question being asked.

Types of Data

In addition to characterizing the function of variables in an analysis, we must determine the type of data contained in the measurement of each variable to select a statistical procedure. To categorize types of data, the first distinction we make is between CONTINUOUS and DISCRETE data.

Continuous data are defined as data that provides the possibility of observing any of an infinite number of equally spaced numerical values between any two points in its range of measurement. Examples of continuous data include blood pressure, serum cholesterol, age, and weight. For each of these variables, we can choose any two numerical values and imagine additional intermediate measurements that would be, at least theoretically, possible to observe between those values. We might, for instance, consider the ages of 35 and 36 years. We could think of different ages between 35 and 36 that are distinguished by the number of days since a person's 35th birthday or the number of hours or minutes since that birthday. Theoretically, there is no limit to how finely we can imagine time being measured. Notice, however, that continuous data do not need to have an infinite range of possible values but rather an infinite number of possible values within their range. That range may, and usually does, have a lower and upper boundary. Age is a good example. The lower boundary is zero, and it is difficult to imagine individuals much older than 120 years.

Discrete data, on the other hand, can have only a finite or limited number of values in their range of measurement. Examples of discrete data include number of pregnancies, stage of disease, and gender. For each of these variables, we can select two values between which it is not possible to imagine other values. For instance, there is no number of pregnancies between two and three pregnancies that we include in our measurements.

In practice, the distinction between continuous and discrete data is often unclear. For one thing, no variables exist for which we can actually measure an infinite number of values.[13] We solve this problem by recognizing that, if a great number of measurements can be made and if the intervals between measurements are uniform, then the measurements are nearly continuous. This, however, creates another source of confusion in that it allows data that are, even theoretically discrete, to be redefined as continuous. For example, the number of hairs on one's scalp is certainly discrete data: We cannot imagine observing a value between 99,999 and 100,000 hairs. Even so, the number of possible numerical values within the entire range of the number of hairs is very great. Can we consider such a variable to be composed of continuous data? Yes, for most purposes that would be entirely appropriate.

Data can be defined further by their scale of measurement. Continuous data are measured on scales, called RATIO or INTERVAL SCALES,[14] which are defined as having a uniform or constant interval between consecutive measurements. As opposed to continuous data, some types of discrete data measurements are made on an ORDINAL SCALE. Data on an ordinal scale have a specific ranking or ordering, as do continuous data, but the interval between consecutive measurements is not necessarily constant. A common sort of variable measured on an ordinal scale is an ordering of the stage of disease. We know, for instance, that stage 2 is more advanced than stage 1, but we cannot assert that the difference between the two stages is the same as the difference between stage 3 and stage 2.

If we are unable to apply any ordering to discrete data, then we say that the data were measured on a NOMINAL SCALE. Examples of characteristics composed of nominal scale discrete data are treatment, gender, race, and eye color. Data that we treat as nominal data include measurements with two categories even though they might be considered to have an innate order, because one is clearly better than the other (*e.g.,* dead vs. alive).

Note that the term nominal variable can be confusing. In its common use, a nominal variable is a characteristic, such as gender or race, that has two or more potential categories. From a statistical point of view, however, one nominal variable is limited to only two categories. Thus, race or eye color should be referred to as nominal data which require more than one nominal variable for inclusion in statistical procedures. The number of nominal variables required is equal to the number of categories of the nominal data minus one.

For purposes of selecting a statistical procedure or interpreting the result of such a procedure, it is important to distinguish between three categories of variables:

1. Continuous variables: includes continuous data, such as age, and discrete data that contain a great number of possible values, such as number of hairs;
2. Ordinal variables: includes ordinal data that can be ordered one higher than the next and with at least three and at most a limited number of possible values, such as stages of cancer;
3. Nominal variables: includes nominal data that cannot be ordered, such as race, and data that can assume only two possible values, such as dead or alive.

---

[13]For example, we might imagine but could not determine blood pressure in picometers of mercury. So, in reality, all data are discrete.

[14]The distinction between the ratio scale and the interval scale is that the former includes a true zero value whereas the latter does not. Certain types of discrete data, such as counts, have uniform intervals between measurements and, therefore, are measured in ratio or interval scales. Other types of discrete data, however, are measured either on an ordinal or a nominal scale.

The order in which those categories are listed indicates the relative amount of information contained in each type of variable. That is, continuous variables contain more information than ordinal variables, and ordinal variables contain more information than nominal variables. Thus, continuous variables are considered to be at a higher level than nominal variables.

Measurements with a particular level of information can be rescaled to a lower level. For example, age (measured in years) is a continuous variable. We could legitimately rescale age to be an ordinal variable by defining persons as being children (0–18 years), young adults (19–30 years), adults (31–45 years), mature adults (46–65 years), or elderly adults (>65 years). We could rescale age further to be a nominal variable. For instance, we might simply divide persons into two categories: young and old or children and adults. We cannot, however, rescale variables to a higher level than the one at which they were actually measured.

When we rescale measurements to a lower level, we lose information. That is, we have less detail about a characteristic if it is measured on a nominal scale than we do if the same characteristic was measured on an ordinal or continuous scale. For example, we know less about a woman when we label her a mature adult or an adult than we do when we say that she is 54 years old. If an individual was 54 years old and we measured age on a continuous scale, we could distinguish that person's age from another individual who is 64 years old. However, if age was recorded on the ordinal scale, we could not recognize a difference in age, such as 54 versus 64, between those individuals.

Loss of information, when rescaled measurements are used in statistical procedures, has the consistent effect, all else being equal, of increasing the Type II error rate. That is to say, rescaling to a lower level reduces statistical power, making it harder to establish statistical significance and, thus, to reject a false null hypothesis. What we gain by rescaling to a lower level is the ability to circumvent making certain assumptions, such as uniform intervals, about the data that are required to perform certain statistical tests. Specific examples of tests that require and those that circumvent such assumptions will be described in greater detail in following chapters in this section.

Thus far, we have reviewed the initial steps that must occur in selecting a statistical procedure. These steps are:

1. Identify one dependent variable and all independent variables, if present, on the basis of the study question.
2. Determine for each variable whether it represents continuous, ordinal, or nominal data.

Having completed these steps, we are ready to begin the process of selecting a statistic.

The Flowchart

The remaining chapters of this section are arranged as branches of a flowchart designed to facilitate selection and interpretation of statistical methods. Most statistical procedures that are frequently encountered in health research have been included.

To use the initial flowchart (Fig. 34.5), you must first determine which of a set of variables is the dependent variable. If the set contains more than one dependent

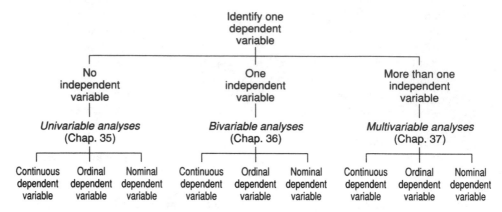

Figure 34.5. Flowchart to determine the chapter and division that discuss statistical procedure relevant to a particular set of variables.

variable, you can analyze the data using one of the dependent variables at a time.[15] If your collection of variables seems to contain more than one dependent variable, the data may address more than one study hypothesis. In that case, the relevant variables for a specific study hypothesis should be considered.

Once a single dependent variable has been identified, you can use the number of independent variables in the investigation to guide you to the chapter that discusses this number of independent variables. Each chapter contains three major divisions. The first is concerned with sets of variables in which the dependent variable is continuous. The second division addresses ordinal dependent variables, and the third addresses nominal dependent variables. Within each division, techniques for continuous, ordinal, and nominal independent variables, if available, are described. Chapter 38 puts together the flowcharts that were discussed in Chapters 35, 36, and 37.

[15]Alternatively you can use multivariate procedures such as discriminant analysis or factor analyses.

35 Univariable Analyses

If a set of measurements contains one dependent variable and no independent variables, the statistical methods used to analyze these measurements are a type of UNIVARIABLE ANALYSIS. Three common uses of univariable analysis methods are found in the health literature. The first use is in descriptive studies (*e.g.,* case series) in which only one sample has been examined. For example, a researcher might present a series of cases of a particular disease, examining various demographic and pathophysiologic measurements on those patients. The purpose of analysis in such a study would be to account for the influence of chance in the measurement of each characteristic.

The second common application of univariable analysis is when a sample is drawn for inclusion in a study. For example, before randomization in a randomized clinical trial, we might want to perform measurements on the entire sample chosen for study. That is, we may want to determine the mean age and percentage of women in the group selected to be randomized before they are assigned to a study or control group.

Usually, in descriptive studies and when examining one sample, the interest is in point estimation and confidence interval estimation rather than statistical significance testing. Tests of hypotheses are possible in the univariable setting, but one must specify, in the null hypothesis, a value for a population's parameter. Often, it is not possible to do this in a univariable analysis. For example, it is difficult to imagine what value would be hypothesized for prevalence of hypertension among individuals in a particular community.[1]

The third application of univariable analysis is one in which such a hypothesized value is easier to imagine. That is the case in which a measurement, such as diastolic blood pressure, is made twice on the same, or very similar, individuals, and the difference between the measurements is of interest. In that application, it is logical to imagine a null hypothesis stating that the difference between measurements is equal to zero. Thus, the difference in diastolic blood pressure measurements is the dependent variable. Even though the difference, by its nature, is a comparison of groups, differences themselves are not compared between any groups. Therefore, there is no independent variable. When comparing two measurements of the same characteristic on the same, or very similar, individuals, we are dealing with a univariable problem. Thus, in an investigation using paired data in which the measurement on each pair constitutes one observation, the data are analyzed using univariable methods. The pairs may consist of data from one individual or from two individuals who are paired before the data are analyzed.

---

[1]At first, it may seem that a null hypothesis might state that the prevalence in a particular community is equal to the prevalence in some other community or the prevalence estimated in another study. It is important to keep in mind, however, that the value suggested for a population's parameter in a null hypothesis must be known without error. That will not be true unless all members of the comparison community were included in the calculation of prevalence.

Continuous Dependent Variable

In univariable analysis of a continuous dependent variable, data are usually assumed to come from a population with a gaussian distribution. Therefore, the mean is commonly used to measure location. The sample's estimate of the population's mean is usually the estimate of primary interest. The flowchart focuses on our interest in the mean. Dispersion of gaussian distributions is measured by the standard deviation or, alternatively, by the standard deviation squared, which is called the VARIANCE.[2] At the bottom of each flowchart is listed the general category of statistical techniques that are most frequently used to calculate confidence intervals or test hypotheses by statistical significance testing.

In Chapter 34 we learned that the first steps in choosing a statistical procedure are:

1. Decide which variable is the dependent variable.
2. Determine how many, if any, independent variables the set of observations contains.
3. Define the type of data represented by the dependent variable as being continuous, ordinal, or nominal.

If we follow the Flowchart Figure 34.5 down to Univariable analyses we can continue by using Figure 35.1. Since we are interested in a continuous dependent variable we are led to the mean. The mean is the point estimate of interest when we have a continuous dependent variable and no independent variable. Next we note "paired tests" enclosed in a box followed by Student's *t* test that is underlined. In this and subsequent components of the flow chart, boxes indicate, if applicable, general categories of statistical methods, and underlines indicate specific procedures that are used for statistical significance testing or calculating confidence intervals. FN[3]

To calculate a confidence interval for the mean of a sample, the STUDENT'S *t* DISTRIBUTION is most often used. The Student's *t* distribution is a standard distribution to which means of continuous dependent variables are converted to make analysis easier. The Student's *t* distribution is like the gaussian distribution, but it requires an additional parameter known as DEGREES OF FREEDOM. The purpose of degrees of

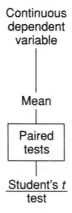

Figure 35.1. Flowchart to select a univariable statistical procedure for a continuous dependent variable (continued from Fig. 34.5).

[2]Estimates of the standard deviation and the variance or other measures of dispersion are not listed in the flowcharts. Estimates of dispersion are usually used to take into account the role of chance in estimating the location of the population's distribution. They are not, by themselves, frequently estimates of primary interest.

freedom in the Student's t distribution is to reflect the role of chance in estimation of the standard deviation.[3]

The Student's t distribution allows us to derive confidence intervals based on the observed mean and the STANDARD ERROR. The standard error measures the spread or dispersion in the means that we would expect if all possible samples of the same size as the one actually obtained were drawn from the population. The standard error of a mean becomes smaller as the sample's size grows larger. More specifically, the standard error is equal to the standard deviation divided by the square root of the sample's size.

The standard error is used with the Student's t distribution in calculating interval estimates for means of continuous variables. The confidence interval for a mean is equal to the sample's estimate of the mean ± the Student's t value for the desired level of confidence multiplied by the standard error. For a 95%, two-tailed estimate, the Student's t value is approximately equal to 2 for sample sizes of 20 or more. By adding and subtracting a value equal to twice the standard error to the point estimate of the mean, one can determine an approximate confidence interval when the sample size is 20 or greater. That is tantamount to saying, with 95% confidence, that the population's mean lies within the interval limited by the sample mean ± two standard errors.[4] For example, if we read in a research report that the mean ± the standard error for serum cholesterol in a sample is equal to 150 ± 15 mg/dL, we can be 95% confident that the population mean lies within the approximate interval from 120 to 180 mg/dL.

As mentioned previously, there is a special case of a univariable analysis in which statistical significance testing is applicable. The most common example is a study in which a continuous dependent variable is measured twice on the same individual. For instance, we might measure blood pressure before and after a patient receives an antihypertensive medication. If our interest is not really in the actual measurements before and after treatment but rather in the difference between those measurements, we have a paired design.[5] This is a univariable problem because the dependent variable is the difference between measurements and no independent variable exists. By using a paired design, we have attempted to remove the influence of variation between subjects in the initial, or baseline, measurement.

A Student's t distribution is used to test hypotheses or construct interval estimates for continuous data from a paired design in the same way it is used for other univariable analyses. Although the statistical procedures used to analyze data collected in a paired design are no different from other univariable procedures, they are often given separate treatment in introductory statistical texts. In those cases, the procedure for examining the mean difference in data from a paired design is called a PAIRED or MATCHED STUDENT'S t TEST.

[3]Use of the Student's t distribution to make interval estimates for means or for statistical significance testing recognizes the fact that the standard deviation is estimated from the sample. That is, the standard deviation is not precisely known. The degrees of freedom for a univariable sample of a continuous variable equals the sample's size minus one.

[4]Other confidence intervals can, likewise, be estimated by considering multiples of the standard error. More than 99% of possible sample estimates of the mean are included within the range of the population mean ± 3 standard errors. This assumes that the population of all possible means has a gaussian distribution.

[5]Another paired design would be a continuous dependent variable measured on two paired individuals who are similar in that they share characteristics thought to influence the magnitude of the dependent variable.

Rather than the sample's estimate of the mean ± the standard error, we often see univariable data presented as the sample mean ± the standard deviation. The sample mean ± the standard error communicates how confident we can be in our estimate of the population's mean. Remember that the standard error is an indicator of the dispersion of sample means that might be obtained by sampling the population repeatedly, each time obtaining a sample of the same size.

The sample mean ± the standard deviation, addresses a different issue. The standard deviation estimates, using the sample's data, the dispersion of measurements or data values in the larger population. That is, the dispersion of the one sample's data is the best estimate we have available of the dispersion in the larger population. Approximately 95% of the data values in a population distribution occur within the range of the population mean ± 2 standard deviations.[6] Therefore, when using univariable statistical procedures for a continuous dependent variable, we are interested in either estimating the location of the population's mean and, thus, in the observed mean of and standard error or alternatively in estimating the dispersion of data values in the population and, thus, in the observed mean and standard deviation.

Ordinal Dependent Variable

Univariable statistical methods for ordinal dependent variables are presented in Figure 35.2.

Unlike continuous variables, we do not assume a particular distribution of population data, such as a gaussian distribution, for ordinal variables. Methods used for ordinal variables are, thus, referred to as DISTRIBUTION-FREE or NONPARAMETRIC. It is important to realize, however, that these procedures are not assumption-free. For example, we continue to assume that our sample is representative of or randomly sampled from some population of interest.

Because we are not assuming a particular distribution of the population's data measured on an ordinal scale, we cannot estimate the population's parameters that summarize the distribution. We might, however, be interested in describing the location of ordinal data along a continuum. We can do that with the MEDIAN. The median is the mid-point of a collection of data, selected so that half the values are

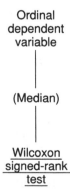

Figure 35.2. Flowchart to select a univariable statistical procedure for an ordinal dependent variable (continued from Fig. 34. 5). In this and subsequent components of the flowchart boxes indicate a general classification of statistical procedures and the underlined procedure indicates the name of the most commonly used procedure for significance testing and calculation of confidence intervals.

[6]About two thirds of the population data occur within the mean ±1 standard deviation, and more than 99% occur within the mean ± 3 standard deviations. To apply these interpretations, we assume that the population's data have a gaussian distribution.

larger and half the values are smaller than the median.[7] The median will equal the mean when the population has a symmetric distribution, as illustrated in Figure 35.3A. If we are interested in testing the null hypothesis that the median equals zero in a univariable analysis, for instance in a study with a paired design, we can use the WILCOXON SIGNED-RANK TEST.

Nominal Dependent Variable

A NOMINAL DEPENDENT VARIABLE represents data in which a condition exists or, by default, that it does not exist. Examples of nominal dependent variables include dead–alive, cured–not cured, and diseased–not diseased. The amount of information contained in a single nominal dependent variable is quite limited compared with continuous dependent variables, such as age, or with ordinal dependent variables, such as stage of disease.

For each measurement or observation of a variable composed of nominal data, we determine only the presence or absence of the condition. For example, we might determine whether an individual in a sample has a particular disease. For a sample consisting of more than one observation, we can estimate the FREQUENCY or the number of times the condition occurs in the population. For instance, we can estimate the number of persons in the population with a particular disease. Most often, we are interested in that frequency relative to the total number of observations. If we divide the number of times a particular condition is observed in a sample by the total number of observations in that sample, we have calculated the PROPORTION of

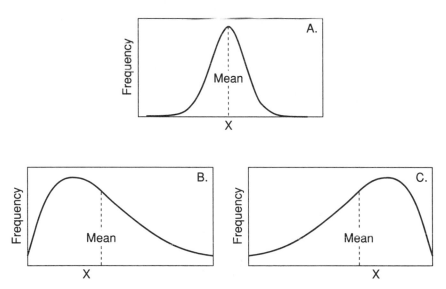

Figure 35.3. Location of the mean for (**A**) symmetric and (**B,C**) asymmetric distributions. X indicates the location of the median.

[7]No theoretical population distribution has the median as its measure of location, but it can be used as an estimate of the mean of a gaussian distribution. The median circumvents an assumption we make when calculating the mean. That assumption is that intervals between measurements in a distribution are known and uniform. Since the median is calculated using only the relative rank or order of the measurements, the same median would be estimated regardless of whether or not those intervals are known or uniform. Therefore, we can use the median to estimate the mean of a population of continuous data.

observations in the sample with the condition. A proportion calculated from the sample's observations is a point estimate of the proportion of the population with the condition. An equivalent way to interpret the sample's proportion is that it estimates the PROBABILITY of the condition occurring in the population. Two commonly encountered proportions or probabilities in health research are prevalence, and case fatality.

Probabilities do not have a gaussian distribution. They are assumed to have either a BINOMIAL or POISSON DISTRIBUTION. A binomial distribution is generally applicable to any probability calculated from nominal data when the observations are independent from one another. By independent, we mean that the result of one observation does not influence the result of another. The binomial distribution is a standard distribution that can be used to calculate P values for statistical significance tests and to calculate confidence intervals.

A Poisson distribution is a special case of a binomial distribution that is used when the nominal event, such as disease or death, is rarely observed and the number of observations is great. The Poisson distribution is computationally simpler than the binomial distribution. It generally provides a good approximation of the binomial distribution when the number of individuals observed with the condition is less than or equal to 5 and the total number of individuals in a sample is greater than or equal to 100.

Statistical significance testing and calculation of confidence intervals for binomial and Poisson distributions are not usually feasible if we wish to perform exact procedures that actually use the binomial or Poisson distributions. Fortunately, we do not often have to use exact procedures.

Calculating confidence intervals or performing statistical significance tests for nominal dependent variables becomes feasible when, under certain conditions, the binomial and Poisson distributions can be approximated by the gaussian distribution. This is often called a NORMAL APPROXIMATION, and it can be done if the number of individuals with a condition is greater than 5 and the number of observations is greater than 10.[8]

Interest in Rates

In statistical terminology, the term RATE is reserved to refer to a ratio in which the denominator included a measure of time. It is important to distinguish a rate from a proportion. Rates, unlike proportions, are altered or affected by the unit of time that is used in measuring the denominator. We say that rates are affected by time. Both rates and proportions include the frequency of events in their numerators. However, a proportion includes only the total number of observations in the denominator. The most common measurement of interest in health research that meets the statistical definition of a rate is the incidence rate.

Because diseases usually occur infrequently per unit of time, rates are often assumed, in univariable analysis, to have a Poisson distribution. As with propor-

---

[8]In a normal approximation to a binomial or Poisson distribution, we only need to estimate the probability of observing the event because the standard error is calculated from that probability. This is unlike using the gaussian distribution for continuous variables when we must make separate estimates of location and dispersion. As a result, it is not necessary or even appropriate to use the Student's *t* distribution to take into account, through degrees of freedom, the precision with which dispersion has been estimated. Rather, the standard normal distribution is used.

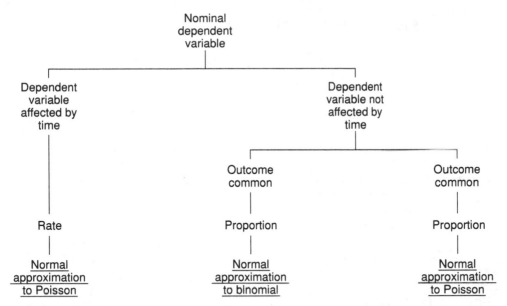

Figure 35.4. Flowchart to select a univariable statistical procedure for a nominal dependent variable (continued from Fig. 34.5).

tions, it is theoretically possible to perform exact procedures on rates, but more commonly, statistical significance tests and determination of interval estimates for rates rely on a normal approximation. Thus, procedures for rates are the same as those used for probabilities, except that statistical significance testing and interval estimates, if performed, use the Poisson distribution or its normal approximation.

Figure 35.4 summarizes the steps or decisions that need to be made when choosing which measurement to use for estimation and for statistical significance testing or calculating confidence intervals with one nominal dependent variable. The underlined procedures indicate those used for statistical significance testing and calculating confidence intervals.

36 Bivariable Analyses

In bivariable analysis, we are concerned with one dependent variable and one independent variable. In addition to determining the type of dependent variable being considered, it is necessary, when choosing an appropriate statistical procedure, to identify the type of data represented by the independent variable. The criteria for classifying independent variables are the same as those previously discussed for dependent variables.

Methods for univariable analysis are largely concerned with calculating confidence intervals rather than statistical significance testing. The reason for that emphasis is that appropriate null hypotheses for univariable analyses are, except for observations from paired samples, difficult to imagine. This limitation does not apply to bivariable or multivariable analyses. In general, the null hypothesis of no association between the dependent and independent variables is relevant to bivariable analyses.

Continuous Dependent Variable

Figure 36.1. summarizes the steps in the flowchart that are needed when we have one continuous dependent variable and one independent variable. In Figure 36.1, note that we do not consider a continuous dependent variable associated with an ordinal independent variable. The reason for this omission is that no statistical procedures are available to compare a continuous dependent variable associated with an ordinal independent variable without converting the continuous variable to an ordinal scale.

Nominal Independent Variable

A nominal independent variable divides dependent variable values into two groups. For example, suppose we measured bleeding time for women who were birth-control pill (BCP) users and nonusers. The dependent variable, bleeding time, is continuous; the independent variable, BCP use–nonuse, is nominal. The nominal independent variable divides bleeding time into a group of bleeding time measurements for BCP users and for BCP nonusers. We have sampled bleeding time from a population that contains a group of BCP users and a group of BCP nonusers.[1]

Two methods of sampling independent variables are important in this example.[2] The first method is NATURALISTIC SAMPLING. In the example of bleeding time, naturalistic sampling would imply that we would randomly sample, for example, 200 women from a large population and then determine who is a BCP user or a BCP

[1]A universal assumption in statistics is that our observations are the result of random sampling. This assumption applies to the dependent variable, but it is not necessarily assumed by statistical tests for sampling of independent variables.

[2]There is actually a third method of sampling independent variables. That method is similar to purposive sampling, but instead of selecting observations that have specific independent variable values, the researcher randomly assigns a value, such as a dose, to each subject. This third method of sampling is used in experimental studies.

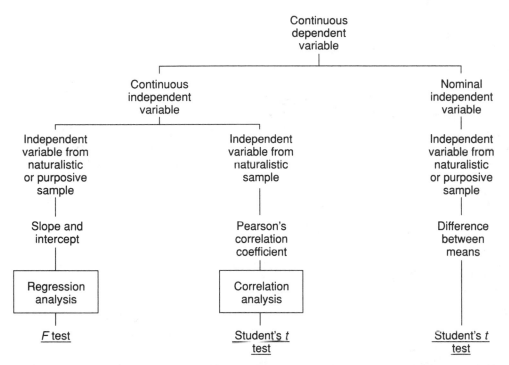

Figure 36.1. Flowchart to select a bivariable statistical procedure for a continuous dependent variable (continued from Fig. 34.5).

nonuser. If our sampling method was unbiased, the relative frequencies of BCP users compared with BCP nonusers in our sample would be representative of the frequency of BCP use in the population.

The second method is PURPOSIVE SAMPLING. If we used a purposive sample to study bleeding time, we might randomly sample 100 women who are BCP users and 100 women who are BCP nonusers. Because the researcher determines the number of observations for each independent variable value, the relative frequency of individuals in the sample with the nominal condition, birth-control pill use, is not representative of the relative sizes of the groups in the population. This is true even if our sampling method is random and unbiased among those who use and those who do not use BCPs. The fact that our sample contains 100 BCP users and 100 BCP nonusers does not suggest that half the women in the population use birth-control pills.

Thus, the distinction between naturalistic and purposive sampling is whether or not the independent variable in the sample is representative of the distribution of that variable in the population. Naturalistic sampling may be used in cohort studies. Purposive sampling is common in case-control studies and randomized clinical trials. As we shall see later in this chapter, the method used to sample the independent variable affects our options for appropriate statistical techniques or the statistical power of the technique chosen.

In bivariable analysis, such as the association between birth-control pill use and bleeding time, we are interested in a way in which we can compare bleeding times between BCP users and nonusers. In the comparison of means, our interest is generally in their difference.[3] For example, we are interested in the difference between mean bleeding times for BCP users and nonusers. The standard error for the difference between means is calculated from estimates of the variances in the two groups being compared.[4] To calculate the standard error for the difference in mean bleeding times, we would combine our estimates of the variance in bleeding times among BCP users and the variance among BCP nonusers. Interval estimates and statistical significance testing involving differences between means use the Student's *t* distribution, as indicated at the bottom right of Figure 36.1.

The appropriateness of using the Student's *t* distribution in statistical significance testing and calculation of confidence intervals is not affected by the method of sampling the independent variable. However, the statistical power of those procedures is greatest when the number of observations is the same for each of the potential categories of the independent variable. That is, we would have the greatest chance of demonstrating statistical significance for a true difference in mean bleeding times among 200 women if we used purposive sampling, selecting 100 BCP users and 100 BCP nonusers.

Continuous Independent Variable

We are often interested in using the measurement of a continuous independent variable to estimate the measurement of a continuous dependent variable[5]. As an example, suppose that we are interested in evaluating the relationship between the dosage of a hypothetical drug for treating glaucoma and intraocular pressure. Specifically, we would like to estimate the intraocular pressures (dependent variable) we expect to be associated in the population with various dosages of the drug (independent variable).

Some types of questions that can be addressed about estimation of the dependent variable depend on how the continuous independent variable was sampled. Regardless of whether naturalistic or purposive sampling was used, however, we can construct a linear or straight-line equation to estimate the mean value of the dependent variable (Y_i) for each value of the independent variable (X_i). In our example, the dependent variable is the mean intraocular pressure, and the independent variable is the dosage of medication. A linear equation in a population is described by two parameters: a SLOPE (α) and an INTERCEPT (β).

$$Y_i = \alpha - \beta X_i$$

The intercept estimates the mean of the dependent variable when the independent variable is equal to zero. Therefore, the intercept for the linear equation for intraocular pressure and dosage would estimate the population's mean intraocular pressure for individuals not receiving the drug. The slope of a linear equation tells us the amount the mean of the dependent variable changes for each unit change in the

[3]The reason for this interest is that differences between means tend to have a gaussian distribution, whereas other arithmetic combinations, such as ratio of means, do not.

[4]Specifically, this standard error is equal to the square root of the sum of the variances of the distributions of each group mean divided by the sum of the sample sizes. Knowing that, we can more fully understand why we cannot use univariable confidence intervals as a reliable surrogate for bivariable tests of inference. Comparison of univariable confidence intervals is equivalent to adding standard errors of two samples. That is not algebraically equivalent to the standard error of differences between means.

[5]The term predict rather than estimate is often used. We have avoided the term predict since it implies the ability to extrapolate from independent data to dependent data even when the dependent data is not known or is outside the range of values indicated in the investigation.

numerical value of the independent variable. For example, the slope of the equation that relates intraocular pressure to the dosage of drug estimates how much intraocular pressure decreases for each unit increase in dosage.

If we are interested in this sort of estimation, we need to calculate two point estimates from our sample's observations: the intercept and the slope. To obtain these estimates, we most often use LEAST SQUARES REGRESSION. This method selects numerical values for the slope and intercept that minimize the distances or, more specifically, the sum of the differences squared between the data observed in the sample and those estimated by the linear equation.[6]

Rather than consider the intercept and the slope separately, however, we can consider the linear equation as a whole as the estimate of interest. To do this, we examine the amount of variation in the dependent variable that we are able to explain using the linear equation divided by the amount of variation that we are unable to explain with the linear equation. In the example of medication to treat elevated intraocular pressure, we would divide the variation in intraocular pressure that is explained by knowing medication dosage by the variation in intraocular pressure that is left unexplained. Then, we can perform statistical significance testing on the null hypothesis that the data contained in the regression equation do not add to our ability to explain the value of the dependent variable (intraocular pressure), given a value of the independent variable (medication dosage). We use the F test to test that null hypothesis in regression analysis, as indicated on the left side of Figure 36.1.

In investigations such as the one examining mean intraocular pressure and dosage of a medication to treat glaucoma, we usually assign dosages that are not representative of all dosages that could have been selected. In other words, we seldom can use naturalistic sampling to investigate a dose-response relationship. It is appropriate to use linear regression methods regardless of whether a naturalistic or a purposive sampling method is used to obtain values of the independent variable. When a representative method of sampling, such as naturalistic sampling, is used to obtain the sample of an independent variable, it is possible to use another category of statistical techniques known as CORRELATION ANALYSIS.

Correlation analysis might be used, for example, if we randomly sampled individuals from a population and measured both their quantity of salt intake and their diastolic blood pressure. Here, both the independent variable (salt intake) and the dependent variable (diastolic blood pressure) have been randomly sampled from the population. The distribution of quantities of salt intake in our naturalistic sample is representative, on average, of the population's distribution of salt intake.

The distinction between the dependent and the independent variables is less important in correlation analysis than it is in other sorts of analyses. The same results are obtained in correlation analysis if those functions are reversed. In our example, it does not matter, from a statistical point of view, whether we consider diastolic blood pressure or salt intake as the dependent variable when performing a correlation analysis.[7]

---

[6]The differences between the observed numerical values of the dependent variables and those estimated by the regression equation are known as RESIDUALS. Residuals indicate how well the linear equation estimates the dependent variable.

[7]When performing regression analyses or correlations, we make a series of assumptions. These are referred to as random sampling of the dependent variable, homogeneity of variances, linear relationship between dependent and independent variables, and independent variable measured with perfect precision.

In correlation analysis, we measure how the dependent and independent variable's values change together. In our example, we would measure how consistently an increase in salt intake is associated with an increase in diastolic blood pressure. The statistic that is calculated to reflect how closely the two variables change together is called their COVARIANCE. The ratio of covariance to the square root of the product of the variances of the individual variables is known as the CORRELATION COEFFICIENT and is symbolized by r. The most commonly used correlation coefficient for two continuous variables is known as PEARSON'S CORRELATION COEFFICIENT.

This correlation coefficient is a point estimate of the strength of the association between two continuous variables. This is an important distinction between regression analysis and correlation analysis. Regression analysis can be used to estimate dependent variable values from independent variable values but does not estimate the strength of the relationship between those variables in the population. Correlation analysis estimates the strength of the relationship in the population but cannot be used to estimate values of the dependent variable corresponding to values of the independent variable.

The correlation coefficient has a range of possible values from −1 to +1. A correlation coefficient of zero indicates no relationship between the dependent and independent variables. Positive correlation coefficients indicate that as the value of the independent variable increases, the value of the dependent variable increases. Negative correlation coefficients indicate that as the value of the independent variable increases, the value of the dependent variable decreases.

Interpreting the strength of association between the dependent and independent variables is facilitated if we square the correlation coefficient to obtain the COEFFICIENT OF DETERMINATION (R^2). If we multiply the coefficient of determination by 100%, it indicates the percentage of variation in the dependent variable that is explained by or attributed to the value of the independent variable. The coefficient of determination can be thought of as a measure for continuous variables parallel to attributable risk percentage for nominal variables[8] because it addresses how much variability in the dependent variable can be attributed to the independent variable. Remember, however, that it is appropriate to use the coefficient of determination only when the independent variable, as well as the dependent variable, is sampled using representative or naturalistic sampling.

One of the most common errors in interpretation of statistical analysis is to use incorrectly the correlation coefficient to make point estimates for a particular population even though the independent variable's values are not sampled by a method that ensures, on average, that the sample will be representative of the population, that is, by naturalistic sampling. We can create an artificially high correlation coefficient by sampling only extreme values of the independent variable.

Ordinal Dependent Variable

In Figure 36.2, note that we do not consider an ordinal dependent variable associated with a continuous independent variable because the continuous independent variable must be converted to the ordinal scale. This is similar to the situation we discussed with a continuous dependent variable included in an analysis with an ordinal independent variable. No statistical procedures are commonly used to com-

---

[8]The term explain is used here because it is widely used. Explain should not imply a cause and relationship correlation is really a form of association.

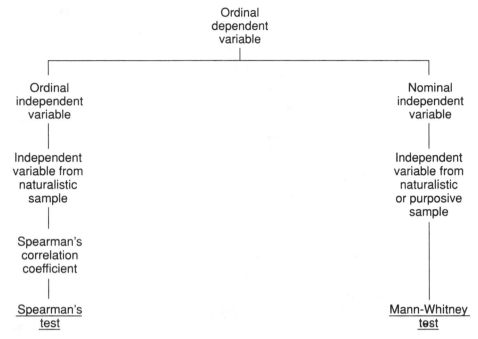

Figure 36.2. Flowchart to select a bivariable statistical procedure for an ordinal dependent variable (continued from Fig. 34.5).

pare an ordinal dependent variable with a continuous independent variable without making such a conversion.

Nominal Independent Variable

As indicated in Figure 36.2, the MANN-WHITNEY TEST is a statistical significance test applicable to a nominal independent variable and an ordinal dependent variable. It is also applicable to a continuous dependent variable converted to an ordinal scale to circumvent some of the assumptions of the Student's t test. The null hypothesis considered in a Mann-Whitney test is that the two groups do not differ in location in the population. Because this is a nonparametric test, no parameter of location is specified in the null hypothesis.

Ordinal Independent Variable

If the independent variable represents ordinal or continuous data converted to an ordinal scale, we can estimate the strength of the association between the dependent and independent variables using a method parallel to correlation analysis. In the case of ordinal variables, the most commonly used correlation coefficient is SPEARMAN'S CORRELATION COEFFICIENT. That coefficient can be calculated without making many of the assumptions necessary to calculate the coefficient described for continuous variables. It is important to remember, however, that any correlation coefficient must be determined from samples in which both the dependent and the independent variables are representative of a larger population. In other words, we must use naturalistic sampling. There is no nonparametric test that releases us from this assumption.

As for a correlation coefficient calculated for two continuous variables, we can perform statistical significance testing and calculation of confidence intervals for Spearman's correlation coefficients using Spearman's test. We can also use the square of the Spearman's correlation coefficient to provide a nonparametric estimate of the coefficient of determination or the percentage of the variation in the dependent variable that is explained by the independent variable. As opposed to Pearson's coefficient of determination, Spearman's coefficient of determination tells us the percentage change in the variable's rank that can be explained by changes in the rank of the independent variable.[9]

Nominal Dependent Variable

Bivariable statistical methods for nominal dependent variables are presented in Figure 36.3.

Nominal Independent Variable: Paired Design

If we are interested in collecting information on a nominal dependent variable and a nominal independent variable, we have the choice of a paired or an unpaired design. If appropriately constructed, a paired design may have more statistical power than a corresponding unpaired design. Remember that pairing is the special type of matching in which both the dependent and independent variables are measured on each individual from a pair of two similar individuals and the observations on the pair are analyzed together. Alternatively, data from the same individual can be used twice in the analysis.

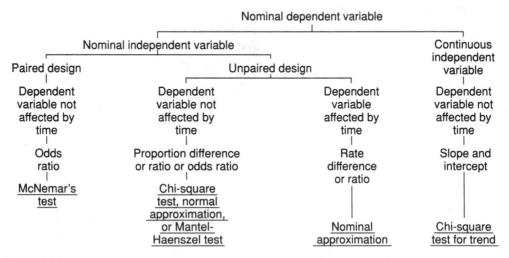

Figure 36.3. Flowchart to select a bivariable statistical procedure for a nominal dependent variable (continued from Fig. 34.5).

[9]Note that if continuous data is converted to ordinal data and a Spearman's correlation coefficient is calculated, it will often be larger than the corresponding Pearson's correlation coefficient.

As indicated in Figure 36.3, the odds ratio is the most common summary value or point estimate used for estimating the strength of the relationship in a paired design. To conduct statistical significance tests on pairs of data, MCNEMAR'S TEST is used. Related methods can be used to calculate confidence intervals for the odds ratio from paired observations.

Nominal Independent Variable: Unpaired Design

In bivariable analysis of an unpaired nominal dependent variable, we first determine whether the dependent variable is affected by time implies that an increase in the length of observation result in a greater probability of observing the outcome. This distinction is especially applicable and important when study subjects are observed for different length of time. If the denomination variable is not affected by time, we may use a proportion and obtain either a difference or a ratio, or alternatively, we can calculate an odds ratio. If the dependent variable is affected by time, we use a rate and obtain either a difference or a ratio.

From a statistical significance testing point of view, the choice of a ratio or a difference between proportions or between rates usually does not matter. In fact, in bivariable analysis, the same statistical significance tests are used regardless of whether the point estimate is a ratio or a difference. This is suggested by the fact that the null hypothesis that a difference is equal to 0 is equivalent to the null hypothesis that a ratio is equal to 1. When a ratio is equal to 1, the numerator must be equal to the denominator; thus, the difference between the numerator and the denominator must be equal to 0.

In bivariable analysis of nominal independent and dependent variables from an unpaired design, we are likely to encounter a variety of statistical significance testing methods. As in univariable analysis of a nominal dependent variable, these methods are of two general types: exact methods and normal approximations. The exact method for bivariable proportions is the FISHER EXACT procedure.[10] Two commonly used approximation methods for proportions are the NORMAL APPROXIMATION and the CHI-SQUARE TEST.[11] Rates are most often analyzed using a normal approximation. Statistical significance tests and calculation of confidence intervals for the odds ratio are usually based on the MANTEL-HAENSZEL CHI, also a normal approximation.

Continuous Independent Variable

When we have a continuous independent variable that is not affected by time and a nominal dependent variable, we are able to consider the possibility that a trend exists for various values of the independent variable. For example, we might be interested in examining the study hypothesis that the proportion of individuals who develop stroke increases in a linear or straight-line fashion as the diastolic blood pressure increases versus the null hypothesis that no linear relationship exists between those variables. This same sort of hypothesis is considered in simple linear regression with the exception that here we have a nominal dependent variable

---

[10]The Fisher exact procedure is used when any of the frequencies predicted by the null hypothesis for a 2×2 table are less than 5.

[11]Actually, the normal approximation and the chi-square procedures are equivalent in bivariable analysis. The square root of the chi-square statistic is equal to the normal approximation statistic.

rather than a continuous dependent variable, as indicated on the right side of Figure 36.3. Rather than a simple linear regression, we perform a CHI-SQUARE TEST FOR TREND.

Even though we have a special name for the test used to investigate the possibility of a linear trend in a nominal dependent variable, we should realize that a chi-square test for trend is very similar to a linear regression. In fact, the point estimates in the most commonly used methods to investigate a trend are a slope and intercept of a linear equation that are identical to the estimates we discussed for linear regression.[12]

We have now examined the commonly used statistical method for analyzing one independent variable and one dependent variable. Often, however, we will be interested in more than one independent variable. In these situations, we will use multivariable techniques, as discussed in the next chapter.[13]

---

[12]Point estimation of the coefficients in a chi-square test for trend is identical to estimation in a simple linear regression. For inference and interval estimation, a slightly different assumption is made that causes confidence intervals to be a little wider and P values to be a little larger in the chi-square test compared with linear regression. That difference decreases as the sample size increases.

[13]Note that when nominal data have more than two categories, more than one nominal variable is required to represent the data. When nominal data are used as independent variables, multivariable analysis, as explained in Chapter 34, is used. When more than one nominal variable is required for the dependent variable, special multivariate techniques, such as discriminant analysis, are needed. These techniques are beyond the scope of this book.

37 Multivariable Analyses

In multivariable statistics, we have one dependent variable and two or more independent variables. The independent variables may be measured on the same scale or on different scales. For example, all the independent variables may be represented by continuous data or, alternatively, some may be represented by continuous data and some may be represented by nominal data. Only nominal and continuous independent variables are indicated in a number of flowcharts that follow. In these situations, ordinal independent variables can be considered in multivariable analysis, but they must first be converted to a nominal scale.[1]

There are three general advantages to using multivariable methods to analyze health research data. First, this approach allows investigation of the relationship between a dependent variable and an independent variable while controlling or adjusting for the effect of other independent variables. This is the method for removing the influence of confounding variables in the analysis of health research data. Thus, multivariable methods are used to adjust for the influence of confounding variables.

For example, if we were interested in diastolic blood pressure for persons receiving various dosages of an antihypertensive drug, we may want to control for the potential confounding effects of age and gender. To do this in the analysis phase of a research project, we would use multivariable analysis with diastolic blood pressure as the dependent variable and with dosage, age, and gender as independent variables.

The second advantage of multivariable statistical methods is that they may allow us to perform statistical significance tests on several variables while maintaining a chosen probability (α) of making a Type I error. In other words, at times we may use multivariable analysis to avoid the multiple comparison problem introduced in Part 1, *Studying a Study*.

To recall the multiple comparison problem, imagine that we have several independent variables that we compare with a dependent variable using a bivariable method such as the Student's t test. Although in each of those bivariable tests we permit only a 5% chance of making a Type I error, the chance that we would commit at least one Type I error among all those comparisons would be somewhat greater than 5%. We call the chance of making a Type I error for any particular comparison the TESTWISE ERROR. The chance of making a Type I error for at least one comparison is known as the EXPERIMENTWISE ERROR. Bivariable analyses control the testwise error rate. Many multivariable methods, on the other hand, are designed to maintain a consistent experimentwise type I error rate. That is, at times multivariable procedures are in-and-of-themselves capable of taking into account multiple comparison issues.

---

[1]Conversion of ordinal scale data to a nominal scale results in a loss of information but needs no justification. Conversion of such data to a continuous scale, however, suggests that the data contain more information than they actually do. This is difficult to justify.

Two types of null hypotheses are examined in most multivariable methods of analysis that are designed to avoid the multiple comparison problem. The first is known as the OMNIBUS NULL HYPOTHESIS. This null hypothesis addresses the relationship between the dependent variable and the entire collection of independent variables as a unit. A drawback of the omnibus null hypothesis, however, is that it does not allow investigation of relationships between the dependent variable and each of the independent variables individually. This is accomplished by the second type of null hypotheses addressed in PAIRWISE or PARTIAL TESTS.

The third advantage of multivariable analysis is that it can be used to compare the separate abilities of two or more independent variables to estimate values of the corresponding dependent variable. For example, suppose we conduct a large cohort study to examine risk factors for coronary heart disease. Among the independent variables we measure are diastolic blood pressure and serum cholesterol levels. We would like to determine whether both variables contribute to the probability of coronary heart disease. Examining their ability to explain who will develop coronary heart disease in bivariable analyses, however, could be misleading if individuals with elevated diastolic blood pressure tend to be the same individuals who have high serum cholesterol. If, on the other hand, we use multivariable methods to compare these risk factors, we would be able to separate their ability to estimate the probability of coronary heart disease from their apparent association with coronary heart disease because of their association with each other.

Because of these advantages of multivariable methods, they are frequently used to analyze health research data. Let us now take a closer look at these methods and the ways they can be interpreted to give us these advantages.

Continuous Dependent Variable

Nominal Independent Variables

In bivariable analysis of a continuous dependent variable and a nominal independent variable, the independent variable has the effect of dividing the dependent variable's values into two subgroups. In multivariable analysis, we have more than one nominal independent variable and, thus, we are able to divide dependent variable values into more than two subgroups. The most common methods to compare means of the dependent variable among three or more subgroups are forms of a general statistical approach called ANALYSIS OF VARIANCE *(ANOVA)*[2] (Fig. 37.1).

The simplest type of ANOVA is one in which a number (K) of nominal independent variables are used to separate the nominal dependent data into k + 1 subgroups or categories. For example, suppose we are interested in only the relationship between fasting blood glucose and race, defined as white, black, or other. Other is the result when the race is not white or black. We now have to consider three (k + 1 = 3) subgroups of race (white, black, and other) for which we determine fasting blood sugar. This type of ANOVA is known as a ONE-WAY ANOVA.[3] The omnibus null hypothesis in a One-way ANOVA is that the means of the

---

[2]It seems incongruous that a method to compare means should be called an analysis of variance. The reason for this name is that ANOVAs examine the variation between subgroups, assuming that the variation within each of the subgroups is the same. If the variance between subgroups exceeds the variation within those groups, the subgroups must differ in location, measured by means.

[3]When k = 1, only one nominal independent variable is being considered. In that case, we are comparing only two subgroups, and the one-way ANOVA is exactly the same as a *t* test for bivariable analysis.

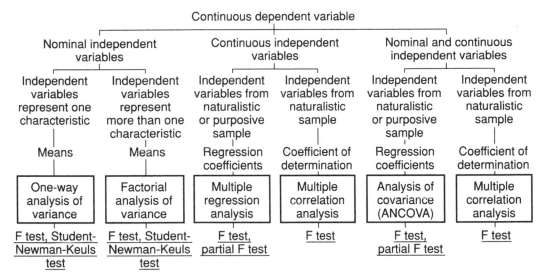

Figure 37.1. Flowchart to select a multivariable statistical procedure for a continuous dependent variable (continued from Fig. 34.5).

$k + 1$ subgroups are all equal to one another. In our example, the omnibus null hypothesis would be that mean fasting blood sugar for whites is the same as for blacks and for persons of other races.

In order to use One-way ANOVA, we need to assume that it is impossible for an individual to be included in more than one category. For example, in health research, we usually regard races as mutually exclusive categories. For each individual, we record a single race. Thus, it is impossible, in this context, for an individual to be considered both white and black.

Now let us imagine that we are interested in both race and gender. When we use both race and gender, the individual characteristics are most often not mutually exclusive from one another. For example, an individual can be of either gender regardless of his or her race. It is necessary, therefore, to have another way in which subgroups can be defined by nominal independent variables when we wish to utilize more than one characteristic. Commonly, the solution is to segregate those characteristics into FACTORS. A factor is a collection of one or more nominal independent variables that each defines mutually exclusive, but topically related, categories or characteristics. For example, suppose we have two independent variables defining race and one independent variable defining gender in our sample of persons for whom we measure fasting blood glucose levels. The three independent variables in this example actually represent two separate factors: race and gender. We can define $(k_{race} - 1) \times (k_{gender} - 1) = 6$ subgroups among which we wish to compare mean fasting blood glucose levels: white males, white females, black males, black females, other males, and other females. The type of ANOVA that considers two or more factors is known as a FACTORIAL ANOVA.

With Factorial ANOVA, we can test the same sort of omnibus null hypothesis tested in a One-way ANOVA. In our example, the null hypothesis would be that mean fasting blood sugar is the same in white females as it is in white males, black females, black males, other females, and other males. In addition, we can test hypotheses about the equality of means of fasting blood sugar between the subgroups within a given factor. That is, we can examine the separate effect of race on mean fasting blood sugar or the effect of gender on that dependent variable. The statistical tests that are used to examine the factors separately are often called tests of MAIN EFFECTS. All these null hypotheses in ANOVAs are tested using an F test.

The results of examining a main effect take into account possible confounding relationships of the other factors. In our example, if we tested the null hypothesis that the fasting blood sugar means for the three race subgroups are all equal by using an ANOVA test of the main effect of race, that test would control for any differences in distribution of genders among the racial groups. Thus, Factorial ANOVA allows us to take advantage of the ability of multivariable analysis to control for confounding variables.

To interpret tests of main effects, it is assumed that the factor has the same relationship with the dependent variable regardless of the level of other factors. That is, we assume that the difference between the fasting blood sugar means in blacks, whites, and other races is the same regardless of whether the individual is a male or a female. This is not always the case. For example, females might have a higher fasting blood sugar than do males among white subjects, but females and males might be similar or, in a greater extreme, males might have higher fasting blood sugars than do females among black subjects. If this sort of relationship exists between factors, we say that an INTERACTION exists between gender and race. In clinical terminology, we might say that a synergy or effect modification exists between race and gender in determining fasting blood sugar levels. In addition to testing for main effects, Factorial ANOVAs can be used to test hypotheses about interactions. Additional interaction variable(s) for race and gender would tell us, for instance, how much more the fasting blood sugar level differs for black women than would be expected by adding the effect of being black to the effect of being female.

We have seen how Factorial ANOVAs allow us to use one of the advantages of multivariable methods by controlling for confounding variables. In our example, we assumed that we were primarily interested in the relationship between race and fasting blood sugar and that we wanted to control for the potential confounding effects of gender. Another way to think about the data presented in this example might be that we consider race and gender both to be factors that could potentially be used to estimate fasting blood sugar level. In this case, rather than looking at the main effect of race while controlling for gender, we would use the factorial ANOVA to examine how race and gender compare and interact in their ability to estimate fasting blood sugar. Factorial ANOVAs would, thus, allow us to examine the separate abilities of race and gender to estimate fasting blood sugar. This is an example of the third advantage of multivariable methods.

In addition, ANOVAs also address the second advantage that dealing with the multiple comparison problem. In ANOVAs, the omnibus null hypothesis maintains an experimentwise Type I error rate equal to α, usually 5%. It is seldom enough, however, to know that differences exist among means within a factor without knowing specifically in which category the means differ. That is, it is not enough to know that mean fasting blood sugar differs by race without knowing which races contribute to the difference. To examine the subgroup means in greater detail, we use pairwise tests.[4] The most widely used pairwise test for sets of obser-

---

[4]In ANOVA, these pairwise tests are often called Á POSTERIORI TESTS. The reason for that terminology is that some pairwise tests, especially the older tests, require a statistically significant test of the omnibus hypothesis before the pairwise test can be used.

vations that include a continuous dependent variable and more than one nominal independent variable is the STUDENT-NEWMAN-KEULS TEST. As indicated in Figure 37.1, this test is used for pairwise statistical significance testing for One-way and Factorial analyses of Variance. This test allows examination of all pairs of subgroup means while maintaining an experimentwise Type I error rate of $\alpha = 0.05$.[5] An algebraic rearrangement of the Student-Newman-Keuls test allows us to calculate confidence intervals for the dependent variable for each value of the independent variables. Note that in flowchart 38.1 the underlined test used for statistical significance tests of the omnibus hypothesis is followed after a comma by the statistical significance test used for pairwise comparisons.

Continuous Independent Variables

When the independent variables in a study are represented by continuous data, we can choose between two approaches that correspond to approaches discussed in Chapter 36 in which we considered regression analysis and correlation analysis. Most often, we are interested in estimating values of the dependent variable corresponding to specific independent variable values. In bivariable analysis, we used linear regression to estimate the value of the dependent variable given the value of the independent variable. When we have more than one continuous independent variable, we use MULTIPLE REGRESSION ANALYSIS.

In multiple regression, the mean of a continuous dependent variable is estimated by a linear equation that is like the one in simple linear regression except that it includes two or more continuous independent variables.

$$Y = \alpha + \beta_1 X_1 + \beta_2 X_2 + \ldots + \beta_k X_k$$

For example, suppose we are interested in estimating plasma cortisol levels based on total white blood cell (WBC) count, body temperature, and urine production in response to a water load. To investigate that relationship, we measure cortisol (μg/dL), WBC count (10^3), temperature (°C), and urine volume (mL) in 20 patients. Using multiple regression, we might estimate the following linear equation:

Cortisol $= -36.8 + 0.8 \times$ WBC $+ 1.2 \times$ temperature $+ 4.7 \times$ urine volume

As in ANOVA, multiple regression allows testing of an omnibus hypothesis that has a Type I error rate equal to α. The hypothesis in multiple regression is that the entire collection of independent variables cannot be used to estimate values of the dependent variable. An F test is used to evaluate the statistical significance of the multiple regression omnibus null hypothesis. Suppose that, in our example, we find a statistically significant F. This implies that, if we know the WBC count, temperature, and urine volume for a particular patient, then we can do better than chance in estimating, the value of that patient's plasma cortisol level.

In addition to interest in the omnibus hypothesis in multiple regression, it is most often desirable to examine relationships between the dependent variable and individual independent variables. One way in which those relationships are reflected is in the regression coefficients associated with the independent variables. REGRES-

---

[5]Other pairwise tests also are available for such comparisons or for different sorts of comparisons among subgroup means. An example of a different type would be when we want to compare a control group with a series of experimental groups.

SION COEFFICIENTS are estimates of the βs in the regression equation. The results of multiple regression analysis allow point estimation and calculation of confidence intervals for those coefficients. As indicated in Figure 37.1, statistical significance testing for individual coefficients involves the PARTIAL F TEST to test the null hypothesis that the coefficient equals zero.

Table 37.1 shows partial F tests for the independent variables used to estimate plasma cortisol. Although the omnibus hypothesis was rejected in this example, we see that only temperature and urine volume have regression coefficients that are statistically significant. In bivariable regression, the regression coefficients estimate the slope of the line estimating values of the dependent variable as a function of the independent variable in the population that was sampled. In multivariable regression, the relationship between the dependent variable and any particular independent variable is not so straightforward. The regression coefficient actually reflects the relationship between the remaining changes in the numerical values of the independent variable associated with changes in the dependent variable of interest after adjustment for the other independent variables. That is, the reported contribution of any particular independent variable in multiple regression is only the contribution over and above the contributions of all other independent variables.

This might be considered both good news and bad news. The good news is that multiple regression coefficients can be used to reflect the relationship between the dependent variable and the independent variable controlling for the effects of the other independent variables. Thus, multiple regression can be used to remove the effect of a continuous confounding variable.

It may be considered bad news that controlling for the effect of other independent variables is synonymous with removing variation in the dependent variable that is associated with the other independent variables. If each of two independent variables, by themselves, are good at explaining the same numerical changes in the dependent variable, both independent variables will appear to be unimportant in explaining changes in the dependent variable in a multiple regression. Sharing of predictive information by independent variables is known as MULTICOLLINEARITY.[6] If multicollinearity is kept in mind, however, multiple regression can be used to examine the separate abilities of the independent variables to explain the dependent variable.

For example, suppose we are interested in cardiac output during exercise. As independent variables, we include the continuous variable energy expended, heart rate, and systolic blood pressure. We know that each of these independent variables is strongly associated with cardiac output. In a multiple regression analysis,

Table 37.1. *Partial* F *Tests on Regression Coefficients Estimated for Independent Variables Used to Predict Plasma Cortisol*

Variable	Coefficient	*F*	*P* value
White blood cell count	0.8	1.44	0.248
Temperature	1.2	4.51	0.050
Urine	4.7	9.51	0.007

[6]Some indication of the existence of shared information by independent variables can be obtained by examining bivariable correlation coefficients for those variables, but the best method to evaluate the existence of multicollinearity is to inspect regression models that include and exclude each independent variable. If regression coefficients change substantially when different models are considered, multicollinearity exists.

however, it would be unlikely that any of them would appear to be statistically significant in their association with the dependent variable. That result is expected because of the large amount of information about cardiac output that is shared by those independent variables.

Calculation of confidence intervals and statistical significance testing for coefficients associated with individual independent variables in multiple regression is parallel to pairwise analyses in ANOVA. In ANOVA, however, pairwise analyses were designed to maintain an experimentwise Type I error rate equal to α. In multiple regression, the testwise Type I error rate equals α, but the experimentwise error rate is influenced by the number of independent variables being considered. The more independent variables examined in multiple regression, the greater the likelihood that at least one regression coefficient will appear to be a statistically significant estimator even though no relationship exists between those variables in the larger population being sampled. Therefore, in multiple regression, statistically significant associations between the dependent variable and independent variables that were not expected to be important before the data were examined should be interpreted with some skepticism.

If all the continuous independent variables in a set of observations are the result of naturalistic sampling from some population of interest, we might be interested in estimating the strength of the association between the dependent variable and the entire collection of independent variables. This is parallel to our interest in bivariable correlation analysis. As indicated in Figure 37.1, in multivariable analysis, the method used to measure the degree of association is called MULTIPLE CORRELATION ANALYSIS. The result of multiple correlation analysis can be expressed either as a multiple coefficient of determination or as its square root, the MULTIPLE CORRELATION COEFFICIENT. It is important to keep in mind that these statistics reflect the degree of association between the dependent variable and the entire collection of independent variables. For instance, suppose that in our example we obtain a multiple coefficient of determination equal to 0.82, meaning that 82% of the variation in plasma cortisol among patients can be explained by knowing WBC count, temperature, and urine volume. The statistically significant F test associated with the test of the omnibus null hypothesis in multiple regression analysis also tests the null hypothesis that the population's multiple coefficient of determination equals zero. Confidence intervals for coefficients of determination can be derived from these same calculations.

Nominal and Continuous Independent Variables

Often, we are faced with a set of observations in which some of the independent variables are continuous and some are nominal. For example, suppose we conducted a study designed to explain cardiac output on the basis of energy output during exercise. Further, we expect the relationship between cardiac output and energy output to be different for the two sexes. In this example, our set of observations would contain cardiac output, a continuous dependent variable; energy output, a continuous independent variable; and gender, a nominal independent variable.

To examine a data set that contains a continuous dependent variable and a mixture of nominal and continuous independent variables, we use an ANALYSIS OF COVARIANCE *(ANCOVA)*. The continuous independent variables in ANCOVA are related to the dependent variable in the same way that continuous independent variables are related to the dependent variable in a multiple regression. The nominal independent variables are related to the dependent variable in the same way nominal independent variables are related to the dependent variable in ANOVA. Therefore, ANCOVA is a hybrid method containing aspects of both multiple regression and ANOVA.

With ANCOVA, we deal with nominal data, such as gender, using an INDICATOR VARIABLE, which is given a numerical value of 0 or 1. Indicator variables allow us to create two different regression lines that differ only by their intercept. An indicator variable for gender would tell us how much the estimate of cardiac output differs between males and females.[7]

Ordinal Dependent Variable

In univariable and bivariable analyses, statistical methods are available to analyze ordinal dependent variables and to allow us to convert continuous dependent variables to an ordinal scale when we could not fulfill the assumptions necessary to use the statistical methods designed for continuous dependent variables. This also is true of multivariable methods for ordinal dependent variables.

Ideally, we would like to have methods for ordinal dependent variables that parallel all the important multivariable methods for continuous dependent variables: ANOVA, ANCOVA, and multiple regression. Unfortunately, this is not the case. The only well-accepted multivariable procedures for ordinal dependent variables are ones that can be used as nonparametric equivalents to certain ANOVA designs. Thus, Figure 37.2 is restricted to methods that can be used with nominal independent variables or, alternatively, with ordinal independent variables. Continuous independent variables must be converted to an ordinal or nominal scale to use these methods.

Methods for ordinal-dependent variable may be used because the dependent variable is measured on an ordinal scale. Alternatively they may be used because the data does not satisfy the assumptions required to utilize the data as continuous data. Let us reconsider the previous example of fasting blood sugar measured among persons of three race categories (black, white, and other) and of both genders. Our interest was in determining the independent effects of race and gender on blood sugar. To analyze the data, we used a factorial ANOVA. If we were concerned about fasting blood sugar satisfying the assumptions of the ANOVA,[8] we could convert the data to an ordinal scale by assigning relative ranks to fasting blood sugar measurements. Then, we could apply the KRUSKAL-WALLIS TEST or alternatively DUNN'S TEST to those converted data. Those test are appropriate for performing statistical significance testing on an ordinal dependent variable and two or more nominal independent variables with either a one-way or factorial design. Nonparametric procedures also are available to make pairwise comparisons among subgroups of the dependent variable.

As indicated in Figure 37.2, when all the independent variables are represented by ordinal data and the dependent variable is also represented by ordinal data, KENDALL'S COEFFICIENT OF CONCORDANCE can be used as a nonparametric multiple correlation analysis.

---

[7]The coefficient of the indicator variable does not allow us to compare the strength of the relationship between gender and cardiac output with other independent variables in the regression equation.

[8]The assumptions for ANOVA and ANCOVA are the same as those previously labeled in the footnote 1 on regression analysis in Chapter 36.

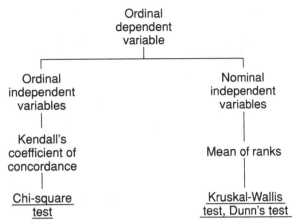

Figure 37.2. Flowchart to select a multivariable statistical procedure for an ordinal dependent variable (continued from Fig. 34.5).

When using multivariable methods designed for ordinal dependent variables to analyze sets of observations that contain a continuous dependent variable which we have converted to an ordinal scale, we should keep in mind a potential disadvantage. The nonparametric procedure has less statistical power than does the corresponding parametric procedure if the assumptions of the parametric procedure are not violated by the continuous dependent variable. This is true for all statistical procedures performed on continuous data converted to an ordinal scale. Thus, if the assumptions of a parametric statistical procedure are fulfilled, it is advisable to use this parametric procedure to analyze a continuous dependent variable rather than a parallel nonparametric procedure.

Nominal Dependent Variable

In health research, we are often interested in outcome measurements such as live–die, cure–not cure, or disease–no disease measured as nominal data. Further, because of the complexity of health phenomena, it is most often desirable to measure several independent variables to consider several separate hypotheses, to control for confounding variables, and to investigate the possibility of synergy or interaction between variables. Consequently, multivariable analyses with nominal dependent variables are frequently used in the analysis of health research data.

We have separated multivariable statistical procedures for nominal dependent variables into two groups: those that are useful when the independent variables are all nominal and those that are useful for a mixture of nominal and continuous independent variables (Fig. 37.3). The analyses in the first group are restricted to nominal independent variables or variables converted to a nominal scale. The analyses in the second group, on the other hand, can be used with nominal and continuous independent variables. There are no well-established methods to consider ordinal independent variables unless they are converted to a nominal scale.

Nominal Independent Variables

When we analyze a nominal dependent variable and two or more nominal independent variables, we are interested in measures that are the same as those of interest in bivariable analysis of a nominal dependent variable and a nominal indepen-

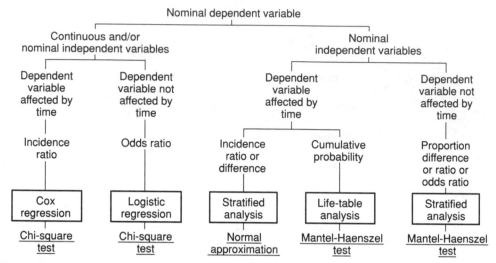

Figure 37.3. Flowchart to select a multivariable statistical procedure for a nominal dependent variable (continued from Fig. 34.5).

dent variable. For example, we might be interested in proportions, rates, or odds. In multivariable analysis of nominal dependent and independent variables, however, we are interested in these measures of disease occurrence while adjusting for the other independent variable(s).

For example, suppose we are interested in comparing the prevalence of lung cancer among coffee drinkers and subjects who do not drink coffee. Here, prevalence of lung cancer is the variable of interest and, therefore, the nominal dependent variable. Coffee drinking (yes or no) is the nominal independent variable. We would want to adjust for the potential confounding effect of cigarette smoking. To do that, we might include another nominal independent variable that identified cigarette smokers versus nonsmokers.

When we have two or more independent variables in a data set and they are all nominal, or are converted to a nominal scale, the general approach to adjust for independent variables is often a STRATIFIED ANALYSIS. As described in Part 1, *Studying a Study,* stratified analysis methods involve separating observations into subgroups defined by values of the nominal independent variables thought to be confounding variables. In our example of lung cancer prevalence and coffee consumption, we would begin a stratified analysis by dividing our observations into two groups: one composed of smokers and one composed of nonsmokers.

Within each subgroup, such as cigarette smokers and nonsmokers, we would calculate a separate estimate of the prevalences of lung cancer for coffee drinkers and nondrinkers. Those separate estimates are known as STRATUM-SPECIFIC POINT ESTIMATES. The stratum-specific point estimates are combined using a particular system of weighting the strata-specific estimates. That is, we would combine the information from each stratum, using a method to determine how much impact each stratum-specific estimate should have on the combined estimate.[9] The

[9]The system of weighting stratum-specific estimates is an important way in which different stratified analysis methods differ. In direct standardization, the weighting system is based on the relative frequencies of each stratum in some reference population. The most useful weighting systems, from a statistical point of view, are those that reflect the precision of stratum-specific estimates.

resulting combined estimate is considered to be an adjusted or standardized point estimate for all strata combined with the effects of the confounding variable removed.

In the flowchart (see Fig. 37.3), we have indicated two types of nominal dependent variables: those that are and those that are not affected by time. Being affected by time implies that the frequency with which a nominal outcome is observed is influenced by the duration of follow-up and different individuals are observed for different periods of time. We examined this type of situation in the discussion of cohort or longitudinal life tables.[10]

Dependent variables that are affected by time can cause problems in interpretation if the groups being compared differ in their lengths of follow-up, which is often the case. These problems can be circumvented if we consider incidence rate as the appropriate estimate for the dependent variable because the incidence rate has a unit of time in the denominator and, thus, takes length of follow-up into account. Unfortunately, incidence rate is a measurement that can be confusing to interpret. Most persons find it difficult to intuitively understand what "cases per person-year" implies. By contrast, it is much easier to understand RISK. Risk is the proportion of persons who develop an outcome over a specified period of time. Thus, risk measures the CUMULATIVE PROBABILITY of developing the outcome.

If we are interested in risk and the data contain observations from persons followed for various periods of time, we must use special statistical procedures to adjust for differences in follow-up. When all independent variables are nominal, the methods we use are types of LIFE-TABLE ANALYSIS. These methods consider periods of follow-up time, such as 1-year intervals, as a collection of nominal independent variables. Each 1-year interval is used to stratify observations in the same way data are stratified by categories of a confounding variable such as age group. Cumulative survival,[11] which is equal to 1 minus the cumulative probability of death, is determined by combining these adjusted probabilities of surviving each time period.

Continuous and Nominal Independent Variables

The stratified analysis approach appeals to many researchers because it appears to be simpler than other analyses. However, this approach does have some shortcomings. Stratified analysis is designed to examine the relationship between a nominal dependent variable and one nominal independent variable while controlling for the effect of nominal confounding variables. It does not allow for a straightforward examination of more than one explanatory variable, investigation of interactions or synergy, consideration of continuous confounding variables without converting them to a nominal scale, or estimation of the importance of confounding variables. These are often features of great interest to health researchers.

Methods of analysis that permit simultaneous investigation of nominal and continuous independent variables and their interactions are parallel in their general

---

[10]Being affected by time also implies that, as the length of follow-up increases, the probability that the event will occur also increases.

[11]Life tables were originally designed to consider the risk of death, but they can be used to calculate the risk of any irreversible outcome that can occur only once.

approach to multiple regression discussed earlier. The methods we use here, however, are different from multiple regression in three ways. The first difference, as
the flowchart indicates (see Fig. 37.3), is that multiple regression is a method of
analyzing continuous dependent variables while we are now concerned with nominal dependent variables. The second difference is that most of the methods for
nominal dependent variables do not use the least squares method used in multiple
regression to find the best fit for the data. Most often, nominal dependent variable
regression coefficients are estimated using the MAXIMUM LIKELIHOOD METHOD.[12]

The third difference is perhaps the most important to health researchers interpreting the results of regression analysis of nominal dependent variables. Although
this type of analysis provides regression coefficient estimates and their standard
errors, the remainder of the information resulting from the analysis is unlike that
in multiple regression. These regressions do not provide us with any estimates parallel to correlation coefficients. Thus, without a coefficient of determination, it is
not possible to determine the percent of variation in the dependent variable that is
explained by the collection of independent variables.[13]

For outcomes affected by time, the most commonly used regression method is
the COX REGRESSION.[14] In this approach, the collection of independent variables
and, if desired, their interactions are used to estimate the incidence rate[15] of the
nominal dependent variable[16] such as the incidence of death. Simple algebraic
combination of the coefficients for a particular Cox regression equation can be used
to estimate and plot the survival curve for a set of independent variable values.
When all the independent variables are nominal, the Cox regression estimates survival curves that are very similar to those resulting from life-table analysis.

Cox regression can in-and-of-itself address our three basic questions of statistics: estimation, inference, and adjustment. The size or magnitude of the difference
between groups can be estimated by using the percentage survival from the end or
right side of the survival curves. Inference or statistical significance testing can be
performed comparing the survival curves. Finally, Cox regression has the advantage of incorporating the adjustment for confounding variables. Thus, the Cox
regression is increasingly used in health research.

As indicated in Figure 37.3, nominal dependent variables that are not affected
by time are frequently analyzed using a multivariable approach called LOGISTIC
REGRESSION.

The dependent variable in logistic regression is the natural logarithm of the odds
of group membership. Thus, odds ratios can be obtained from logistic regression.
We can, therefore, view logistic regression as a method of adjusting odds ratios for
nominal and continuous confounding variables.

Now that we have completed our overview of univariable, bivariable, and multivariable analyses, let us put the process together and see how we can use the combined flowchart.

---

[12]The maximum likelihood method chooses estimates for regression coefficients to maximize the
likelihood that the data observed would have resulted from sampling a population with those coefficients.

[13]A surrogate for the coefficient of determination has been proposed, but its usefulness is not well
accepted among statisticians.

[14]This method is also known as PROPORTIONAL HAZARDS REGRESSION.

[15]The term HAZARD is most often used as a synonym for incidence in the Cox model.

[16]Actually, Cox regression predicts the natural logarithm of the ratio of the incidence adjusted for
the independent variables divided by the incidence unadjusted for those variables.

38 Flowchart Summary

In this chapter, we reproduce the entire flowchart that is required for selecting a statistic. This summary flowchart can be used in two ways. One way is to start at the top as we have done previously beginning with Figure 38.1 and trace the flowchart down to discover what types of statistical procedures are appropriate for a particular investigation. To use the flowchart this way, you must first use Figure 38.1 to identify one dependent variable and then 0, 1, or more than 1 independent variables. Next, you must decide the type of data represented by the dependent variable (*i.e.* continuous, ordinal, or nominal). After you make these decisions, you will encounter a figure number that will guide you to the next flowchart element that is applicable to your data.

Each of the subsequent flowchart components is constructed in a similar way. If your data contain independent variables, you will need to identify the type of data represented by each one.[1] If special restrictions are applicable to statistical procedures, you will need to decide if the data satisfy the restrictions. If no statistical procedures are available for the type of data represented by one or more of the variables, it is often possible to convert the variable or variables to a lower level scale and consult the flowchart for an option that is consistent with the converted variable(s).

Following down the flowchart, you will come to a summary measurement or point estimate that is useful for your data. These are followed if applicable by a general classification of statistical procedures that are enclosed in a box. At the very bottom, you will encounter the name of the procedures that are most commonly used for both statistical significance testing and calculation of confidence intervals on data sets like the one you are examining. These are underlined.

When using the flowchart, note the following:

1. Additional conditions that need to be satisfied to use a type of statistical procedure are shown immediately after the type of independent variables.
2. Terms enclosed in a box indicate a general classification of statistical procedures.
3. Procedures with a line under them are used for statistical significance testing or calculation of confidence intervals.
4. When "or" is used it indicates that either test is acceptable for addressing the same question; however, the test listed first has more statistical power, or is used more frequently, or both.
5. When a comma alone appears between two statistical significance tests, the first test is used to evaluate the omnibus null hypothesis, whereas the second test is used in pairwise comparisons.

---

[1]Remember that, for statistical purposes, a nominal variable refers to only two categories of a characteristic. If a characteristic has k categories, k − 1 nominal variables will be needed. If more than one nominal variable is needed to represent the independent variable then multivariable analysis is needed.

The flowchart, starting at the top, is applicable to researchers who are interested in selecting a statistical procedure for a set of data. More often, as readers of the health research literature, we are interested in checking that a procedure selected by others is an appropriate one. The flowchart can be used to assist in that process by first finding the name of the selected procedure at the bottom of the flowchart and tracing the flowchart backward to determine whether the procedure is a logical choice for the data set being analyzed.

Let us consider an example of how to use the flowchart of statistics in Figure 38.1 through Figure 38.10. Together these figures represent the overall flowchart presented in Chapters 34 through 37. To see how the flowchart can be used, consider the following research study.

> A randomized clinical trial of a new prenatal vitamin supplement is designed to test the hypothesis that the new supplement will reduce the chance that the mother will deliver a second child with spina bifida. The study was conducted by randomizing 500 women who had previously delivered a child with spina bifida to the new treatment study group and 500 other women who had previously delivered a child with spina bifida to the conventional treatment control group. All women were in their first trimester of pregnancy. The study and control groups were similar except that the control group had an average age of 32 years compared to 28 years for the study group. Maternal age is believed to be a risk factor for spina bifida.

To use the flowchart, we start with Figure 38.1. The first step is to identify one dependent variable. The dependent variable is the characteristic of primary interest for which the investigation is trying to estimate a value or test a hypothesis. In this investigation, we are testing the hypothesis that the new prenatal vitamins will prevent spina bifida. The presence or absence of spina bifida is the dependent variable.

Moving down the flowchart in Figure 38.1, we come to the next question that must be addressed: How many independent variables does this investigation include? The independent variables represent all the other data that we wish to include in the analysis. In this study, we need to include treatment (vitamin supplement or conventional treatment) and age. Age is included because it is a potential confounding variable. Thus, we have more than one independent variable and can move down Figure 38.1 to multivariable analysis. The next question will require us to select one of the following figures (Figs. 38.2 through 38.10) that display the complete flowchart.

The next question is, "What type of dependent variable do we have?" Because the presence or absence of spina bifida is the dependent variable, we have one nominal dependent variable. This brings us to the end of Figure 38.1 and leads us to Figure 38.10. At the bottom of Figure 38.1 are references to Figures 38.2 through 38.10. Thus, Figure 38.1 should guide you to one of the subsequent flowcharts.

Turning to Figure 38.10, we see all the methods we have discussed for one nominal dependent variable. We now ask whether this investigation has only nominal independent variables or whether it has both continuous and nominal independent variables. In this investigation, the independent variables are treatment group and age. The treatment group has only two categories; therefore, it is a nominal variable. Age is a continuous variable having an unlimited number of equally spaced categories. Thus, having both nominal and continuous variables, we can proceed down the left side of the flowchart in Figure 38.10.

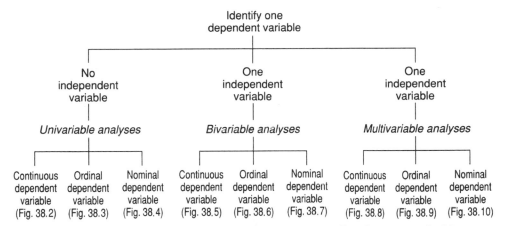

Figure 38.1. Master flowchart to determine which of the subsequent flowcharts are applicable to a particular data set. The figure's number at the bottom of the flowchart refers you to subsequent flowcharts.

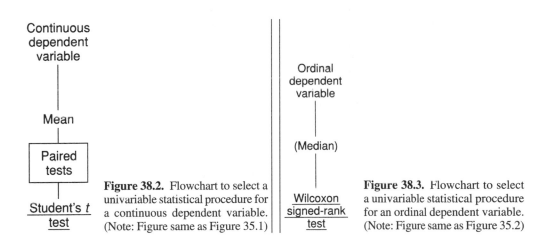

Figure 38.2. Flowchart to select a univariable statistical procedure for a continuous dependent variable. (Note: Figure same as Figure 35.1)

Figure 38.3. Flowchart to select a univariable statistical procedure for an ordinal dependent variable. (Note: Figure same as Figure 35.2)

Now we need to decide whether the dependent variable is affected by time. Being affected by time implies that there are different periods of follow-up and that the longer the observation continues the more likely it is that the outcome will occur. This is often the situation in randomized clinical trials. However, here we are only assessing outcome at the time of birth. Thus, there is only one assessment point, and the dependent variable is not affected by time.

This leads us to the odds ratio as our estimate of the strength of the relationship between treatment group and the occurrence of spina bifida. Proceeding down the flowchart we come to the general category of statistical techniques known as LOGISTIC REGRESSION (enclosed in the box). As indicated by the underlined chi-square test, statistical significance testing and confidence intervals are performed using a chi-square method.

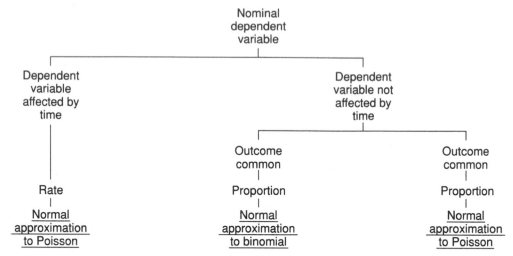

Figure 38.4. Flowchart to select a univariable statistical procedure for a nominal dependent variable.

Having worked through the flowchart starting at the top, we have seen the type of investigation in which logistic regression can be used. When logistic regression has been used in an investigation, you should appreciate the conditions under which its use is appropriate. Thus, you can use the flowchart in reverse. When you read in the health literature that a statistical procedure has been used, you can look through Figures 38.2 through 38.10 and locate that procedure such as logistic regression. Then you can move up the flowchart and identify the types of data and any special conditions that are necessary for its use.

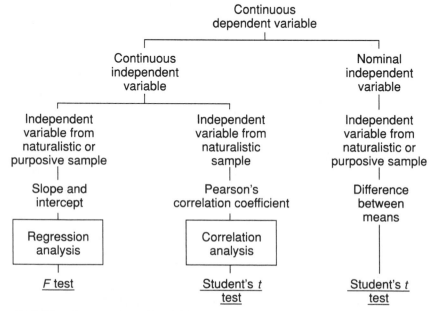

Figure 38.5. Flowchart to select a bivariable statistical procedure for a continuous dependent variable.

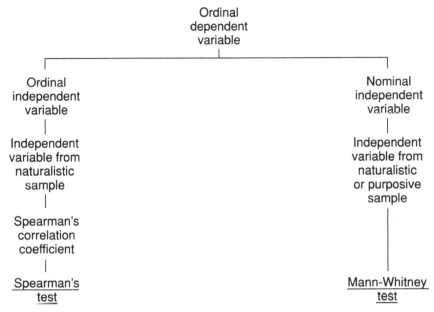

Figure 38.6. Flowchart to select a bivariable statistical procedure for an ordinal dependent variable.

The flowchart is designed to be a practical guide to help you identify and understand the use of the most common statistical procedures. Used along with the previous questions checklists, you should be ready to venture forth to make reading the health research literature a regular part of your professional practice.

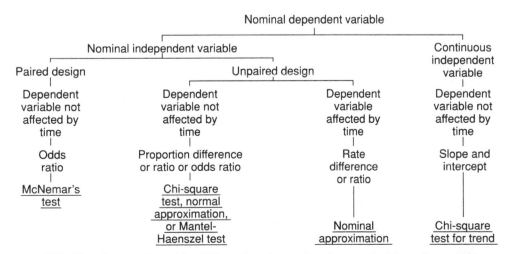

Figure 38.7. Flowchart to select a bivariable statistical procedure for a nominal dependent variable.

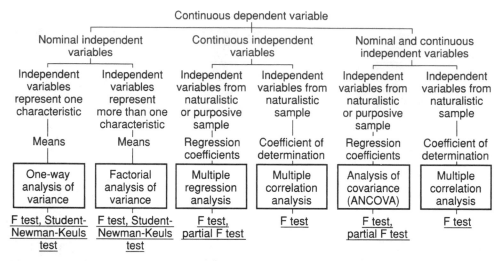

Figure 38.8. Flowchart to select a multivariable statistical procedure for a continuous dependent variable.

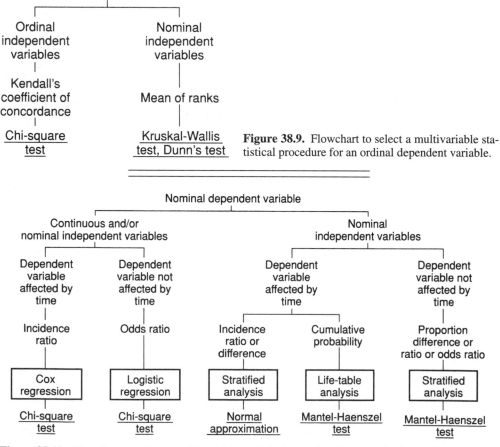

Figure 38.9. Flowchart to select a multivariable statistical procedure for an ordinal dependent variable.

Figure 38.10. Flowchart to select a multivariable statistical procedure for a nominal dependent variable.

Glossary

Accuracy   Without systematic error or bias; on average the results approximate those of the phenomenon under study.

Actual Differences or Changes   Differences or changes in the measurement of occurrence which reflect differences or changes in the phenomenon under study as opposed to artifactual changes.

Actuarial Survival   The actuarial survival is an estimate of life expectancy based on a cohort or longitudinal life table. The 5-year actuarial survival estimates the probability of surviving 5 years based on the limited number of individuals actually followed for 5 years.

Adjusted Number-Needed-to-Treat   A summary measurement that can be derived from an expected utility decision analysis that takes into account the utilities as well as the probabilities of the outcome. Measures the number of individuals, on average, who need to receive the better alternative in order to obtain one additional QALY.

Adjustment   Techniques used after the collection of data to take into account or control for the effect of known or potential confounding variables. (*Synonym:* control for, take into account, standardize)

Affected by Time   A measurement is affected by time if an increase in the duration of observation results in a greater probability of observing the outcome and individuals are observed for different lengths of time.

Aggregate Effects   The overall impact of a recommendation or practice guideline on the entire population of individuals to whom it is directed.

Alternative Hypothesis   In statistical significance testing, the actual choices are between the null hypothesis and an alternative hypothesis. The alternative hypothesis states that a difference or association exists.

Analysis   The comparison of the outcome of the study and control groups. Includes issues of estimation, inference, and adjustment.

Analysis of Covariance (ANCOVA)   Statistical procedures for analysis of data that contain a continuous dependent variable and a mixture of nominal and continuous independent variables.

Analysis of Variance (ANOVA)   Statistical procedures for analysis of data that contain a continuous dependent variable and more than one nominal independent variable. ANOVA procedures include one-way and factorial ANOVA.

Analytical Study   All types of investigations that include a comparison group within the investigation itself (*e.g.,* case-control, cohort, and randomized clinical trials).

Artifactual Differences or Changes   Differences or changes in measures of occurrence that result from the way the disease or condition is measured, sought, or defined.

Assessment   The determination of the outcome of the study and control groups.

Assessment Bias   A generic term referring to any type of bias in the assessment process.

Assignment   The selection of individuals for study and control groups.

Association   A relationship among two or more characteristics or other measurements beyond what would be expected by chance alone. When used to establish criterion number 1 of contributory cause, association implies that the two characteristics occur in the same individual more often than expected by chance alone.

Attributable Risk Percentage   The percentage of the risk among those with the risk factor that is associated with the risk factor. If a cause-and-effect relationship exists, attributable risk is the percentage of a disease that can be expected to be eliminated among those with the risk factor, if the effect of the risk factor can be completely eliminated. (*Synonym:* attributable risk, attributable risk [exposed], etiological fraction [exposed], percentage risk reduction, protective efficacy ratio)

Averaging Out   The process of obtaining overall expected utilities for a decision tree by adding together the expected utilities of each of the potential outcomes included in the decision tree.

Base-Case Estimate   The estimate that is used in a decision-making investigation which reflects the investigators best available or best guess estimate of the relevant value of a particular variable. High and low estimates reflect the extremes of the realistic range of values around the base-case estimate for a particular variable.

Baseline Measurement   The numerical value of a characteristic at the beginning of a study.

Bayes' Theorem   A mathematical formula that can be used to calculate post-test probabilities (or odds) based on pretest probabilities (or odds) and the sensitivity and specificity of a test.

Bayesian   An approach to statistics that takes into account the probability (or odds) of a disease or a study hypothesis when analyzing and interpreting the data in the investigation.

Bias   A condition that produced results which depart from the true values in a consistent direction. (*Synonym:* systematic error)

Binomial Distribution   A mathematical distribution that is used to calculate probabilities for populations composed of nominal data.

Biological Plausibility   An ancillary, adjunct, or supportive criteria of cause and effect which implies that the relationship is consistent with a known biological mechanism.

Bivariable Analysis   Statistical analysis in which there is one dependent variable and one independent variable.

Blind Assessment   The evaluation of the outcome for individuals without the individual who makes the evaluation knowing whether the study subjects were in the study group or the control group. (*Synonym:* masked assessment)

Blind Assignment   Occurs when individuals are assigned to a study group and a control group without the investigator or the subjects being aware of the group to which they are assigned. When both investigator and subjects are "blinded" or "masked," the study is sometimes referred to as a double-blind model. (*Synonym:* masked assignment)

Carry-Over Effect   A phenomenon that may occur in a cross-over study when the initial therapy continues to have an effect after it is no longer being administered. A "wash-out" period is often used to minimize the potential for a carry-over effect.

Case-Control Study   A study that begins by identifying individuals with a disease (cases) and individuals without a disease (controls). The cases and controls are identified without knowledge of an individual's exposure or nonexposure to factors being investigated. (*Synonym:* retrospective study)

Case Fatality   The number of deaths due to a particular disease divided by the number of individuals diagnosed with the disease at the beginning of the time interval. The case fatality estimates the probability of eventually dying from the disease. A case fatality rate includes, in addition, the number of person-years as a unit of time in the denominator.

Case-Mix Bias   A form of selection bias that may be created when treatments are selected by clinicians to fit characteristics of individual patients.

Chance Node   A circle in a decision tree that indicates that once a decision is made, there are two or more outcomes that may occur by a chance process. These potential outcomes are displayed to the right of the chance node.

Chi-Square Distribution   A standard mathematical distribution that can be used to calculate P values and confidence intervals in a variety of statistical procedures for nominal dependent variables.

Chi-Square Test   A statistical significance test that can be used to calculate a P value for a nominal independent and a nominal dependent variable. The chi-square test is one of a large number of uses of the chi-square distribution.

Chi-Square Test for Trend   A statistical significance test that is used for a nominal dependent variable and an ordinal or continuous independent variable.

Coefficient of Determination (R^2)   The square of a correlation coefficient. This statistic indicates the proportion of the variation in one variable (the dependent variable) that is explained by knowing a value of one or more other variables (the independent variables).

Cohort   A group of individuals who share a common exposure, experience, or characteristic. (*See:* cohort study, cohort effect)

Cohort Effect   A change in rates that can be explained by the common experience or characteristic of a group or cohort of individuals. A cohort effect implies that current rates should not be directly extrapolated into the future.

Cohort Study   A study that begins by identifying individuals with and without a factor being investigated. These factors are identified without knowledge of which individuals have or will develop disease. Cohort studies may be concurrent or nonconcurrent. (*Synonym:* prospective study)

Concurrent Cohort Study   A cohort study in which an individual's group assignment is determined at the time that the study begins and the study and control group participants are followed forward in time to determine if the disease occur. (*Synonym:* prospective cohort study)

Confidence Interval (95%)   In statistical terms, the interval of numerical values within which one can be 95% confident the population value being estimated lies. (*Synonym:* interval estimate)

Confidence Limits   The upper and lower extremes of the confidence interval.

Confounding Variable   A characteristic or variable that is distributed differently in the study and control groups and that affects the outcome being assessed. A confounding variable may be due to chance or bias. When it is due to bias in the assignment process, the resulting error is also called a selection bias. (*Synonym:* confounder)

Continuous Data   A type of data with an unlimited number of equally spaced potential values (*e.g.,* diastolic blood pressure, cholesterol).

Contributory Cause   Contributory cause is established when all three of the following have been established: (1) the existence of an association between the cause and the effect; (2) the cause precedes the effect in time; and (3) altering the cause alters the probability of occurrence of the effect.

Control Group   A group of subjects used for comparison with a study group. Ideally, the control group is identical to the study group except that it does not possess the characteristic or has not been exposed to the treatment under study. (*Synonym:* reference group)

Controlled Clinical Trial   *See:* Randomized Clinical Trial

Convenience Sample   A subset from a population that is assembled because of the ease of collecting the data without regard for the degree to which the sample is random or representative of the population of interest.

Conventional Care   The current level of intervention accepted as routine or standard care.

Correlation   A statistic used for studying the strength of an association between two variables, each of which has been sampled using a representative or naturalistic method from a population of interest.

Correlation Analysis   A class of statistical procedures that is used to estimate the strength of the relationship between a continuous dependent variable and a continuous independent variable when both the dependent variable and the independent variable are selected by naturalistic sampling.

Correlation Coefficient   An estimate of the strength of the association between a dependent variable and an independent variable when both are obtained using naturalistic sampling.

Cost-and-Effectiveness Studies   The type of decision analysis study that compares the cost of achieving a common unit of effectiveness, such as a life saved or a diagnosis made.

Cost-Benefit Analysis   The type of decision-making investigation that converts effectiveness as well as cost into monetary terms. Benefit in a cost-benefit analysis refers to net effectiveness, that is, the favorable minus the unfavorable outcomes.

Cost-Consequence Analysis   A type of cost-effectiveness analysis in which harms, benefits, and costs are measured or described but not directly combined or compared.

Cost Effective   An alternative is considered cost effective if the increase in effectiveness is considered worth the increase in cost; if the decreased effectiveness is considered worth the substantial reduction in costs; or if there is reduced cost plus increased effectiveness.

Cost-Effectiveness Analysis   The type of decision-making investigation in which costs are considered as well as harms and benefits.

Cost-Effectiveness Ratios   The average cost per QALY obtained. The comparison alternative in a cost-effectiveness ratio is not usually specified but should generally be considered to be the do-nothing alternative.

Cost QALY Graph   A graph that includes cost on the Y axis and QALYs on the X axis and includes four quadrants with different interpretations related to cost effectiveness. The intersection of the X and Y axis represents the do-nothing comparison alternative.

Cost Savings   A reduction in cost that may be accompanied by a reduction or an increase in effectiveness.

Cost-Utility Analysis   The type of cost-effectiveness analysis that measures and combines benefits, harms, and costs taking into account the probabilities and the utilities. Cost-utility investigations often use QALYs as the measure of effectiveness and thus may be called cost-effectiveness analysis using QALYs.

Covariance   The statistic that is calculated to estimate how closely a dependent and an independent variable change together.

Cox Regression   A statistical procedure for a nominal dependent variable and a mixture of nominal and continuous independent variables that can be used when the independent variable is affected by time. (*Synonym:* proportional hazard regression)

Credibility Intervals   A term used in decision-making investigations to present the results in a form that parallels confidence intervals. The Monte Carlo method may be used to generate credibility interval by performing large numbers of simulations using the investigations own decision-making model.

Cross-Over Study   A type of paired design in which the same individual receives a study and a control therapy and an outcome is assessed for each therapy.

Cross-Sectional Study   A study that identifies individuals with and without the condition or disease under study and the characteristic or exposure of interest at the same point in time. The independent and the dependent variable are measured at the same point in time. A cross-section study may not be regarded as a special type of case-control study.

Cumulative Survival   The estimate of survival derived for a life-table analysis calculated by combining the probabilities from each time interval.

Database Research   Investigations done based on previously collected data. May be used as a synonym for nonconcurrent cohort study when a study group and a control group are identified based on prior characteristics contained in a database.

Database Studies   *See:* Nonconcurrent Cohort Studies

Decision Analysis   As used in decision-making investigations, refers to the type of investigations in which benefits and harms are included but not costs. Often used generically to refer to all quantitative decision making.

Decision-Making Model   A diagram or written description of the steps involved in each of the alternatives being considered in a decision-making investigation. A decision tree is a common method of presenting the decision-making model.

Decision Node   A square in a decision tree that indicates that a choice needs to be made. (*Synonym:* choice node)

Decision Tree   A graphic display of the decision alternatives, including the choices that need to be made and the chance events that occur.

Declining Exponential Approximation of Life Expectancy (DEALE)   A specialized life-expectancy measure which incorporates life expectancy related to a disease as well as life expectancy based on age and other demographic factors derived from a cross-sectional life table.

Dependent Variable   Generally, the outcome variable of interest in any type of research study. The outcome that one intends to explain or estimate.

Descriptive Epidemiology   An investigation that provides data on one group of individuals and does not include a comparison group at least within the investigation itself. (*Synonym:* description study, case series)

Direct Cause   A contributory cause that is the most directly known cause of a disease (*e.g.,* hepatitis B virus is a direct cause of hepatitis B infection, and contaminated needles are an indirect cause). The direct cause is dependent on the current state of knowledge and may change as more immediate mechanisms are discovered.

Discordant Pairs   In a case-control study, the pairs in which the study and controls differ in their exposure or nonexposure to the potential risk factor.

Discounted Present Value   The amount of money that needs to be invested today to pay a bill of a particular size at a particular time in the future.

Discounting   A method used in decision-making investigations to take into account the reduced importance of benefits, harms, and also costs that occur at a later period of time compared to those that occur immediately.

Discrete Data   Data with a finite or limited number of categories or potential values. Discrete data may be further classified as either nominal or ordinal data.

Disease-Adjusted Life Expectancy (DALE)   A life-expectancy measure which incorporates morbidity as well as mortality.

Dispersion   Spread of data around a measure of central tendency, such as a mean.

Distribution   Frequencies or relative frequencies of all possible values of a characteristic. Population and sample distributions can be described graphically or mathematically. One purpose of statistics is to estimate parameters of population distributions.

Distributional Effects   A term used in decision-making investigations that indicates that the average results do not take into account the distributions of the adverse and favorable outcomes among subgroups with different demographic characteristics.

Dominant Alternative   An alternative is dominant when a recommendation can be made on the basis of probabilities alone. That is, one alternative is preferred regardless of the utilities that are attached to particular favorable and unfavorable outcomes.

Do-Nothing Approach   The comparison alternative in decision-making investigations in which only supportive care is used, i.e., care which is not aimed at altering prognosis. This type of care is the same as conventional care only when no effective intervention exists.

Dose-Response Relationship   A dose-response relationship is present if changes in levels of an exposure are associated with changes in the frequency of the outcome in a consistent direction. A dose-response relationship is an ancillary or supportive criterion for contributory cause.

Ecological Fallacy   The type of error that can occur when the existence of a group association is used to imply the existence of a relationship that does not exist at the individual level.

Effect   An outcome that is brought about, at least in part, by an etiological factor known as the cause.

Effect of Observation   A type of assessment bias that results when the process of observation alters the outcome of the study.

Effect Size   A summary measure of the magnitude of the difference or association found in the sample.

Effectiveness   The extent to which a treatment produces a beneficial effect when implemented under the usual conditions of clinical care for a particular group of patients. In the context of cost effectiveness, effectiveness incorporates desirable outcomes as well as undesirable outcomes.

Efficacy   The extent to which a treatment produces a beneficial effect when assessed under the ideal conditions of an investigation. Efficacy is to therapy what contributory cause is to etiology of disease.

End-Point   An outcome in a cohort study or randomized clinical trial which terminates the follow-up for an individual patient. In a case-control study, may refer to the prior characteristic being assessed.

Estimate   A value or interval of values calculated from sample observations that are used to approximate a corresponding population value or parameter. Obtaining an estimate is one of the primary goals of statistical methods. (*See:* Interval Estimate, Point Estimate)

Exclusion Criteria   Conditions which preclude entrance of candidates into an investigation even if they meet the inclusion criteria.

Expected Utility   The results of multiplying the probability times the utility of a particular outcome. (*Synonym:* quality adjusted probability)

Expected Utility Decision Analysis   The type of decision analysis that considers probabilities and utilities but does not explicitly incorporate life expectancy.

Expected Value   A measure that incorporates cost as well as benefit and harm into a decision tree. The outcome is then measured in monetary terms.

Experimentwise Error   The probability of making a type I error for at least one comparison in an analysis that involves more than one comparison.

Exploratory Meta-Analysis   A meta-analysis in which there is not a specific hypothesis and all potentially relevant investigations are included.

Extrapolation   Conclusions drawn about the meaning of the study for a target population. The target population may be similar to those included in the investigation or may include types of individuals or a range of data not represented in the study sample.

***F* distribution**   A standard distribution that can be used to calculate P values and confidence intervals in ANOVA, ANCOVA, multiple regression, and multiple correlation analysis procedures.

Factor   A term used in ANOVA procedures to separate a collection of characteristics that define mutually exclusive but topically related categories, such as race. Statistical significance tests on factors are called tests of main effects in a factorial ANOVA.

Fail-Safe-N   The number of studies which must be omitted from a meta-analysis before the results would no longer be statistically significant. These additional studies are assumed to be of the same average size as the included studies and have, on average, an effect size of 0 for differences or 1 for ratios.

False Negative   An individual whose result on a test is negative but who has the disease or condition as determined by the final outcome gold standard.

False Positive   An individual whose result on a test is positive but who does not have the disease or condition as determined by the gold standard.

Final Outcome   An outcome that occurs at the completion of a decision option. This outcome is displayed at the right end of a decision tree.

Fisher Exact Procedure   A method for calculating P values for data with one nominal dependent and one nominal independent variable when any of the frequencies predicted by the null hypothesis are less than 5.

Fixed Costs   Costs which do not vary with modest increases or decreases in the volume of services provided. Space and personnel costs are considered examples of fixed costs, which partly explain why institutional decision making does not always conform to the recommendations of cost-effectiveness analysis.

Folding Back the Decision Tree   A process in which probabilities are multiplied together to obtain a probability of a particular outcome known as a path probability. Calculations of path probabilities assume that the probability of each of the outcomes that occur along the path is independent of the other probabilities along the same path.

Funnel Diagram   A graphical method for assessing whether publication bias is likely to be present in a meta-analysis.

Gaussian Distribution   A distribution of data assumed in many statistical procedures. The gaussian distribution is a symmetrical, continuous, bell-shaped curve with its mean value corresponding to the highest point on the curve. (*Synonym:* normal distribution)

Gold Standard   The criterion used to unequivocally define the presence and absence of a condition or disease under study.

Group Association   The situation in which a characteristic and a disease both occur more frequently in one group of individuals compared with another. Group association does not necessarily imply that individuals with the characteristic are the same ones who have the disease. (*Synonym:* ecological association, ecological correlation)

Group Matching   A matching procedure used during assignment in an investigation that selects study and control individuals in such a way that the groups have a nearly equal distribution of a particular variable or variables. (*Synonym:* frequency matching)

Guideline   In practice guidelines, the term indicates a recommendation for (or against) an intervention except under specified exceptions.

Healthy Worker Effect   A tendency for workers in an occupation to be healthier than the general population of individuals of the same age.

Historical Control   A control group from an earlier period of time that is used to compare outcome(s) with a study group in an investigation.

Homogeneous   When used in the context of a meta-analysis, homogeneous refers to investigations which can be combined into a single meta-analysis because the study characteristics being examined do not substantially affect the outcome.

Human Capital   An approach to converting effectiveness to monetary terms that uses the recipient's ability to contribute to the economy.

Hypothesis-Driven Meta-Analysis   A meta-analysis in which a specific hypothesis is used as the basis for inclusion or exclusion of investigations for the meta-analysis.

Incidence Rate   The rate at which new cases of disease occur per unit of time. The incidence rate is theoretically calculated as the number of individuals who develop the disease over a period of time divided by the total person-years of observation. (*Synonym:* hazard)

Inclusion Criteria   Conditions which must be met by all potential candidates for entrance into an investigation.

Incremental Cost-effectiveness Ratio   The cost of obtaining one additional QALY using one alternative compared with the use of the conventional alternative or, if specified, another alternative.

Independence   Two events or two tests are independent if the results of the first do not influence or affect the results of the second.

Independent Variable   Variables being measured to determine the corresponding measurement of the dependent variable in any type of research study. Independent variables define the conditions under which the dependent variable is to be examined.

Indicator Variable   A variable that is used to represent the value of a nominal variable in ANCOVA. An indicator variable tells us how much the estimate of the continuous dependent variable differs between levels of the indicator variable.

Indirect Cause   A contributory cause that acts through a biological mechanism that is more closely related to the disease than it is to the direct cause (e.g., contaminated needles are an indirect cause of hepatitis B; the hepatitis B virus is a direct cause). (*See:* Direct Cause)

Inference   In statistical terminology, inference is the logical process that occurs during statistical significance testing in which conclusions concerning a population are obtained based on data from a random sample of the population. (*See:* Statistical Significance Test)

Influence Diagram   An alternative to decision trees that displays the factors that influence events.

Intention to Treat   A method for data analysis in a randomized clinical trial in which individual outcomes are analyzed according to the group to which they have been randomized even if they never received the treatment to which they were assigned.

Interaction   Occurs when the outcome resulting from more than one variable is altered by the level of the variables. Interaction between variables may be more than additive or less than additive. (*Synonym:* effect modification, synergy)

Intercept   The intercept estimates the mean of the dependent variable when the independent variables are equal to zero.

Interobserver Variation   Variation in measurement by different individuals.

Interpretation   The drawing of conclusions about the meaning of any differences found between the study group and the control group for those included in the investigation.

Interval Estimate   *See:* Confidence Interval

Intervention Modeling   As used here, a method for utilizing all the independent variables found to be statistically significant in a regression analysis as the basis for simulations. These simulations examine the impact of the intervention on a target population made up of individuals similar to the subjects included in the investigation or, alternatively, to populations with different distributions of the independent variables.

Intraobserver Variation   Variation in measurements by the same person at different times.

Kendall's Coefficient of Concordance   An estimate of the degree of correlation. This estimate can be used when the dependent variable and all the independent variables are ordinal.

Koch's Postulates   A set of criteria developed for demonstrating cause and effect that was extensively applied to infectious disease. Koch's postulates include necessary cause.

Kruskal-Wallis Test   A statistical significance test that can be used when there is an ordinal dependent variable and two or more nominal independent variables. Dunn's test may be used as an alternative test.

Lead-Time Bias   Overestimation of survival time due to earlier diagnosis of disease. Actual time of death does not change when lead-time bias is present despite the earlier time of diagnosis.

Least Squares Regression   A method of regression analysis that selects numerical values for the slope and intercept which minimize the sum of the squared differences between the data observed in the sample and those estimated by the regression equation.

Length Bias   The tendency of a screening test to more frequently detect individuals with a slowly progressive disease compared with individuals with a rapidly progressive disease.

Life Expectancy   The average number of years of remaining life from a particular age based on the probabilities of death in each age group in one particular year. Life expectancy assumes a stationary population and the same probabilities of death in subsequent years, or it is not an accurate prediction of the average number of years of remaining life.

Life Table (Cross-Sectional or Current)   A technique that uses mortality data from one year's experience and applies the data to a stationary population to calculate life expectancies.

Life-Table Method (Cohort or Longitudinal)   A method for organizing data that allows examination of the experience of one or more groups of individuals over time when some individuals are followed for longer periods of time than others. (*Synonym:* Kaplan-Meier, Cutler-Ederer life tables)

Likelihood Ratio of Negative Test   A ratio of the probability of a negative test if the disease is present to the probability of a negative test if the disease is absent.

Likelihood Ratio of Positive Test   A ratio of the probability of a positive test if the disease is present to the probability of a positive test if the disease is absent.

Linear Extrapolation   A form of extrapolation that assumes, often incorrectly, that levels of a variable beyond the range of the data will continue to operate in the same manner that they operate in the investigation. Linear extrapolation is often used to extrapolate beyond the data by extending the straight-line relationship obtained from an investigation.

Linear Regression   A form of regression analysis in which there is only one dependent and one independent variable.

Location   A measure of central tendency of a distribution. Means and medians are examples of measures of location.

Logistic Regression   A multivariable method used when there is a nominal dependent variable and a nominal and/or continuous independent variable that are not affected by time.

Main Effect   A term used in factorial ANOVA to indicate statistical tests used to examine each factor separately.

Mann-Whitney Test   A statistical significance test that is used for an ordinal dependent variable and a nominal independent variable.

Mantel-Haenszel Chi   A method that can be used for statistical significance testing and calculation of confidence intervals for an odds ratio in bivariable or multivariable analysis.

Marginal Cost   The impact on costs of greatly increasing the scale of operation of an intervention so that economies of scale and diseconomies of scale may impact on the costs. Distinguished from incremental cost which relates to the cost of one additional unit.

Markov Analysis   A method of analysis used in decision-making investigations to take into account recurrent events such as recurrence of previous disease or development of a second episode of disease.

Masked   *See:* Blinded

Matched Test   A type of statistical significance test that is used to analyze data from a paired design.

Matching   An assignment procedure in which study and control groups are chosen to ensure that a particular variable is the same in both groups. Pairing is a special type of matching in which study group or control group subjects are analyzed together.

Maximum Likelihood Regression   A regression method that chooses estimates for the regression coefficients to maximize the likelihood that the data observed would have resulted from sampling a population with those coefficients.

McNemar's Test   A statistical significance test for paired data when there is one nominal dependent and one nominal independent variable.

Mean   Sum of the measurements divided by the number of measurements being added together. The "center of gravity" of a distribution of observations. A special type of average.

Median   The mid-point of a distribution. The median is chosen so that half the data values occur above and half occur below the median.

Meta-analysis   A series of methods for systematically combining information from more than one investigation to draw a conclusion which could not be drawn solely on the basis of the single investigations.

Monte Carlo Simulation   A method used in cost-effectiveness analysis and other applications that repeatedly samples the same population to derive a large number of samples whose distribution can be used to calculate point estimates and confidence ranges.

Mortality Rate   A measure of the incidence of death. This rate is calculated as the number of deaths over a period of time divided by the product of the number of individuals times the period of follow-up.

Multicollinearity   Sharing of information among independent variables, which helps to estimate the value of the dependent variable.

Multiple Correlation Analysis   Statistical methods used with one continuous dependent variable and nominal and continuous independent variables when all variables are obtained by naturalistic sampling.

Multiple Regression Analysis   Statistical methods used with one continuous dependent variable and more than one continuous independent variable.

Multivariable Analysis   A statistical analysis in which there is one dependent variable and more than one independent variable.

Multivariate Analysis   A statistical analysis in which there is more than one dependent variable. Commonly but incorrectly used as a synonym for multivariable analysis.

Mutually Exclusive   Categories are mutually exclusive if any one individual can only be included in one category.

N-of-One Study   An investigation using one individual designed to establish a cause-and-effect relationship.

Natural Experiment   A special type of cohort study in which the study and control groups' outcomes are compared with their own outcomes before and after a change is observed in the exposure of the study group.

Natural History Study   A type of descriptive epidemiological study that provides data on the course of a disease among a group of individuals over a period of time.

Naturalistic Sample   A set of observations obtained from a population in such a way that the sample distribution of independent variable values is representative of their distribution in the population.

Necessary Cause   A characteristic is a necessary cause if its presence is required to bring about or cause the disease.

Nominal Data   A type of data with named categories. Nominal data may have more than two categories that cannot be ordered (*e.g.*, race, eye color). Nominal data are represented by more than one nominal variable if there are more than two potential categories.

Nonconcurrent Cohort Study   A cohort study in which an individual's group assignment is determined before the investigator is aware of the outcome even though the outcome has already occurred. A nonconcurrent cohort study uses a previously collected database. (*Synonym:* retrospective cohort study, database research)

Nonparametric Statistics   Statistical procedures that do not make assumptions about the distribution of parameters in the population being sampled. Nonparametric statistical methods are not free of assumptions such as the assumption of random sampling. They are most often used for ordinal data but may be used for continuous data converted to an ordinal scale. (*Synonym:* distribution-free)

Normal Approximation   A statistical method that can be used to calculate approximate probabilities for binomial and Poisson distributions using the standard normal distribution.

Normal Distribution   *See:* Gaussian Distribution

Null Hypothesis   The assertion that no true association or difference between variables exists in the larger population from which the study samples are obtained.

Number-Needed-to-Treat   The reciprocal of the difference in risk. The number of patients, similar to the study patients, who need to be treated to obtain one fewer bad outcome or one more good outcome.

Observational Study   An investigation in which the assignment is conducted by observing the subjects who meet the entry and exclusion criteria. Case-control and cohort studies are observational studies

Observed Assignment   Refers to the method of assignment of individuals to study and control groups in observational studies when the investigator does not intervene to perform the assignment.

Odds   A ratio in which the numerator contains the number of times an event occurs and the denominator includes the number of times the event does not occur.

Odds Ratio   A ratio measuring the degree or strength of an association applicable to all types of studies employing nominal data but usually applied to case-control and cross-sectional studies. The odds ratio for case-control and cross-sectional studies is measured as the odds of having the risk factor if the condition is present divided by the odds of having the risk factor if the condition is not present.

Omnibus Null Hypothesis   A null hypothesis that addresses the relationship between the dependent variable and the entire collection of independent variables as a unit.

One-Tailed Test   A statistical significance test in which deviations from the null hypothesis in only one direction are considered. Use of a one-tailed test implies that the investigator does not consider a true deviation in the opposite direction to be possible.

Option   Used in practice guidelines to indicate that the evidence does not support a clear recommendation or that inadequate data are available to make a recommendation.

Ordinal Data   A type of data with a limited number of categories with an inherent ordering of the categories from lowest to highest. Ordinal data, however, say nothing about the spacing between categories (*e.g.,* stage 1, 2, 3, and 4 cancer).

Outcome   The phenomenon being measured in the assessment process of an investigation. In case-control studies, outcome is a prior characteristic; in cohort studies and randomized clinical trials, the outcome is a future event which occurs subsequent to the assignment.

Outcome Studies   A generic term which refers to investigations of the results of therapeutic interventions regardless of the type of investigation used.

Outcomes Profile   The type of decision analysis that measures the benefits and harms but does not directly compare them. (*Synonym:* balance sheet)

Outliers   An investigation included in a meta-analysis or a subject in a single investigation whose results are substantially different from the vast majority of studies or subjects, suggesting a need to examine the situation to determine why such an extreme result has occurred.

Overmatching   The error which occurs when investigators attempt to study a factor closely related to a characteristic by which the groups have been matched or paired.

***P* Value**   The probability of obtaining data at least as extreme as the data obtained in the investigation's sample set if the null hypothesis was true. The *P* value is considered the "bottom line" in statistical significance testing.

Paired Design   A study design in which the data are analyzed using the difference between the measurements on the two members of a pair.

Pairing   A special form of matching in which each study individual is coupled or paired with a control group individual and their outcomes are compared. When pairing is used, special statistical methods called matching methods should be used. These methods may increase the statistical power of the study.

Parameter   A value that summarizes the distribution of a large population. One purpose of statistical analysis is to estimate a population's parameters from the sample's observations.

Partial Test   A statistical significance test of a null hypothesis that addresses the relationship between the dependent variable and one of the independent variables. (*Synonym:* pairwise test)

Path Probability   The probability of a final outcome in a decision-making investigation. Path probabilities are calculated by multiplying the probabilities of each of the outcomes that follow chance nodes and that lead to a final outcome.

Pearson's Correlation Coefficient   The correlation coefficient that may be used when the dependent variable and the independent variable are both continuous and both have been obtained by naturalistic sampling.

Person-Years   A person-year is equivalent to one person observed for a period of 1 year. Person-years are used as a measure of total observation time in the denominator of a rate.

Perspective   The perspective of an investigation asks how extensively one should consider the impact of the benefits, harms, and costs. (*See:* social perspective, and user perspective)

Plateau Effect　A flat portion of a life-table curve at the right end of the curve that may reflect the fact that very few individuals remain in the investigation rather than indicating cure.

Point Estimate　A single value calculated from sample observations that is used as the estimate of the population value, or parameter.

Poisson Distribution　A special case of a binomial distribution that can be used when the nominal event, such as disease or death, is rarely observed and the number of observations is great.

Population　A large group often but not necessarily comprising individuals. In statistics, one attempts to draw conclusions about a population by obtaining subsets or samples made up of individuals from the larger population.

Population-Attributable Risk Percentage　The percentage of the risk in a community, including individuals with and without a risk factor, that is associated with exposure to a risk factor. Population attributable risk does not necessarily imply a cause-and-effect relationship. (*Synonym:* attributable fraction [population], attributable proportion [population], etiological fraction [population])

Positive-if-All-Positive　A screening strategy in which a second test is administered to all those who have a positive result on the initial test. The results are labeled positive if both tests are positive. Also called serial or consecutive testing; however, these terms may cause confusion.

Positive-if-One-Positive　A screening strategy in which two or more tests are administered to all individuals and the initial screening is labeled as positive if one or more tests produce positive results. Also called parallel or alternative testing; however, these terms can cause confusion.

Power　The ability of an investigation to demonstrate statistical significance when a true association or difference of a specified strength exists in the population being sampled. Power equals one minus the Type II error. (*Synonym:* statistical power, resolving power)

Practice Guidelines　A set of recommendations for using or not using available interventions in clinical or public health practice. Practice guidelines may recommend standards, guidelines, or options and may be based only on considerations of harms and benefits or may also include costs.

Precise　Without random error, without variability from measurement to measurement of the same phenomenon. (*Synonym:* reproducibility, reliability)

Predictive Value of a Negative Test　The proportion of individuals with a negative test who do not have the condition or disease as measured by the gold standard. This measure incorporates the prevalence of the condition or disease. Clinically, the predictive value of a negative test is the probability that an individual does not have the disease if the test is negative. (*Synonym:* post-test probability after a negative test)

Predictive Value of a Positive Test　The proportion of people with a positive test who actually have the condition or disease as measured by the gold standard. This measure incorporates the prevalence of the condition or disease. Clinically, the predictive value of a positive test is the probability that an individual has the disease if the test is positive. (*Synonym:* post-test probability after a positive test)

Pretest Probability　The probability of disease before the results of a test are known. Pretest probability may be derived from disease prevalence alone when screening for disease or may also include the clinical symptoms with which a patient presents.

Prevalence   The proportion of persons with a particular disease or condition at a point in time. Prevalence can also be interpreted as the probability that an individual selected at random from the population of interest will be someone who has the disease or condition.

Primary End-Point   Used to refer to the outcome measurement in a study which is used to calculate the sample's size. It should be a frequently occurring and biologically important end-point. (*See:* Secondary End-Point)

Probability   A proportion in which the numerator contains the number of times an event occurs, and the denominator includes the number of times an event occurs plus the number of times it does not occur.

Proportion   A fraction in which the numerator contains a subset of the individuals contained in the denominator.

Proportionate Mortality Ratio   A fraction in which the numerator contains the number of individuals who die of a particular disease over a period of time and the denominator contains the number of individuals dying from all diseases over the same period of time.

Prospective Study   *See:* Cohort Study

Protocol Deviant   An individual in a randomized clinical trial whose treatment differs from that which the person would have received if his or her treatment had followed the rules contained in the investigation's protocol.

Proximal Cause   A legal term that implies an examination of the time sequence of cause and effect to examine the element in the constellation of causal factors that was most closely related in time to the outcome.

Pruning the Decision Tree   The process of reducing the complexity of a decision tree by combining outcomes and removing potential outcomes which are considered extremely rare, inconsequential, or both.

Publication Bias   The tendency to not publish small studies which do not demonstrate a statistically significant difference between groups.

Purposive Sample   A set of observations obtained from a population in such a way that the sample's distribution of independent variable values is determined by the researcher and not necessarily representative of their distribution in the population.

QALY Decision Analysis   The form of decision analysis that uses QALYs as the outcome measure. (*Synonym:* QALY study)

Quality-Adjusted Life-Years (QALYs)   A measure which incorporates probabilities, utilities, and life expectancies.

Random Error   Error which is due to the workings of chance, which can either operate in the direction of the study hypothesis or in the opposite direction.

Random Sampling   A method of obtaining a sample that ensures that each individual in the larger population has a known, but not necessarily equal, probability of being selected for the sample.

Randomization   A method of assignment in which individuals have a known, but not necessarily equal, probability of being assigned to a particular study or control group. As distinguished from random sampling, the individuals being randomized may or may not be representative of a large population. (*Synonym:* random assignment)

Randomized Clinical Trial   An investigation in which the investigator assigns individuals to study and control groups using a process known as randomization. (*Synonym:* controlled clinical trial, experimental study)

Range   The difference between the highest and lowest data values in a population or sample.

Range of Normal   *See:* Reference Interval

Rate   Commonly used to indicate any measure of disease or outcome occurrence. From a statistical point of view, rates are those measures of disease occurrence that include time in the denominator (*e.g.,* incidence rate).

Ratio   A fraction in which the numerator is not necessarily a subset of the denominator as opposed to a proportion.

Real Rate of Return   Discounting of cost is designed to take into account the fact that money invested rather than spent is expected to increase in value, on average, at a rate that approximates the rate of return for invested capital in the overall economy, that is, the rate above and beyond inflation.

Recall Bias   An assessment bias that occurs when individuals in one group are more likely to remember past effects than individuals in another of the study or control groups. Recall bias is especially likely when a case-control study involves serious disease and the characteristics under study are commonly occurring, subjectively remembered events.

Receiver-Operator Curve (ROC)   A technique for assisting in identifying a separating or cutoff line used to define the limits of the reference interval.

Reference Case   In decision-making investigations, this is the accepted method for presenting the data using the social perspective, best guess, or baseline estimates for variables, a 3% discount rate, and a series of other generally accepted assumptions.

Reference Group   The group of presumably disease-free individuals from which a sample of individuals is drawn whose measurements on a test are used to establish a reference interval. (*Synonym:* reference population)

Reference Interval   The test results obtained from a reference sample group which reflects the variation among those who are free of the disease. (*Synonym:* range of normal)

Reference Sample Group   The sample used to represent the population of individuals who are believed to be free of the disease. The characteristics of the sample chosen may affect the reference interval derived from the reference sample group.

Regression Coefficient   In a regression analysis, an estimate of the amount that the dependent variable changes in value for each change in the corresponding independent variable.

Regression Techniques   A series of statistical methods useful for describing the association between one dependent variable and one or more independent variables. Regression techniques are often used to perform adjustment for confounding variables.

Regression to the Mean   A statistical principle based on the fact that unusual events are unlikely to recur. By chance alone, measurements subsequent to an unusual measurement are likely to be closer to the mean.

Relative Risk   A ratio of the probability of developing the outcome in a specified period of time if the risk factor is present divided by the probability of developing the outcome in that same period of time if the risk factor is not present. The relative risk is a measure of the strength or degree of association applicable to cohort and randomized clinical trials. In case-control studies, the odds ratio often can be used to approximate the relative risk.

Reporting Bias   An assessment bias that occurs when individuals in one group are more likely to report past events than individuals in another of the study or control groups. Reporting bias is especially likely to occur when one group is under disproportionate pressure to report confidential information.

Reproducibility   *See:* Precision

Retrospective Study   *See:* Case-Control Study

Risk   The probability of an event occurring during a specified period of time. For the risk of disease, the numerator of risk contains the number of individuals who develop the disease during the time period; the denominator contains the number of disease-free persons at the beginning of the time period. (*Synonym:* absolute risk, cumulative probability)

Risk Factor   A characteristic or factor that has been shown to be associated with an increased probability of developing a condition or disease. A risk factor does not necessarily imply a cause-and-effect relationship. In this book, a risk factor implies that at least an association has been established on an individual level.

Risk Neutral   Decision-making investigations are risk neutral if the choice of alternatives is governed by the probabilities and utilities and is not influenced by the tendency to either gamble to achieve a desired outcome (risk seeking) or to avoid an alternative that poses the possibility of losing an acceptable current condition (risk avoiding).

Robust   A statistical procedure is robust if its assumptions can be violated without substantial effects on its conclusions.

Rule of 3   The number of individuals who must be observed to be 95% confident of observing at least one case of an adverse effect is three times the denominator of the true probability of occurrence of the adverse effect.

Run-In Period   Preinvestigation observation of patients usually designed to ensure that they are appropriate candidates for entrance into a randomized clinical trial, especially with regard to their adherence to therapy.

Sample   A subset of a larger population obtained for investigation to draw conclusions or make estimates about the larger population.

Sampling Error   An error introduced by chance differences between the estimate obtained in a sample and the true value in the larger population from which the sample was drawn. Sampling error is inherent in the use of sampling methods and is measured by the standard error.

Secondary End-Point   An end-point which is of interest and importance, such as death, but which occurs too infrequently to use to calculate the sample's size.

Selection Bias   A bias in assignment that occurs when the study and control groups are chosen so that they differ from each other by one or more factors that affect the outcome of the study. A special type of confounding variable that results from study design rather than chance. (*See:* Confounding Variable)

Self-Selection Bias   A bias related to screening that may occur when volunteers are used in an investigation. The bias results from differences between volunteers and the larger population of interest, i.e., the target population.

Sensitivity   The proportion of those with the disease or condition, as measured by the gold standard, who are positive by the test being studied. (*Synonym:* positive-in-disease)

Sensitivity Analysis   A method used in decision-making investigations that alters one or more factors from their best guess or baseline estimates and examines the impact on the results. One-way, multiple-way, best-case/worst-case sensitivity analyses, and threshold analyses are special types of sensitivity analyses.

Simple Random Sample   A random sample in which the sample is drawn to represent the overall larger population without stratification to ensure greater representation of particular groups within the population.

Slope   The regression coefficient in linear regression analysis. The slope of a linear equation in linear regression estimates the amount that the mean of the dependent variable changes for each unit change in the numerical value of the independent variable.

Social Perspective   The perspective that takes into account all health-related impacts of the benefits, harms, and cost regardless of who experiences these outcomes. The social perspective is considered the appropriate perspective for decision-making investigations.

Spearman's Correlation Coefficient   A correlation coefficient that can be obtained in a bivariable analysis when the dependent variable and the independent variable are both ordinal and are obtained through naturalistic sampling.

Specificity   The proportion of those without the disease or condition, as measured by the gold standard, who are negative by the test being studied. (*Synonym:* negative-in-health)

Standard   Used in practice guidelines to indicate that the intervention is either routinely indicated or routinely contraindicated.

Standard Deviation   A commonly used measure of the spread of dispersion of data. The standard deviation squared is known as the *variance*.

Standard Distributions   Distribution for which statistical tables have been developed. Use of standard distributions, when chosen appropriately, simplify the calculation of P values and confidence intervals.

Standard Error   The spread or dispersion of point estimates, such as the mean obtained from all possible samples of a specified size. The standard error is equal to the standard deviation divided by the square root of the sample size. (*See:* sampling error)

Standardization (of a Rate)   An effort to take into account or adjust for the effects of a factor such as age or sex on the obtained rates (*See:* Adjustment).

Standardized Mortality Ratio   A ratio in which the numerator contains the observed number of deaths and the denominator contains the number of deaths that would be expected based on a comparison population. A standard mortality ratio implies that indirect standardization has been used to control for confounders. Note that the terms standardized mortality ratio and proportionate mortality ratio are not synonymous.

Stationary Population   A population often defined as 100,000 births, which experiences no entry or exit from the population except for birth or death.

Statistic   A value calculated from sample data that is used to estimate a value or parameter in the larger population from which the sample was obtained.

Statistical Significance Test   A statistical technique for determining the probability that the data observed in a sample, or more extreme data, could occur by chance if there is no such difference or association in the larger population (*i.e.,* if the null hypothesis is true). (*Synonym:* inference, hypothesis testing)

Stratification   In general, stratification means to divide into groups. Stratification often refers to a process to control for differences in confounding variables by making separate estimates for groups of individuals who have the same values for the confounding variable. A purposive sampling method that is designed to oversample rare categories of an independent variable.

Stratified Analysis   Statistical procedures that can be used when there is a nominal dependent variable and more than one nominal independent variable. Stratified analysis produce stratum-specific point estimates.

Stratum   When data are stratified or divided into groups using a characteristic such as age, each age group is known as a stratum.

Student-Newman-Keuls Test   A pairwise statistical significance test for a continuous dependent variable and more than one independent variable.

Student's *t* Distribution   A standard distribution that is used to obtain *P* values and confidence intervals for a continuous dependent variable. The Student's *t* distribution is used to obtain the Student's *t* test of statistical significance.

Study Group   In a cohort or randomized clinical trial, a group of individuals who possess the characteristics or who are exposed to the factors under study. In case-control or cross-sectional study, a group of individuals who have developed the disease or condition being investigated.

Study Hypothesis   An assertion that an association or difference exists between two or more variables in the population sampled. A study hypothesis can be one-tailed (considering associations or differences in one direction only) or two-tailed (not specifying the direction of the association or difference).

Study Population   The population of individuals from which samples are obtained for inclusion in an investigation.

Subgroup Analysis   Examination of the relationship between variable(s) in smaller subgroups, such as gender or age groups obtained from the original study and control groups.

Subjective Probabilities   Probabilities that are obtained based on perceived probabilities.

Sufficient Cause   A characteristic is a sufficient cause if its presence in-and-of-itself will bring about or cause the disease.

Supportive Criteria   When contributory cause cannot be established, additional criteria can be used to develop a judgment regarding the existence of a contributory cause. These include strength of association, dose-response relationship, consistency of the relationship, and biological plausibility. (*Synonym:* adjunct, ancillary criteria)

Surrogate End-Point   The use of test results instead of clinical outcome measures to assess the outcomes of an investigation. Proper use of surrogate end-points requires a strong association between the surrogate end-point and a relevant clinical outcome.

Survival Plot   A graphic display of the results of a longitudinal life table.

Target Population   The group of individuals to whom one wishes to apply or extrapolate the results of an investigation. The target population may be, and often is, different from the study population from which the sample used in an investigation is obtained.

Test-Based Confidence Interval   Confidence intervals derived from the process of statistical significance tests on a particular set of data.

Test-wise Error   The probability of making a Type I error for any one particular comparison.

Time Frame The point in the course of the disease when the alternatives are being applied. When considering disease that is already fully developed, prevention may not be an available alternative because it is not within the time frame of the investigation.

Time Horizon The follow-up period of time used to determine which potential outcomes that occur in the future will be included in a model for a decision-making investigation. (*Synonym:* analysis horizon)

True Negative An individual who does not have the disease or condition, as measured by the gold standard, and has a negative test result.

True Positive An individual who has the disease or condition, as measured by the gold standard, and has a positive test result.

Two-Tailed Test A statistical significance test in which deviations from the null hypothesis in either direction are considered. Use of a two-tailed test implies that the investigator was willing to consider deviations in either direction before data were collected.

Type I Error An error that occurs when data demonstrate a statistically significant result when no true association or difference exists in the population. The alpha level is the size of the Type I error which will be tolerated (usually 5%).

Type II Error An error that occurs when the sample's observations fail to demonstrate statistical significance when a true association or difference actually exists in the larger population(s). The beta level is the size of the Type II error that will be tolerated. (*See:* Power)

Unbiased Lack of systematic error. *See:* Bias

Univariable Analysis Statistical analysis in which there is one dependent variable and no independent variable.

User Perspectives Perspectives that take into account the impacts of benefits, harms, and cost as they affect a particular user of the decision-making investigation. User perspectives include payer, provider, and patient perspectives.

Utility A measure of the worth or value of a particular health state measured on a scale of 0 to 1. Utilities are measured on the same scale as probabilities in order to multiply utilities times probabilities in decision-making investigations. A variety of methods exist for measuring utilities, including the rating scale, time trade-off, and reference gamble methods.

Valid A measurement is valid if it is appropriate for the question being addressed and is accurate and precise.

Variable Generally refers to a characteristic for which measurements are made in a study. In strict statistical terminology, a variable is the representation of those measurements in an analysis. Continuous or ordinal scale data are expressed using one variable as are nominal data with only two categories. However, nominal data with more than two categories must be expressed using more than one variable.

Variance Variance is the mean square deviation of data from the mean. (*See:* standard deviation)

Weighting A method used in adjustment to take into account the relative importance of a specific stratum. Each stratum is given a weight prior to combining its data.

Wilcoxon Signed-Rank Test   A statistical significance test that can be used for univariable analysis of an ordinal dependent variable.

Willingness to Pay   An approach to converting effectiveness to monetary terms that uses past choices made in specific situations to estimate how much society is willing to pay to obtain a specific outcome.

Subject Index

Page numbers followed by f refer to figures; those followed by t refer to tables; and those followed by n refer to footnotes.